Board Review Series

Gross Anatomy

4th edition

Board Review Series

Gross Anatomy
4th edition

Kyung Won Chung, Ph.D.

David Ross Boyd Professor and Vice Chairman
Course Director, Medical Gross Anatomy
Department of Cell Biology
College of Medicine
University of Oklahoma Health Sciences Center
Oklahoma City, Oklahoma

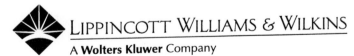

LIPPINCOTT WILLIAMS & WILKINS
A **Wolters Kluwer** Company
Philadelphia · Baltimore · New York · London
Buenos Aires · Hong Kong · Sydney · Tokyo

Editor: Elizabeth A. Nieginski
Editorial Director: Julie P. Martinez
Development Editor: Virginia Barishek
Managing Editor: Marette Magargle-Smith
Marketing Manager: Kelley Ray

351 West Camden Street
Baltimore, Maryland 21201-2436 USA

530 Walnut Street
Philadelphia, Pennsylvania 19106 USA

The publisher is not responsible (as a matter of product liability, negligence, or otherwise) for any injury resulting from any material contained herein. This publication contains information relating to general principles of medical care which should not be construed as specific instructions for individual patients. Manufacturers' product information and package inserts should be reviewed for current information, including contraindications, dosages, and precautions.

Printed in the United States of America

ISBN# 0-683-30727-4

The publishers have made every effort to trace the copyright holders for borrowed material. If they have inadvertently overlooked any, they will be pleased to make the necessary arrangements at the first opportunity.

We'd like to hear from you! If you have comments or suggestions regarding this Lippincott Williams & Wilkins title, please contact us at the appropriate customer service number listed below, or send correspondence to **book_comments@lww.com**. If possible, please remember to include your mailing address, phone number, and a reference to the book title and author in your message. To purchase additional copies of this book call our customer service department at **(800) 638-3030** or fax orders to **(301) 824-7390**. International customers should call **(301) 714-2324**.

00 01 02
1 2 3 4 5 6 7 8 9 10

Dedication

To My Wife, Young Hee,

and

Our Sons and Daughters-in-law

Harold M. Chung, M.D.
John M. Chung, M.D.
Kathie E. Cho, M.D.
Anna J. Chen, M.D.

Contents

Sun.

Sat.

Mon.

viii

Preface to the Fourth Edition

This concise review of human anatomy is designed for medical and dental students, and it is intended primarily to help the students prepare for the United States Medical Licensing Examination Step 1 as well as other examinations. It presents the essentials of human anatomy in the form of condensed descriptions and simple illustrations. The text is tightly outlined with related Board-type questions following each section. I have attempted to include all Board-relevant information without introducing a vast amount of material or entangling students in a web of details. However, because this book is in summary form, students are encouraged to consult a standard textbook for a comprehensive study of difficult concepts and fundamentals.

Organization

As with the previous editions, the fourth edition begins with a brief introduction to the skeletal, muscular, nervous, and circulatory systems. Following are chapters on regional anatomy, which include the upper limb, lower limb, thorax, abdomen, perineum and pelvis, back and head and neck.

I believe that anatomy is a visual science of the configuration of the body, and thus the success of learning and understanding it depends largely on the quality of dissection and the illustrations of the human structure. Many of the illustrations are simple schematic drawings used to enhance the student's understanding of the descriptive text. A few of the illustrations are more complex, attempting to exhibit important anatomical relationships. The considerable number of tables of muscles will prove particularly useful as a summary and review. In addition, several summary charts for muscle innervation and action, cranial nerves, autonomic ganglia, and foramina of the skull are included in order to highlight and summarize pertinent aspects of the system.

Test questions at the end of each chapter are designed to emphasize important information and hence lead to a better understanding of the material. These questions also serve as a self-evaluation to help the student uncover areas of weakness. Answers and explanations are provided after the questions.

Features of the new edition

• The upper and lower extremities have been organized as a dual approach: 1) the regional description of structures and their relationships and 2) an understanding of the major systems of the limbs and the continuity of the musculoskeletal, nervous, and vascular systems.

• Test questions reflect the guidelines set forth by the National Board of Medical Examiners and questions measure the basic anatomical knowledge as well as the student's ability to interpret their observations and solve clinical problems.

• Clinically oriented questions are drastically increased because their fundamental utility is based on the relationship of anatomy to clinical medicine.

• A Comprehensive Examination serves as a practice exam and self-assessment tool to help the student diagnose weaknesses prior to beginning a review of the subject. It also serves as self-examination upon completion of the review book prior to the Board examination.

• Some illustrations have been rearranged, redrawn, and new ones have been added.

• More radiograms, computer tomograms, and magnetic resonance images are included in the text and used for test questions to aid in the study of anatomical structures and their relationships, which are essential in clinical practice.

• The clinical application of anatomical knowledge is included throughout the book as clinical considerations. More clinical considerations and clinical questions have been added and expanded for this edition.

Kyung Won Chung

Acknowledgments

I wish to express my sincere thanks to the many medical students, colleagues, and friends who have made valuable suggestions regarding the preparation of the 4th edition. My appreciation is extended to Ms. Diane Abeloff, Medical Illustrator, for her book, Medical Art, Graphics for Use, which was used for illustrations with a little modification in some cases, and to Shawn C. Schlinke, M.D., and Wayne Heim for their excellent illustrations and full cooperation. I am deeply indebted to Martha Cushman, Development Editor, for her critical advice and constructive suggestions for improvement of the text, and to Ae-Son Om, Ph.D. and Iantha Harney, M.D. for their copyediting during the preparation of this edition. Finally, I greatly appreciate and enjoy the privilege of working with the Lippincott Williams & Wilkins staff–Elizabeth Nieginski, Acquisitions Editor; Julie Scardiglia, Editorial Director; and Marette Magargle-Smith, Managing Editor—for their constant guidance, enthusiasm, and unfailing support throughout the production of this book.

1

Introduction

Skeleton and Joints

I. Bones
–are calcified connective tissue consisting of cells (**osteocytes**) in a matrix of ground substance and collagen fibers.

–serve as a **reservoir** for **calcium** and **phosphorus** and act as **levers** on which muscles act to produce the movements permitted by joints.

–contain internal soft tissue, the **marrow,** where blood cells are formed.

–are classified, according to shape, into long, short, flat, irregular, and sesamoid bones; and according to their developmental history into endochondral and membranous bones.

A. Long bones
–include the clavicle, humerus, radius, ulna, femur, tibia, fibula, metacarpals, and phalanges.

–develop by **replacement of hyaline cartilage plate** (endochondral ossification).

–have a shaft (**diaphysis**) and two ends (**epiphyses**). The **metaphysis** is a part of the diaphysis adjacent to the epiphyses.

1. Diaphysis
–forms the **shaft** (central region) and is composed of a thick tube of **compact bone** that encloses the **marrow cavity**.

2. Metaphysis
–is a part of the diaphysis, the growth zone between the diaphysis and epiphysis during bone development.

3. Epiphyses
–are **expanded articular ends,** separated from the shaft by the epiphyseal plate during bone growth, and composed of a **spongy bone** surrounded by a thin layer of compact bone.

B. Short bones
–include the carpal and tarsal bones and are approximately cuboid shaped.

–are composed of **spongy bone** and **marrow** surrounded by a thin outer layer of **compact bone**.

C. Flat bones

–include the ribs, sternum, scapulae, and bones in the vault of the skull.
–consist of **two layers** of **compact bone** enclosing **spongy bone** and **marrow** space (**diploë**).
–have articular surfaces that are covered with fibrocartilage.
–grow by replacement of connective tissue.

D. Irregular bones

–include bones of mixed shapes such as bones of the skull, vertebrae, and coxa.
–contain mostly **spongy bone** enveloped by a thin outer layer of **compact bone**.

E. Sesamoid bones

–**develop in** certain **tendons** and reduce friction on the tendon, thus protecting it from excessive wear.
–are commonly found where tendons cross the ends of long bones in the limbs, as in the wrist and the knee (i.e., patella).

II. Joints

–are places of union between two or more bones.
–are innervated as follows: The nerve supplying a joint also supplies the muscles that move the joint and the skin covering the insertion of such muscles (**Hilton's law**).
–are classified on the basis of their structural features into fibrous, cartilaginous, and synovial types.

A. Fibrous joints (**synarthroses**)

–are joined by fibrous tissue, have **no joint cavities**, and permit little movement.

1. Sutures

–are connected by fibrous connective tissue (i.e., like uniting a wound with stitches).
–are found between the flat bones of the skull.

2. Syndesmoses

–are connected by fibrous connective tissue.
–occur as the inferior tibiofibular and tympanostapedial syndesmoses.

B. Cartilaginous joints

–have **no joint cavity** and are united by cartilage.

1. Synchondroses (primary cartilaginous joints)

–are united by **hyaline cartilage.**
–**permit no movement** but growth in the length of the bone.
–include epiphyseal cartilage plates (the union between the epiphysis and the diaphysis of a growing bone) and spheno-occipital and manubriosternal synchondroses.

2. Symphyses (secondary cartilaginous joints)

–are joined by **fibrocartilage** and are slightly movable joints.
–include the pubic symphysis and the intervertebral disks.

C. Synovial (**diarthrodial**) joints

–permit a great degree of free movement, and are classified according to the shape of the articular surfaces and axes of movement.

–are characterized by four features: **joint cavity, articular (hyaline) cartilage, synovial membrane** (which produces synovial fluid), and **articular capsule.**

1. **Plane (gliding) joints**

   –are united by two flat articular surfaces and allow simple **gliding** or **sliding** of one bone over the other.
   –occur in the proximal tibiofibular, intertarsal, intercarpal, intermetacarpal, carpometacarpal, sternoclavicular, and acromioclavicular joints.

2. **Hinge (ginglymus) joints**

   –resemble **door hinges** (i.e., spool-like surface fits into a concave surface) and permit movement around one axis (uniaxial) at right angles to the bones, allowing **flexion** and **extension** only.
   –occur in the elbow, ankle, and interphalangeal joints.

3. **Pivot (trochoid) joints**

   –are formed by a central bony pivot turning within a bony ring.
   –allow **rotation only** (movement around one longitudinal axis) [uniaxial].
   –occur in the superior and inferior radioulnar joints and in the atlantoaxial joint.

4. **Ellipsoidal joints**

   –have reciprocal elliptical convex and concave articular surfaces.
   –allow movement in two directions (biaxial) at right angles to each other.
   –allow flexion and extension and abduction and adduction but *no axial rotation.*
   –occur in the **wrist** (radiocarpal), **atlanto-occipital,** and **metacarpophalangeal joints.**

5. **Condylar joints**

   –have two convex condyles (knuckles) articulating with two concave condyles. The shape of the articulation is **ellipsoidal.**
   –allow movement in two directions (biaxial), including flexion and extension.
   –occur in the knee (tibiofemoral) and temporomandibular joints.

6. **Saddle (sellar) joints**

   –resemble a saddle on a horse's back.
   –allow movement in several directions (biaxial), including flexion and extension, abduction and adduction, and circumduction, but *no axial rotation.*
   –occur in the **carpometacarpal** joint of the **thumb** and between the **femur and patella.**

7. **Ball-and-socket (spheroidal) joints**

   –are formed by the reception of a globular (ball-like) head into a cup-shaped cavity and allow movement in many directions (multiaxial).
   –allow flexion and extension, abduction and adduction, medial and lateral rotations, and circumduction.
   –occur in the **shoulder** and **hip joints.**

Muscular System

I. Muscle

–consists predominantly of **contractile cells** and produces the **movements** of various parts of the body by contraction.
–occurs in three types:

A. Skeletal muscle

–is under voluntary control and makes up about 40% of the total body mass.
–has two attachments, an **origin** (which is usually the more fixed and proximal attachment), and an **insertion** (which is the more movable and distal attachment).
–is enclosed by **epimysium,** a thin layer of connective tissue. Smaller bundles of muscle fibers are surrounded by **perimysium.** Each muscle fiber is enclosed by **endomysium.**

B. Cardiac muscle

–consists of striated muscle fibers and forms the **myocardium,** the middle layer of the heart.
–is innervated by the autonomic nervous system but contracts spontaneously without any nerve supply.
–includes specialized myocardial fibers that form the cardiac **conducting system.**

C. Smooth muscle

–is generally arranged in two layers, **circular** and **longitudinal,** in the walls of many visceral organs.
–is innervated by the autonomic nervous system, regulating the size of the lumen of a tubular structure.
–undergoes rhythmic contractions called **peristaltic waves** in the walls of the gastrointestinal (GI) tract, uterine tubes, ureters, and other organs.

II. Structures Associated with Muscles

A. Tendons

–are **fibrous bands of dense connective tissue** that connect muscles to bones or cartilage.
–are supplied by sensory fibers extending from muscle nerves.

B. Ligaments

–are **fibrous bands or sheets** connecting bones or cartilage or are folds of peritoneum serving to support and strengthen joints, muscles, and visceral structures.

C. Raphe

–is the line of union of symmetrical structures by a fibrous or tendinous band such as the pterygomandibular, pharyngeal, and scrotal raphes.

D. Aponeuroses

–are **flat fibrous sheets** or **expanded broad tendons** that attach to muscles and serve as the means of origin or insertion of a flat muscle.

E. Retinaculum
–is a fibrous band that holds a structure in place.

F. Bursae
–are **flattened sacs of synovial membrane** that contain a viscid fluid for moistening the bursa wall to facilitate movement by minimizing friction.
–are found where a tendon rubs against a bone, ligament, or other tendon.
–are prone to fill with fluid when infected, and may communicate with an adjacent joint cavity.

G. Synovial tendon sheaths
–are **tubular sacs** filled with synovial fluid that wrap **around the tendons**.
–occur where tendons pass under ligaments or retinacula and through osseofibrous tunnels, thus facilitating movement by reducing friction.
–have linings, like synovial membrane, that respond to infection by forming more fluid and by proliferating more cells, causing adhesions and thus restriction of movement of the tendon.

H. Fascia
–is a **fibrous sheet that envelops the body** under the skin and invests the muscles.
–may **limit the spread of pus** and extravasated fluids such as urine and blood.

1. Superficial fascia
–is a **loose connective tissue** between the dermis and the deep (investing) fascia, and has a fatty superficial layer and a membranous deep layer.
–contains fat, cutaneous vessels, nerves, lymphatics, and glands.

2. Deep fascia
–is a **sheet of fibrous tissue** that invests the muscles and helps support them by serving as an elastic sheath or stocking, providing origins and insertions for muscles and forming retinacula and fibrous sheaths for tendons.
–forms potential **pathways for infection** or extravasation of fluids.
–has no sharp distinction from epimysium.

Nervous System

I. Divisions of the Nervous System
–The nervous system is divided anatomically into the **central nervous system** (CNS), consisting of the brain and spinal cord, and the **peripheral nervous system** (PNS), consisting of 12 pairs of cranial nerves and 31 pairs of spinal nerves, and their associated ganglia.
–The nervous system is divided functionally into the **somatic nervous system,** which controls primarily voluntary activities, and the **visceral (autonomic) nervous system,** which controls primarily involuntary activities.
–It is composed of **neurons** and **neuroglia,** which are non-neuronal cells such as astrocytes, oligodendrocytes, and microglia.
–It controls and integrates the activity of various parts of the body.

II. Neurons

–are the structural and functional units of the nervous system (neuron doctrine).

–are specialized for the reception, integration, transformation, and transmission of information.

A. Components of neurons

–Neurons consist of **cell bodies** (perikaryon or soma) and their processes, **dendrites** and **axons.**

1. **Cell bodies** are located in the gray matter of the CNS, and their collections are called **ganglia** in the PNS and **nuclei** in the CNS.

2. **Dendrites** (dendron means "tree") are usually short and highly branched and **carry impulses toward the cell body.**

3. **Axons** are usually single and long, have fewer branches (collaterals), and **carry impulses away from the cell body.**

B. Classification of neurons

1. **Unipolar (pseudounipolar) neurons**

   –have one process, which divides into a central branch that functions as an axon, and a peripheral branch that serves as a dendrite.

   –are called pseudounipolar because they were originally bipolar. The two processes fuse during development to form a single process that bifurcates at a distance from the cell body.

   –are sensory neurons of the PNS and found in spinal and cranial nerve ganglia.

2. **Bipolar neurons**

   –have two processes, one dendrite and one axon, and are found in the **olfactory epithelium,** the **retina,** and the **inner ear.**

3. **Multipolar neurons**

   –have **several dendrites** and one axon and are most common in the CNS (e.g., motor cells in anterior and lateral horns of the spinal cord, autonomic ganglion cells).

C. Ganglion

–is a collection of neuron cell bodies outside the CNS, and a **nucleus** is a collection of neuron cell bodies within the CNS.

D. Other components of the nervous system

1. **Cells that support neurons**

   –include **Schwann cells** and **satellite cells** in the PNS.

   –are called **neuroglia** in the CNS and are composed mainly of three types: **astrocytes; oligodendrocytes,** which play a role in myelin formation and transport of material to neurons; and **microglia,** which phagocytose waste products of nerve tissue.

2. **Myelin**

   –is the fat-like substance forming a sheath around certain nerve fibers.

   –is formed by **Schwann cells** in the PNS and **oligodendrocytes** in the CNS.

3. Synapses

–are the **sites of functional contact** of a neuron with another neuron, an effector (muscle, gland) cell, or a sensory receptor cell.

–are classified by the site of contact as **axodendritic, axoaxonic,** or **axosomatic** (between axon and cell body).

–subserve the transmission of nerve impulses, commonly from the axon terminals (presynaptic elements) to the plasma membranes (postsynaptic elements) of the receiving cell. In most cases, the impulse is transmitted by means of neurotransmitters released into a **synaptic cleft** that separates the presynaptic from the postsynaptic membrane.

III. Central Nervous System (CNS)

A. Brain

–is enclosed within the cranium, or brain case.

–has a **cortex,** which is the **outer part** of the cerebral hemispheres and is composed of **gray matter.** This matter consists largely of the nerve cell bodies, dendrites, and neuroglia.

–has an interior part composed of **white matter,** which consists largely of axons forming tracts or pathways, and ventricles, which are filled with cerebrospinal fluid (CSF).

B. Spinal cord

–is **cylindrical,** occupies approximately the upper two-thirds of the vertebral canal, and is enveloped by the meninges.

–has cervical and lumbar enlargements for the nerve supply of the upper and lower limbs, respectively.

–has centrally located **gray matter,** in contrast to the cerebral hemispheres, and peripherally located **white matter**.

–grows more slowly than the vertebral column during fetal development, and hence its terminal end gradually shifts to a higher level.

–has a conical end known as the **conus medullaris,** and ends at the level of L2 (or between L1 and L2) in the adult and at the level of L3 in the newborn.

C. Meninges

–consist of three layers of connective tissue membranes (**pia, arachnoid,** and **dura mater**) that surround and protect the brain and spinal cord.

–contain the **subarachnoid space,** which is the interval between the arachnoid and pia mater, filled with CSF.

IV. Peripheral Nervous System (PNS)

A. Cranial nerves

–consist of **12 pairs** and are connected to the brain rather than to the spinal cord.

–have **motor fibers** with cell bodies located within the CNS and **sensory fibers** with cell bodies that form sensory ganglia located outside the CNS.

–emerge from the ventral aspect of the brain (except for the trochlear nerve, cranial nerve IV).

–contain all four functional components of the spinal nerves and three additional components (see Nervous System: IV C; Chapter 8).

B. Spinal nerves (Figure 1-1)

–consist of **31 pairs:** 8 cervical, 12 thoracic, 5 lumbar, 5 sacral, and 1 coccygeal.

–are formed from dorsal and ventral roots; each dorsal root has a ganglion that is within the intervertebral foramen.

–are connected with the sympathetic chain ganglia by **rami communicantes.**

–contain sensory fibers with cell bodies in the dorsal root ganglion [general somatic afferent (GSA) and general visceral afferent (GVA) fibers]; motor fibers with cell bodies in the anterior horn of the spinal cord [general somatic efferent (GSE) fibers]; and motor fibers with cell bodies in the lateral horn of the spinal cord [general visceral efferent (GVE) fibers] between T1 and L2.

–are divided into the **ventral and dorsal primary rami.** The ventral primary rami enter into the formation of plexuses (i.e., cervical, brachial, and lumbosacral); the dorsal primary rami innervate the skin and deep muscles of the back.

C. Functional components in peripheral nerves (Figures 1-2 and 1-3)

1. General somatic afferent (GSA) fibers

–transmit pain, temperature, touch, and proprioception from the body to the CNS.

2. General somatic efferent (GSE) fibers

–carry motor impulses to skeletal muscles of the body.

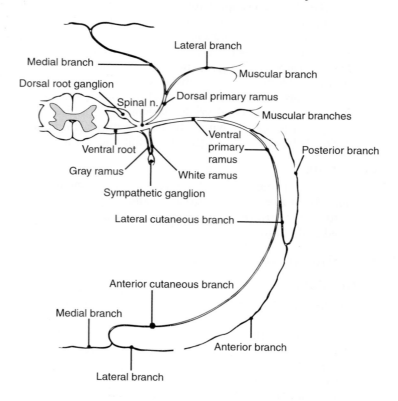

Figure 1-1. Typical spinal nerve.

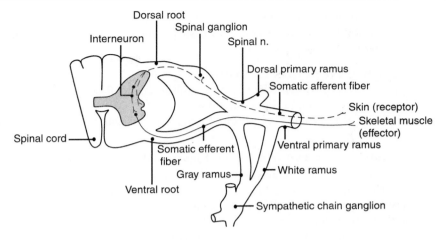

Figure 1-2. General somatic afferent and efferent nerves.

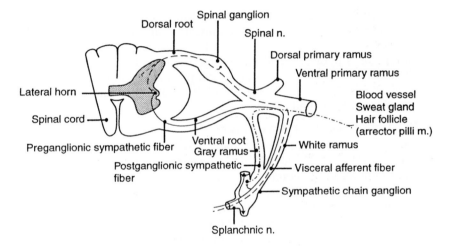

Figure 1-3. General visceral efferent (autonomic) and afferent nerves.

3. General visceral afferent (GVA) fibers
  –convey sensory impulses from visceral organs to the CNS.

4. General visceral efferent (GVE) fibers (autonomic nerves)
  –transmit motor impulses to smooth muscle, cardiac muscle, and glandular tissues.

5. Special somatic afferent (SSA) fibers
  –convey special sensory impulses of vision, hearing, and equilibration to the CNS.

6. Special visceral afferent (SVA) fibers
  –transmit smell and taste sensations to the CNS.

7. Special visceral efferent (SVE) fibers
  –conduct motor impulses to the muscles of the head and neck.

–arise from branchiomeric structures such as muscles for mastication, muscles for facial expression, and muscles for elevation of the pharynx and movement of the larynx.

V. Autonomic Nervous System

–is divided into the **sympathetic** (thoracolumbar outflow), **parasympathetic** (craniosacral outflow), and enteric divisions.

–is composed of two neurons, preganglionic and postganglionic, which are GVE neurons.

A. Sympathetic nerve fibers (see Figure 1-3)

–have preganglionic nerve cell bodies that are located in the lateral horn of the thoracic and upper lumbar levels (L2 or L1–L3) of the spinal cord.

–have **preganglionic fibers** that pass through ventral roots, spinal nerves, and white rami communicantes. These fibers enter adjacent sympathetic chain ganglia, where they synapse or travel up or down the chain to synapse in remote ganglia or run further through the splanchnic nerves to synapse in collateral ganglia, located along the major abdominal blood vessels.

–have **postganglionic fibers** from the chain ganglia that return to spinal nerves by way of gray rami communicantes and supply the skin with secretory fibers to sweat glands, motor fibers to smooth muscles of the hair follicles (arrectores pilorum), and vasomotor fibers to the blood vessels.

–function primarily in **emergencies,** preparing individuals for fight or flight and thus increase heart rate, inhibit GI motility and secretion, and dilate pupils and bronchial lumen.

B. Parasympathetic nerve fibers

–comprise the preganglionic fibers that arise from the brainstem (cranial nerves III, VII, IX, and X) and sacral part of the spinal cord (second, third, and fourth sacral segments).

–are, with few exceptions, characterized by **long preganglionic fibers** and **short postganglionic fibers.**

–are distributed to the walls of the visceral organs and glands of the digestive system but not to the skin or to the periphery.

–decrease heart rate, increase GI peristalsis, and stimulate secretory activity.

–function primarily in **homeostasis,** tending to promote quiet and orderly processes of the body.

C. Enteric division

–consists of enteric ganglia and plexus of the GI tract, including the myenteric (Auerbach's) and submucosal (Meissner's) plexuses.

–plays an important role in the control of GI motility and secretion.

Circulatory System

I. Vascular System

–functions to transport vital materials between the external environment and the internal fluid environment of the body. It carries **oxygen, nutrients, waste products,** including **carbon dioxide, hormones, defense elements,** and **cells** involved in **wound healing.**

–consists of the **heart** and **vessels** (arteries, capillaries, veins) that transport blood through all parts of the body.

–includes the **lymphatic vessels,** a set of channels that begin in the tissue spaces and return excess tissue fluid to the bloodstream.

A. Circulatory loops

1. Pulmonary circulation

–pumps blood from the right ventricle to the lungs through the pulmonary arteries and returns it to the left atrium of the heart through the pulmonary veins.

2. Systemic circulation

–pumps blood from the left ventricle through the aorta to all parts of the body and returns it to the right atrium through the superior and inferior venae cavae and the cardiac veins.

B. Fetal circulation (Figure 1-4)

1. The fetus

–has blood that is oxygenated in the placenta rather than in the lungs.

–has three shunts that partially bypass the lungs and liver:

a. Foramen ovale

–is an opening in the **septum secundum.**

–usually closes functionally at birth, but with anatomic closure occurring later.

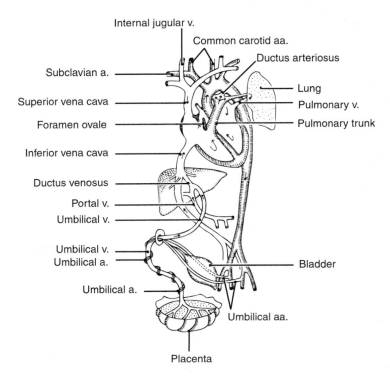

Figure 1-4. Fetal circulation.

–shunts blood from the right atrium to the left atrium, partially by-passing the lungs (pulmonary circulation).

b. Ductus arteriosus

–is derived from the sixth aortic arch and connects the bifurcation of the pulmonary trunk.

–closes functionally soon after birth, with anatomic closure requiring several weeks.

–becomes the **ligamentum arteriosum,** which connects the left pulmonary artery (at its origin from the pulmonary trunk) to the concavity of the arch of the aorta.

–shunts blood from the pulmonary trunk to the aorta, partially bypassing the lungs (pulmonary circulation).

c. Ductus venosus

–shunts oxygenated blood from the umbilical vein (returning from the placenta) to the inferior vena cava, partially bypassing the liver (portal circulation).

–joins the left branch of the portal vein to the inferior vena cava and is obliterated to become the **ligamentum venosum** after birth.

2. Umbilical arteries

–carry blood to the placenta for reoxygenation before birth.

–become **medial umbilical ligaments** after birth, after their distal parts have atrophied.

3. Umbilical veins

–carry **highly oxygenated blood** from the placenta to the fetus.

–consists of the right vein, which is obliterated during the embryonic period, and the left vein, which is obliterated to form the **ligamentum teres hepatis** after birth.

C. Heart

–is a hollow, muscular, **four-chambered organ** that pumps blood through the pulmonary and systemic circulations.

–receives venous blood from the body in the right atrium and then passes it into the right ventricle, which pumps it to the lungs for oxygenation.

–receives the oxygenated blood from the lungs in the left atrium and passes it to the left ventricle, which pumps it through the aorta to supply the tissues of the body.

–is regulated in its pumping rate and strength by the autonomic nervous system, which controls a pacemaker (i.e., **sinoatrial node**).

D. Blood vessels

–carry blood to the lungs, where carbon dioxide is exchanged for oxygen.

–carry blood to the intestines, where nutritive materials in fluid form are absorbed; and to the endocrine glands, where hormones pass through the vessel walls and are distributed to target cells.

–transport the waste products of tissue fluid to the kidneys, intestines, lungs, and skin, where they are excreted.

–are of four types: arteries, veins, capillaries, and sinusoids:

1. **Arteries**
   –carry blood away from the heart and distribute it to all parts of the body.
   –have thicker and stronger walls than do veins.
   –consist of three main types: **elastic arteries, muscular arteries,** and **arterioles.**

2. **Veins**
   –carry blood toward the heart from all parts of the body.
   –consist of the **pulmonary veins,** which return oxygenated blood to the heart from the lungs, and the **systemic veins,** which return deoxygenated blood to the heart from the rest of the body.
   –contain valves that prevent the reflux of blood. Valves are numerous in the veins of the limbs, but are absent in the small veins and in the venae cavae as well as in the hepatic, renal, uterine, and ovarian veins.
   –have **venae comitantes,** which are veins or pairs of veins that closely accompany an artery in such a manner that the pulsations of the artery aid venous return; they are often found in the medium-sized vessels of the arm, forearm, and leg.

3. **Capillaries**
   –are composed of endothelium and its basement membrane and connect the arterioles to the venules.
   –are the **exchange sites** where oxygen and nutritive materials from oxygenated blood diffuse across the endothelial wall of the arteriolar end of the capillary into the tissue spaces, whereas metabolic waste products and carbon dioxide diffuse from the tissue spaces into the blood through the wall of the venous end.
   –are absent in the cornea, epidermis, and hyaline cartilage.
   –may not be present in some areas where the arterioles and venules have direct connections. These **arteriovenous anastomoses** (arteriovenous shunts) bypass the capillaries and are especially numerous in the skin of the nose, lips, fingers, and ears, where they conserve body heat.

4. **Sinusoids**
   –are wider and more irregular than capillaries.
   –substitute for capillaries in the liver, spleen, red bone marrow, carotid body, adenohypophysis, suprarenal cortex, and parathyroid glands.
   –have walls that consist largely of phagocytic cells.
   –form a part of the **reticuloendothelial system,** which is concerned chiefly with phagocytosis and antibody formation.

5. **Portal system**
   –is a system of vessels in which blood traveling through one capillary bed passes through a second capillary network before it returns to the systemic circulation.
   –consists of the **hepatic portal system,** in which blood from the intestinal capillaries passes through the hepatic portal vein and then hepatic capillaries (sinusoids) to the hepatic veins; and the **hypophyseal portal system** in which blood from the hypothalamic capillaries passes through the hypophyseal portal veins and then the pituitary capillary sinusoids to the hypophyseal veins.

II. Lymphatic System

–provides an important **immune mechanism** for the body.

–is involved in the **metastasis** of cancer cells.

–provides a route for transporting fat and large protein molecules absorbed from the intestine to the hepatic portal system.

A. Lymphatic vessels

–serve as one-way drainage toward the heart and return lymph to the bloodstream through the **thoracic duct** (the largest lymphatic vessel), or the right lymphatic duct.

–are not generally visible in dissections but are the major route by which carcinoma metastasizes.

–function to **absorb large protein molecules** and transport them to the bloodstream because the molecules cannot pass through the walls of the blood capillaries back into the blood.

–carry lymphocytes from lymphatic tissues to the bloodstream.

–have **valves** to ensure the flow of lymph away from the tissues and toward the venous system, and are constricted at the sites of valves, showing a **beaded appearance**.

–are absent in the brain, spinal cord, eyeballs, bone marrow, splenic pulp, hyaline cartilage, nails, and hair.

B. Lymphatic capillaries

–begin blindly in most tissues, collect tissue fluid, and join to form large collecting vessels that pass to regional lymph nodes.

–**absorb lymph** from tissue spaces and transport it back to the venous system.

–are called **lacteals** in the villi of the small intestine, where they absorb emulsified fat.

C. Lymph nodes

–are organized collections of lymphatic tissue permeated by lymphatic channels, and have fibroelastic capsules from which connective tissue trabeculae extend into the substance of the organ.

–have a **cortex** (outer part), which contains collections of lymphatic cells called **germinal centers,** and a **medulla** (inner part), which contains cords of lymphatic cells.

–produce **lymphocytes** and **plasma cells.**

–**trap bacteria** drained from an infected area and contain reticuloendothelial cells and phagocytic cells (**macrophages**) that ingest these bacteria.

–serve as **filters.** (Thus, the cancer cells in lymph vessels migrate or metastasize to lymph nodes and tend to remain within them, proliferating and gradually destroying them.)

–are hard and often palpable when there is a metastasis and are enlarged and tender during infection.

D. Lymph

–is a clear, watery fluid that is collected from the intercellular spaces.

–contains no cells until lymphocytes are added in its passage through the lymph nodes. Its constituents are similar to those of blood plasma (e.g., proteins, fats, lymphocytes).

–often contains fat droplets (called **chyle**) when it comes from intestinal organs.

–is filtered by passing through several lymph nodes before entering the venous system.

Review Test

Directions: Each of the numbered items or incomplete statements in this section is followed by answers or by completions of the statement. Select the **one** lettered answer or completion that is **best** in each case.

1. Which of the following fibrous sheets or bands would most likely cover the body under the skin and invest the muscles?

(A) Tendon
(B) Fascia
(C) Synovial tendon sheath
(D) Aponeurosis
(E) Ligament

2. If parasympathetic nerves are damaged, which of the following muscles would most likely be affected?

(A) Muscles in the hair follicles
(B) Muscles in blood vessels
(C) Muscles that act at the elbow joint
(D) Muscles in the gastrointestinal (GI) tract
(E) Muscles enclosed by epimysium

3. Which blood vessel or group of vessels carries richly oxygenated blood to the heart?

(A) Superior vena cava
(B) Pulmonary arteries
(C) Pulmonary veins
(D) Ascending aorta
(E) Coronary sinus

4. Axons of the neurons

(A) carry impulses toward the cell bodies
(B) carry impulses away from the cell bodies
(C) carry only motor impulses
(D) are several in number for multipolar neurons
(E) are found primarily in the gray matter

5. Which of the following structures shunts blood from the pulmonary trunk to the aorta, partially bypassing the lungs?

(A) Placenta
(B) Umbilical artery
(C) Ductus arteriosus
(D) Foramen ovale
(E) Ductus venosus

6. Which of the following structures contains cell bodies of unipolar or pseudounipolar neurons?

(A) Ventral horn of the spinal cord
(B) Lateral horn of the spinal cord
(C) Dorsal horn of the spinal cord
(D) Dorsal root ganglion
(E) Sympathetic chain ganglion

7. Synapses are most likely absent in or on which of the following structures?

(A) Anterior horn
(B) Dorsal root ganglia
(C) Sympathetic chain ganglia
(D) On dendrites
(E) On cell bodies

8. Which of the following structures would most likely be absent in the spinal cord at the L4 spinal cord level?

(A) Dorsal horn
(B) Lateral horn
(C) Ventral horn
(D) Gray matter
(E) White matter

9. The pivot (trochoid) joint is found in which of the following joints?

(A) Atlanto-occipital joint
(B) Atlanto-axial joint
(C) Carpometacarpal joint of the thumb
(D) Proximal tibiofibular joint
(E) Intervertebral disks

10. A patient presents with a loss of sensation to the skin over the shoulder. Injury to which of the following nerve cells would most likely affect the conduction of sensory information to the central nervous system (CNS)?

(A) Multipolar neurons
(B) Bipolar neurons
(C) Unipolar or pseudounipolar neurons
(D) Neurons in the ventral horn
(E) Neurons in sympathetic chain ganglia

Answers and Explanations

1-B. The fascia is a fibrous sheet or band that covers the body under the skin and invests the muscles.

2-D. Smooth muscles in the gastrointestinal (GI) tract are innervated by both parasympathetic and sympathetic nerves. Smooth muscles in the wall of the blood vessels and arrector pili muscles in hair follicles are innervated only by sympathetic nerves. Muscles act at the elbow joint and muscles enclosed by epimysium are skeletal muscles that are innervated by somatic motor [general somatic efferent (GSE)] nerves.

3-C. Pulmonary veins return oxygenated blood to the heart from the lungs. Pulmonary arteries carry deoxygenated blood from the heart to the lungs for oxygen renewal. The ascending aorta carries oxygenated blood from the left ventricle to all parts of the body. The superior vena cava and coronary sinus carry deoxygenated blood to the right atrium.

4-B. The axons of the neurons carry impulses away from the cell bodies, and dendrites carry impulses to the cell bodies. The axons contain sensory or motor fibers. Multipolar neurons have several dendrites and one axon. The gray matter of the central nervous system (CNS) consists largely of neuron cell bodies, dendrites, and neuroglia, whereas the white matter consists largely of axons and neuroglia.

5-C. The ductus arteriosus shunts blood from the pulmonary trunk to the aorta, partially bypassing the lungs. The ductus venosus shunts oxygenated blood from the umbilical vein to the inferior vena cava, without bypassing the liver. The foramen ovale shunts blood from the right atrium to the left atrium, partially bypassing the lungs. The umbilical artery carries blood to the placenta for reoxygenation before birth, and the placenta supplies oxygenated blood to the fetus.

6-D. Ventral, lateral, and dorsal horns, as well as sympathetic chain ganglia, contain multipolar neurons.

7-B. Dorsal root ganglia consist of cell bodies of the unipolar or pseudounipolar neurons and have no synapses. Axosomatic and axodentritic synapses are the most common, but axoaxonal and dendrodendritic contacts are also found in many nerve tissues.

8-B. The lateral horns are found in the gray matter of the spinal cord between T1 and L2 and also between S2 and S4.

9-B. The atlanto-occipital joints are the ellipsoidal (condyloid) joint, the carpometacarpal joint of the thumb is the saddle (sellar) joint, the proximal tibiofibular joint is plane (gliding) joint, and the intervertebral joint is the secondary cartilaginous (symphysis) joint.

10-C. Sensation from the skin is carried by general somatic afferent (GSA) fibers and their cells are unipolar or pseudounipolar types and located in the dorsal root ganglia.

2
Upper Limb

Bones and Joints

I. Bones (Figure 2-1)

A. Clavicle (collarbone)

–is a **commonly fractured bone** that forms the **pectoral (shoulder) girdle** with the **scapula,** which connects the upper limb to the axial skeleton (sternum).

–is **the first bone to begin ossification** during fetal development, but it is the last one to **complete ossification,** at about age 21 years.

–is the only long bone to be **ossified intermembranously.**

–has the medial two-thirds tilted convex forward and the lateral one-third flattened with a marked concavity.

–is the only skeletal connection of the shoulder girdle to the trunk, articulating with the sternum at the sternoclavicular joint and with the scapula at the acromioclavicular joint.

B. Scapula (shoulder blade)

–is a **triangular** flat bone.

1. Spine of the scapula

–is a triangular-shaped process that continues laterally as the **acromion.**

–divides the dorsal surface of the scapula into the upper **supraspinous** and lower **infraspinous fossae.**

–provides an origin for the deltoid muscle and an insertion for the trapezius muscle.

2. Acromion

–is the lateral end of the spine and articulates with the clavicle.

–provides an origin for the deltoid muscle and an insertion for the trapezius muscle.

3. Coracoid process

–provides the origin of the coracobrachialis and biceps brachii muscles and the insertion of the pectoralis minor muscle.

–provides an attachment site for the coracoclavicular, coracohumeral, and coracoacromial ligaments, as well as the costocoracoid membrane.

19

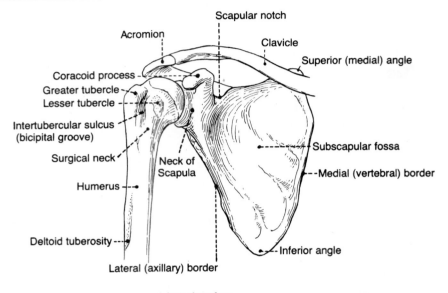

Anterior view

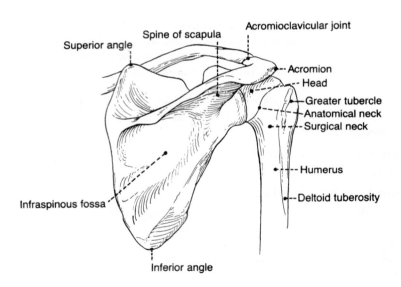

Posterior view

Figure 2-1. Pectoral girdle and humerus.

4. Scapular notch

–is bridged by the superior transverse scapular ligament and is converted into a foramen, which permits passage of the **suprascapular nerve.**

5. Glenoid cavity

–articulates with the head of the **humerus.**
–is deepened by a fibrocartilaginous lip **(glenoid labrum).**

6. **Supraglenoid and infraglenoid tubercles**

    –provide origins for the tendons of the long heads of the biceps brachii and triceps brachii muscles, respectively.

C. **Humerus** (see Figure 2-1)

1. **Head**

    –has a smooth, rounded, articular surface and articulates with the scapula at the **glenohumeral joint.**

2. **Anatomical neck**

    –is an indentation distal to the head of the humerus that provides for the attachment of the articular capsule.

3. **Greater tubercle**

    –lies on the lateral side of the humerus, just lateral to the anatomical neck.
    –provides attachments for the supraspinatus, infraspinatus, and teres minor muscles.

4. **Lesser tubercle**

    –lies on the anterior medial side of the humerus, just distal to the anatomical neck.
    –provides an insertion for the subscapularis muscle.

5. **Intertubercular (bicipital) groove**

    –lies between the greater and lesser tubercles and lodges the tendon of the long head of the biceps brachii muscle.
    –is bridged by the **transverse humeral ligament,** which restrains the tendon of the long head of the biceps brachii.
    –provides insertions for the pectoralis major on its **lateral lip,** the teres major on its **medial lip,** and the latissimus dorsi on its **floor.**

6. **Surgical neck**

    –is a narrow area distal to the tubercles that is a **common site of fracture.**
    –is in contact with the axillary nerve and the posterior humeral circumflex artery.

7. **Deltoid tuberosity**

    –is a V-shaped roughened area on the lateral aspect of the midshaft that marks the insertion of the deltoid muscle.

8. **Spiral groove**

    –is a groove for the radial nerve, separating the origin of the lateral head of the triceps above and the origin of the medial head below.

9. **Trochlea**

    –is shaped like a spool and has a deep depression (between two margins) that articulates with the **trochlear notch of the ulna.**

10. **Capitulum**

    –is globular in shape and articulates with the **head of the radius.**

11. **Olecranon fossa**

    –is a depression above the trochlea on the posterior aspect of the humerus that houses the **olecranon** of the ulna on full extension of the forearm.

12. Coronoid fossa

–is a depression above the trochlea on the anterior aspect of the humerus that accommodates the **coronoid process** of the ulna on flexion of the elbow.

13. Radial fossa

–is a depression above the capitulum on the anterior aspect that is occupied by the **head of the radius** during full flexion of the elbow joint.

14. Medial epicondyle

–projects from the trochlea and is larger and more prominent than the lateral epicondyle.

–provides attachment sites for the ulnar collateral ligament, the pronator teres muscle, and the common tendon of the flexor muscles of the forearm.

15. Lateral epicondyle

–projects from the capitulum and provides the origin of the supinator and extensor muscles of the forearm.

D. Radius (Figure 2-2)

–is shorter than the ulna and is situated lateral to the ulna.

–is characterized by displacement of the hand dorsally and radially when fractured at its distal end **(Colles' fracture).**

1. Head (proximal end)

–articulates with the **capitulum** of the humerus and the **radial notch** of the ulna and is surrounded by the **annular ligament.**

2. Distal end

–articulates with the **proximal row of carpal bones,** including the scaphoid, lunate, and triquetral bones but excluding the pisiform bone.

3. Radial tuberosity

–is an oblong prominence just distal to the neck and provides an attachment site for the biceps brachii tendon.

4. Styloid process

–is located on the distal end of the radius and is about 1 cm distal to that of the ulna and provides insertion of the brachioradialis muscle.

–can be palpated in the proximal part of the anatomical snuff-box between the extensor pollicis longus and brevis tendons.

E. Ulna (see Figure 2-2)

1. Olecranon

–is the curved projection on the back of the elbow that provides an attachment site for the triceps tendon.

2. Coronoid process

–is located below the trochlear notch and provides an attachment site for the brachialis.

3. Trochlear notch

–receives the trochlea of the humerus.

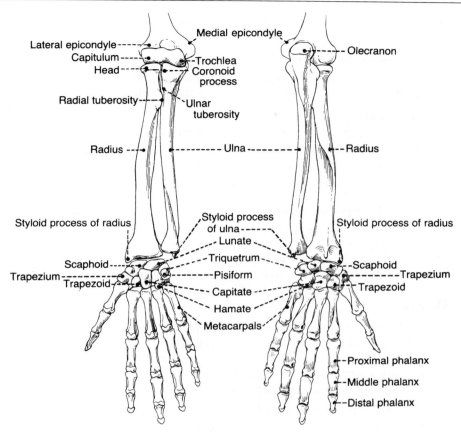

Figure 2-2.   Bones of the forearm and hand.

4. **Ulnar tuberosity**

   –is a roughened prominence distal to the coronoid process that provides an attachment site for the brachialis.

5. **Radial notch**

   –accommodates the head of the radius.

6. **Head (distal end)**

   –articulates with the articular disk of the **distal radioulnar joint** and has a styloid process.

F. **Carpal bones** (see Figure 2-2)

   –are arranged in two rows of four (lateral to medial): **S**caphoid, **L**unate, **T**riquetrum, **P**isiform, **T**rapezium, **T**rapezoid, **C**apitate, and **H**amate (mnemonic device: **S**andra **L**ikes **T**o **P**at **T**om's **T**wo **C**old **H**ands). ("Trapezium" precedes "trapezoid" alphabetically.)

   1. **Proximal row (lateral to medial): scaphoid, lunate, triquetrum, and pisiform**

      –except for the pisiform, articulates with the radius and the articular disk (the ulna has no contact with the carpal bones). The pisiform is said to be a sesamoid bone contained in the flexor carpi ulnaris tendon.

2. **Distal row (lateral to medial): trapezium, trapezoid, capitate, and hamate**

G. Metacarpals

–are miniature long bones consisting of **bases** (proximal ends), **shafts** (bodies), and **heads** (distal ends). Heads form the knuckles of the fist.

H. Phalanges

–are miniature long bones consisting of **bases, shafts,** and **heads.** The heads of the proximal and middle phalanges form the knuckles.
–occur in fingers (three each) and thumb (two).

II. Joints and Ligaments (see Figures 2-1 and 2-2)

A. Acromioclavicular joint

–is a synovial **plane joint** between the acromion and the clavicle. Its articular surfaces are covered by fibrous cartilages.
–allows a gliding movement when the scapula rotates.
–is reinforced by the **coracoclavicular ligament,** which consists of the conoid and trapezoid ligaments.

B. Sternoclavicular joint

–is a double synovial **plane (gliding) joint** and united by the fibrous capsule.
–allows elevation and depression, protraction and retraction, and circumduction of the shoulder.
–is reinforced by the anterior and posterior sternoclavicular, interclavicular, and costoclavicular ligaments.

C. Shoulder (glenohumeral) joint

–is a multiaxial synovial **ball-and-socket (spheroidal) joint** between the glenoid cavity of the scapula and the head of the humerus. Both articular surfaces are covered with hyaline cartilage.
–has a cavity that is deepened by the fibrocartilaginous **glenoid labrum** and communicates with the subscapular bursa.
–allows abduction and adduction, flexion and extension, and circumduction and rotation.
–is surrounded by the **fibrous capsule** that is attached superiorly to the margin of the glenoid cavity and inferiorly to the **anatomical neck** of the humerus. The capsule is reinforced by the **rotator (musculotendinous) cuff,** the superior, middle, and inferior **glenohumeral ligaments,** and the **coracohumeral** and **transverse humeral ligaments.**
–is innervated by the axillary, suprascapular, and lateral pectoral nerves.
–receives blood from branches of the suprascapular, anterior and posterior humeral circumflex, and scapular circumflex arteries.
–may be subject to inferior or anterior **dislocation,** which stretches the fibrous capsule, avulses the glenoid labrum, and may injure the axillary nerve.

1. **Rotator (musculotendinous) cuff**

–is formed by the tendons of the subscapularis, **supraspinatus, infraspinatus, and teres minor muscles.**
–fuses with the joint capsule and strengthens it.
–converges on the greater and lesser tubercle of the humerus.

–keeps the head of the humerus in the glenoid fossa during movements and thus **stabilizes** the shoulder joint.

2. **Ligaments of the shoulder joint**

   a. **Glenohumeral ligaments**

      –extend from the **supraglenoid tubercle** to the upper part of the lesser tubercle of the humerus **(superior glenohumeral ligament),** to the lower anatomical neck of the humerus **(middle glenohumeral ligament),** and to the lower part of the lesser tubercle of the humerus **(inferior glenohumeral ligament).**

   b. **Transverse humeral ligament**

      –extends between the greater and lesser tubercles.
      –holds the tendon of the long head of the biceps in the intertubercular groove.

   c. **Coracohumeral ligament**

      –extends from the coracoid process to the greater tubercle of the humerus.

   d. **Coracoacromial ligament**

      –extends from the coracoid process to the acromion.

3. **Bursae around the shoulder**

   –form a **lubricating mechanism** between the rotator cuff and the coracoacromial arch during movement of the shoulder joint.

   a. **Subacromial bursa**

      –lies between the coracoacromial arch (acromion and coracoacromial ligament) and the supraspinatus muscle.
      –usually communicates with the subdeltoid bursa.
      –protects the supraspinatus tendon against friction with the acromion.

   b. **Subdeltoid bursa**

      –lies between the deltoid muscle and the shoulder joint capsule and usually communicates with the subacromial bursa.
      –facilitates the movement of the deltoid muscle over the joint capsule and the supraspinatus tendon.

   c. **Subscapular bursa**

      –lies between the subscapularis tendon and the neck of the scapula.
      –communicates with the synovial cavity of the shoulder joint.

D. **Elbow joint**

   –forms a synovial **hinge (ginglymus) joint,** the **humeroradial joint** between the capitulum of the humerus and the head of the radius and **humeroulnar joint** between the trochlea of the humerus and the trochlear notch of the ulna.
   –allows flexion and extension.
   –also includes the **proximal radioulnar (pivot) joint,** within a common articular capsule. This allows supination and pronation.
   –is innervated by the musculocutaneous, median, radial, and ulnar nerves.
   –receives blood from the anastomosis formed by branches of the brachial artery and recurrent branches of the radial and ulnar arteries.

–is reinforced by the following ligaments:

1. **Annular ligament**

   –is a fibrous band that forms nearly four-fifths of a circle around the head of the radius; the **radial notch** forms the remainder.

   –forms a collar around the head of the radius and prevents withdrawal of the head of the radius from its socket.

   –fuses with the radial collateral ligament and blends with the articular capsule.

2. **Radial collateral ligament**

   –extends from the lateral epicondyle to the anterior and posterior margins of the radial notch of the ulna and the annular ligament of the radius.

3. **Ulnar collateral ligament**

   –is **triangular** and is composed of anterior, posterior, and oblique bands.

   –extends from the medial epicondyle to the coronoid process and the olecranon of the ulna.

E. **Proximal radioulnar joint**

   –forms a synovial **pivot (trochoid) joint** in which the head of the radius articulates with the radial notch of the ulna.

   –allows **pronation** and **supination.**

F. **Distal radioulnar joint**

   –forms a synovial **pivot joint** between the head of the ulna and the ulnar notch of the radius.

   –allows **pronation** and **supination.**

G. **Wrist (radiocarpal) joint**

   –is an **ellipsoidal joint** formed superiorly by the radius and the articular disk and inferiorly by the proximal row of carpal bones (scaphoid, lunate, and triquetrum), exclusive of the pisiform.

   –has a capsule that is strengthened by radial and ulnar collateral ligaments and dorsal and palmar radiocarpal ligaments.

   –allows flexion and extension, abduction and adduction, and circumduction.

H. **Midcarpal joint**

   –forms a synovial **plane joint** between the proximal and distal rows of carpal bones.

   –allows gliding and sliding movements.

   –is a compound articulation: laterally the scaphoid articulates with the trapezium and trapezoid, forming a **plane joint;** and medially the scaphoid, lunate, and triquetrum articulate with the capitate and hamate, forming an **ellipsoidal joint.**

I. **Carpometacarpal joints**

   –form **saddle (sellar) joints** between the carpal bone (trapezium) and the first metacarpal bone, allowing flexion and extension, abduction and adduction, and circumduction.

   –also form **plane joints** between the carpal bones and the medial four metacarpal bones, allowing a simple gliding movement.

J. Metacarpophalangeal joints

–are **condyloid joints** that allow flexion and extension as well as abduction and adduction.

–are supported by a palmar ligament and two collateral ligaments.

K. Interphalangeal joints

–are **hinge joints** that allow flexion and extension.

–are supported by a palmar ligament and two collateral ligaments.

Cutaneous Nerves, Superficial Veins, and Lymphatics

I. Cutaneous Nerves (Figure 2-3)

A. Supraclavicular nerve

–arises from the cervical plexus (C3, C4) and innervates the skin over the upper pectoral, deltoid, and outer trapezius areas.

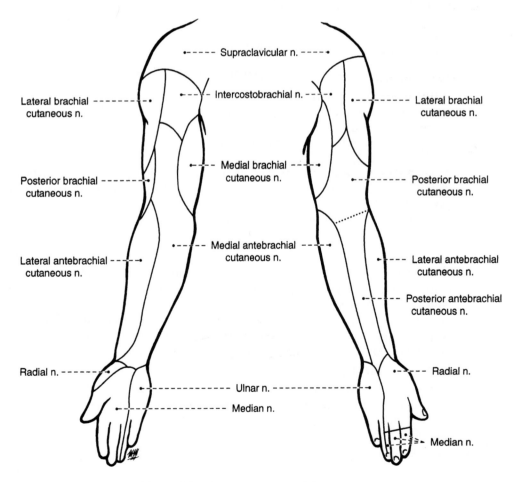

Figure 2-3. Cutaneous nerves of the upper limb.

B. **Medial brachial cutaneous nerve**

–arises from the medial cord of the brachial plexus and innervates the medial side of the arm.

C. **Medial antebrachial cutaneous nerve**

–arises from the medial cord of the brachial plexus and innervates the medial side of the forearm.

D. **Lateral brachial cutaneous nerve**

–arises from the axillary nerve and innervates the lateral side of the arm.

E. **Lateral antebrachial cutaneous nerve**

–arises from the musculocutaneous nerve and innervates the lateral side of the forearm.

F. **Posterior brachial and antebrachial cutaneous nerves**

–arise from the radial nerve and innervate the posterior sides of the arm and forearm, respectively.

G. **Intercostobrachial nerve**

–is the lateral cutaneous branch of the second intercostal nerve and emerges from the second intercostal space by piercing the intercostal and serratus anterior muscles.

–may communicate with the medial brachial cutaneous nerve.

II. **Superficial Veins of the Upper Limb** (Figure 2-4)

A. **Cephalic vein**

–begins as a radial continuation of the dorsal venous network and runs on the lateral side.

–is often connected with the basilic vein by the median cubital vein in front of the elbow.

–ascends along the lateral surface of the biceps, pierces the brachial fascia, and lies in the deltopectoral triangle with the deltoid branch of the thoracoacromial trunk.

–pierces the costocoracoid membrane of the clavipectoral fascia and empties into the axillary vein.

B. **Basilic vein**

–arises from the dorsal venous arch of the hand and accompanies the medial antebrachial cutaneous nerve on the posteromedial surface of the forearm and passes anterior to the medial epicondyle.

–pierces the deep fascia of the arm and joins the two **brachial veins,** the venae comitantes of the brachial artery, to form the **axillary vein** at the lower border of the teres major muscle.

C. **Median cubital vein**

–connects the cephalic vein to the basilic vein over the cubital fossa.

–lies superficial to the **bicipital aponeurosis,** and thus separates it from the brachial artery, which can be punctured during intravenous injections and blood transfusions.

D. **Median antebrachial vein**

–arises in the palmar venous network, ascends on the front of the forearm, and terminates in the median cubital or the basilic vein.

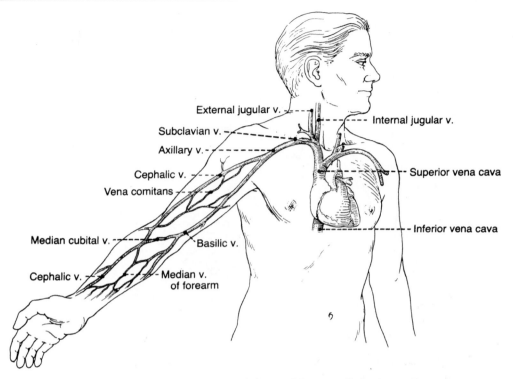

Figure 2-4. Venous drainage of the upper limb.

E. Dorsal venous network
—receives dorsal digital veins by means of dorsal metacarpal veins.
—also receives palmar digital veins by means of intercapitular and palmar metacarpal veins.
—continues proximally as the **cephalic vein** (radial part) and as the **basilic vein** (ulnar part).

III. Superficial Lymphatics and Axillary Lymph Nodes

A. Lymphatics of the finger
—drain into the plexus on the dorsum and palm of the hand.

B. Medial group of lymphatic vessels
—accompanies the basilic vein, passes through the cubital or supratrochlear nodes, and ascends to enter the **lateral axillary nodes,** which drain first into the **central axillary nodes** and then into the **apical axillary nodes.**

C. Lateral group of lymphatic vessels
—accompanies the cephalic vein and drains into the **lateral axillary nodes** and also into the **deltopectoral** (infraclavicular) **node,** which then drain into the **apical nodes.**

D. Axillary lymph nodes (Figure 2-5)

1. Central nodes
—lie near the base of the axilla between the lateral thoracic and subscapular veins; receive lymph from the lateral, pectoral, and posterior groups of nodes; and drain into the apical nodes.

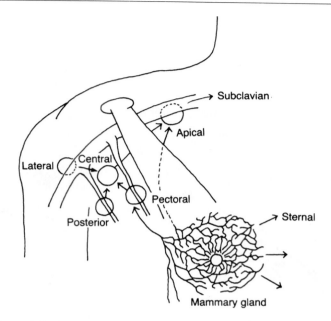

Figure 2-5. Lymphatic drainage of the breast and axillary lymph nodes.

2. Lateral nodes

–lie posteromedial to the axillary veins, receive lymph from the upper limb, and drain into the central nodes.

3. Subscapular (posterior) nodes

–lie along the subscapular vein, receive lymph from the posterior thoracic wall and the posterior aspect of the shoulder, and drain into the central nodes.

4. Pectoral (anterior) nodes

–lie along the inferolateral border of the pectoralis minor muscle; receive lymph from the anterior and lateral thoracic walls, including the breast; and drain into the central nodes.

5. Apical nodes

–lie at the apex of the axilla medial to the axillary vein and above the upper border of the pectoralis minor muscle, receive lymph from all of the other axillary nodes (and occasionally from the breast), and drain into the subclavian trunks.

Pectoral Region and Axilla

I. Fasciae of the Pectoral and Axillary Regions

A. Clavipectoral fascia

–extends between the coracoid process, the clavicle, and the thoracic wall.
–envelops the subclavius and pectoralis minor muscles.

B. **Costocoracoid membrane**

–is a part of the clavipectoral fascia between the first rib and the coracoid process and covers the deltopectoral triangle.

–is pierced by the **cephalic vein,** the **thoracoacromial artery,** and the **lateral pectoral nerve.**

C. **Pectoral fascia**

–covers the pectoralis major muscle, is attached to the sternum and clavicle, and is continuous with the axillary fascia.

D. **Axillary fascia**

–is continuous anteriorly with the pectoral and clavipectoral fasciae, laterally with the brachial fascia, and posteromedially with the fascia over the latissimus dorsi and serratus anterior muscles.

–ascends and invests the pectoralis minor as the suspensory ligament of the axilla that forms the hollow of the armpit when the arm is abducted.

E. **Axillary sheath**

–is a fascial prolongation of the prevertebral layer of the deep cervical fascia into the axilla, enclosing the axillary vessels and the brachial plexus.

II. **Breast and Mammary Gland** (Figure 2-6)

A. **Breast**

–consists of mammary gland tissue, fibrous and fatty tissue, blood and lymph vessels, and nerves.

–extends from the second to sixth ribs and from the sternum to the midaxillary line.

–is divided into the upper and lower lateral and medial quadrants.

–has mammary glands, which lie in the **superficial fascia.**

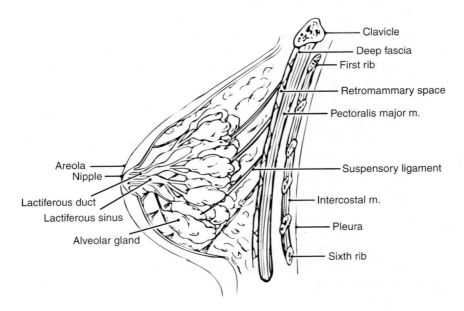

Figure 2-6. Breast.

–is supported by the **suspensory ligaments (Cooper's ligaments),** which are strong fibrous processes that run from the dermis of the skin to the deep layer of the superficial fascia through the breast.

–has a **nipple,** which usually lies at the level of the fourth intercostal space.

–has an **areola,** which is a ring of pigmented skin around the nipple.

–has blood circulation supplied by the **medial mammary** branches of the anterior perforating branches of the internal thoracic artery, the **lateral mammary** branches of the lateral thoracic artery, and the **pectoral** branches of the thoracoacromial trunk.

–is innervated by the anterior and lateral cutaneous branches of the second to sixth intercostal nerves.

–is possible to have presence of more than one pair of breasts (polymastia) and more than one pair of nipples (polythelia).

B. Mammary gland

–is a **modified sweat gland** located in the fatty superficial fascia.

–has the **axillary tail,** a small part of the mammary gland that extends superolaterally sometimes through the deep fascia to lie in the axilla.

–is separated from the deep fascia covering the underlying muscles by an area of loose areolar tissue known as the **retromammary space,** which allows the breast some degree of movement over the pectoralis major muscle.

–has 15 to 20 lobes of glandular tissue, which are separated by fibrous septa that radiate from the nipple. Each lobe opens by a **lactiferous duct** onto the tip of the nipple, and each duct enlarges to form a **lactiferous sinus,** which serves as a reservoir for milk during lactation.

–usually warrants radial incisions to avoid spreading any infection and damaging the lactiferous ducts.

C. Lymphatic drainage (see Figure 2-5)

–removes lymphatic fluid from the lateral quadrants into the axillary nodes and the medial quadrants into the parasternal (internal thoracic) nodes.

–drains primarily (75%) to the **axillary** nodes, more specifically to the **pectoral (anterior)** nodes (including drainage of the nipple).

–follows the perforating vessels through the pectoralis major muscle and the thoracic wall to enter the **parasternal (internal thoracic) nodes,** which lie along the internal thoracic artery.

–also drains to the apical nodes and may connect to lymphatics draining the opposite breast and to lymphatics draining the anterior abdominal wall.

–is of great importance in view of the frequent development of cancer and subsequent dissemination of cancer cells through the lymphatic stream.

III. Axilla

–is a pyramidal region between the upper thoracic wall and the arm.

A. Boundaries of the axilla

1. **Medial wall:** upper ribs and their intercostal muscles and serratus anterior muscle

2. **Lateral wall:** humerus

3. **Posterior wall:** subscapularis, teres major, and latissimus dorsi muscles

4. **Anterior wall:** pectoralis major and pectoralis minor muscles

5. **Base:** axillary fascia

6. **Apex:** interval between the clavicle, scapula, and first rib

B. Contents of the axilla

–include the axillary vasculature, branches of the brachial plexus, lymph nodes, and areolar tissue.

IV. Muscles of the Pectoral Region and Axilla (Figure 2-7; Table 2-1)

Table 2–1. Muscles of the Pectoral Region and Axilla

Muscle	Origin	Insertion	Nerve	Action
Pectoralis major	Medial half of clavicle; manubrium and body of sternum; upper six costal cartilages	Lateral lip of intertubercular groove of humerus	Lateral and medial pectorals	Flexes, adducts, and medially rotates arm
Pectoralis minor	Third, fourth, and fifth ribs	Coracoid process of scapula	Medial (and lateral) pectoral	Depresses scapula; elevates ribs
Subclavius	Junction of first rib and costal cartilage	Inferior surface of clavicle	Nerve to subclavius	Depresses lateral part of clavicle
Serratus anterior	Upper eight ribs	Medial border of scapula	Long thoracic	Rotates scapula upward; abducts arm and elevates it above the horizontal

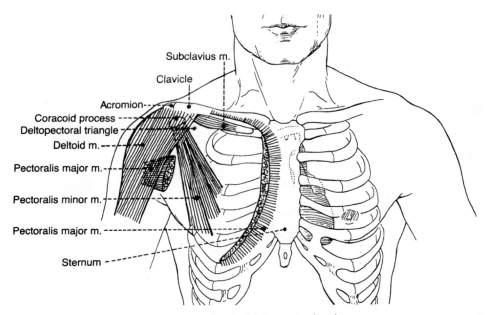

Figure 2-7. Muscles of the pectoral region.

V. Brachial Plexus (see Figure 2-15)

–is described in terms of its formation, branches from the roots, trunks and cords, and distribution (see Nerves: I)

VI. Axillary Artery and Vein (see Figure 2-15)

–are described in terms of their courses and branches (or tributaries) [see Blood Vessels: II, VI C]

VII. Axillary Lymph Nodes (see Cutaneous Nerves, Superficial Veins, and Lymphatics: III D; see Figure 2-5)

Shoulder Region

I. Muscles of the Shoulder Region (Figure 2-8; Table 2-2)

II. Structures of the Shoulder Region (Figure 2-9)

A. Quadrangular space

–is bounded superiorly by the teres minor and subscapularis muscles, inferiorly by the teres major muscle, medially by the long head of the triceps, and laterally by the surgical neck of the humerus.

Table 2–2. Muscles of the Shoulder

Muscle	Origin	Insertion	Nerve	Action
Deltoid	Lateral third of clavicle, acromion, and spine of scapula	Deltoid tuberosity of humerus	Axillary	Abducts, adducts, flexes, extends, and rotates arm medially and laterally
Supraspinatus	Supraspinous fossa of scapula	Superior facet of greater tubercle of humerus	Suprascapular	Abducts arm
Infraspinatus	Infraspinous fossa	Middle facet of greater tubercle of humerus	Suprascapular	Rotates arm laterally
Subscapularis	Subscapular fossa	Lesser tubercle of humerus	Upper and lower subscapular	Adducts and rotates arm medially
Teres major	Dorsal surface of inferior angle of scapula	Medial lip of intertubercular groove of humerus	Lower subscapular	Adducts and rotates arm medially
Teres minor	Upper portion of lateral border of scapula	Lower facet of greater tubercle of humerus	Axillary	Rotates arm laterally
Latissimus dorsi	Spines of T7–T12 thoraco-lumbar fascia, iliac crest, ribs 9–12	Floor of bicipital groove of humerus	Thoracodorsal	Adducts, extends, and rotates arm medially

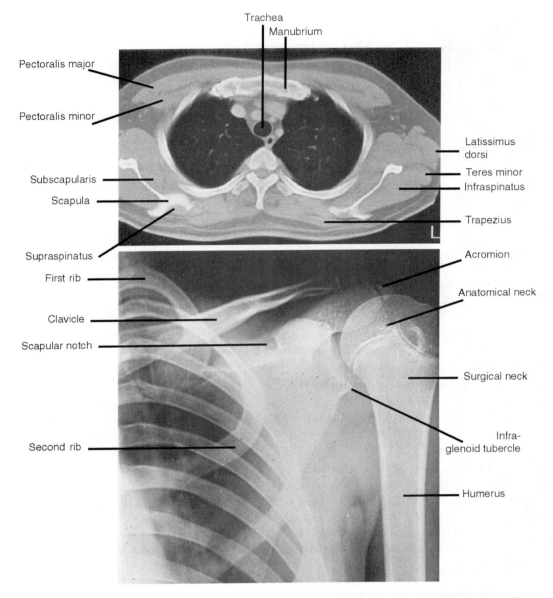

Figure 2-8. Views of the shoulder region. (*A*) Transverse computed tomography (CT) image through the shoulders and upper thorax. (*B*) Radiograph of the shoulder region in an 11-year-old boy.

–transmits the **axillary nerve** and the **posterior humeral circumflex vessels.**

B. Triangular space (upper)

–is bounded superiorly by the teres minor muscle, inferiorly by the teres major muscle, and laterally by the long head of the triceps.

–contains the **circumflex scapular vessels.**

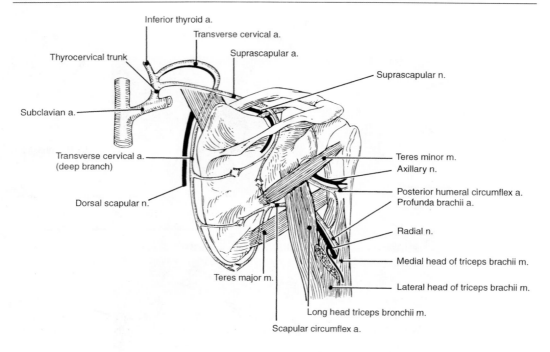

Figure 2-9. Structures of the shoulder region.

C. Triangular space (lower)
–is formed superiorly by the teres major muscle, medially by the long head of the triceps, and laterally by the medial head of the triceps.
–contains the **radial nerve** and the **profunda brachii (deep brachial) artery.**

D. Triangle of auscultation
–is bounded by the upper border of the latissimus dorsi muscle, the lateral border of the trapezius muscle, and the medial border of the scapula; its floor is formed by the rhomboid major muscle.
–is most prominent when the shoulders are drawn forward.
–is the site at which **breathing sounds** are heard most clearly.

III. Arteries

A. Suprascapular artery (see Blood Vessels: I A)

B. Dorsal scapular or descending scapular artery (see Blood Vessels: I B)

C. Arterial anastomoses around scapula
–occur between three groups of arteries: (1) suprascapular, descending scapular, and circumflex scapula arteries; (2) acromial and posterior humeral circumflex arteries; and (3) descending scapular and posterior intercostal arteries.

IV. Nerves

A. Suprascapular nerve (C5–C6) [see Nerves: I B 1]

B. Dorsal scapular nerve (see Nerves: I A 1)

V. Shoulder Joint and Associated Structures

A. Shoulder joint (see Bones and Joints: II C)

B. Acromioclavicular joint (see Bones and Joints: II A)

Arm and Forearm

I. Structures of the Arm and Forearm

A. Brachial intermuscular septa

–extend from the brachial fascia, which is a portion of the deep fascia enclosing the arm.

–consist of medial and lateral intermuscular septa, which divide the arm into the anterior compartment **(flexor compartment)** and the posterior compartment **(extensor compartment).**

B. Cubital fossa

–is a V-shaped interval on the anterior aspect of the elbow that is bounded laterally by the **brachioradialis** muscle and medially by the **pronator teres** muscle.

–has an upper limit that is an imaginary horizontal line connecting the epicondyles of the humerus, with a floor formed by the brachialis and supinator muscles.

–has a lower end where the brachial artery divides into the radial and ulnar arteries, with a fascial roof strengthened by the bicipital aponeurosis.

–contains (from lateral to medial) the **R**adial nerve, **B**iceps tendon, **B**rachial artery, and **M**edian nerve (mnemonic device: **R**on **B**eats **B**ad **M**en).

C. Bicipital aponeurosis

–originates from the medial border of the biceps tendon.

–lies on the brachial artery and the median nerve and passes downward and medially to blend with the deep fascia of the forearm.

D. Interosseous membrane of the forearm

–is a broad sheet of **dense connective tissue** that extends between the radius and the ulna. Its proximal border and the oblique cord (which extends from the ulnar tuberosity to the radius) form a gap through which the posterior interosseous vessels pass.

–is pierced (distally) by the anterior interosseous vessels.

–provides extra surface area for attachment of the deep extrinsic flexor, extensor, and abductor muscles of the hand.

E. Characteristics of the arm and forearm

1. Carrying angle

–is formed laterally by the axis of the arm and forearm when the elbow is extended, because the medial edge of the trochlea projects more inferiorly than its lateral edge.

–is wider in women than in men and disappears when the forearm is flexed or pronated.

2. Pronation and supination

–occur at the **proximal** and **distal radioulnar joints** and have unequal strengths, with supination being the stronger.

–are movements in which the upper end of the radius nearly rotates within the annular ligament.

a. Supination. The palm faces forward (lateral rotation).

b. Pronation. The radius rotates over the ulna, and thus the palm faces backward (medial rotation about a longitudinal axis, in which case the shafts of the radius and ulna cross each other).

II. Muscles of the Arm (Table 2-3)

Table 2–3. Muscles of the Arm

Muscle	Origin	Insertion	Nerve	Action
Coracobrachialis	Coracoid process	Middle third of medial surface of humerus	Musculocutaneous	Flexes and adducts arm
Biceps brachii	Long head, supraglenoid tubercle; short head, coracoid process	Radial tuberosity of radius	Musculocutaneous	Flexes arm and forearm, supinates forearm
Brachialis	Lower anterior surface of humerus	Coronoid process of ulna and ulnar tuberosity	Musculocutaneous	Flexes forearm
Triceps	Long head, infraglenoid tubercle; lateral head, superior to radial groove of humerus; medial head, inferior to radial groove	Posterior surface of olecranon process of ulna	Radial	Extends forearm
Anconeus	Lateral epicondyle of humerus	Olecranon and upper posterior surface of ulna	Radial	Extends forearm

III. Muscles of the Anterior Forearm (Table 2-4)

IV. Muscles of the Posterior Forearm (Table 2-5)

V. Nerves of the Arm and Forearm

–include the musculocutaneous, median, radial, and ulnar nerves (see Nerves: II).

VI. Arteries of the Arm and Forearm

–include the brachial, radial, and ulnar arteries and their branches (see Blood Vessels: III–V).

Table 2–4. Muscles of the Anterior Forearm

Muscle	Origin	Insertion	Nerve	Action
Pronator teres	Medial epicondyle and coronoid process of ulna	Middle of lateral side of radius	Median	Pronates forearm
Flexor carpi radialis	Medial epicondyle of humerus	Bases of second and third metacarpals	Median	Flexes forearm, flexes and abducts hand
Palmaris longus	Medial epicondyle of humerus	Flexor retinaculum, palmar aponeurosis	Median	Flexes forearm and hand
Flexor carpi ulnaris	Medial epicondyle (humeral head); medial olecranon, and posterior border of ulna (ulnar head)	Pisiform, hook of hamate, and base of fifth metacarpal	Ulnar	Flexes forearm; flexes and adducts hand
Flexor digitorum superficialis	Medial epicondyle, coronoid process, oblique line of radius	Middle phalanges of finger	Median	Flexes proximal interphalangeal joints, flexes hand and forearm
Flexor digitorum profundus	Anteromedial surface of ulna, interosseous membrane	Bases of distal phalanges of fingers	Ulnar and median	Flexes distal interphalangeal joints and hand
Flexor pollicis longus	Anterior surface of radius, interosseous membrane, and coronoid process	Base of distal phalanx of thumb	Median	Flexes thumb
Pronator quadratus	Anterior surface of distal ulna	Anterior surface of distal radius	Median	Pronates forearm

Hand

I. Structures of the Hand (Figures 2-10 and 2-11)

A. Extensor retinaculum

–is a thickening of the antebrachial fascia on the back of the wrist, is subdivided into compartments, and places the extensor tendons beneath it.

–extends from the lateral margin of the radius to the styloid process of the ulna, the pisiform, and the triquetrum.

–is crossed superficially by the superficial branch of the radial nerve.

B. Palmar aponeurosis

–is a triangular fibrous layer overlying the tendons in the palm, and is continuous with the palmaris longus tendon, the thenar and hypothenar fasciae, the flexor retinaculum, and the palmar carpal ligament.

–protects the superficial palmar arterial arch, the palmar digital nerves, and the long flexor tendons.

Table 2–5. Muscles of the Posterior Forearm

Muscle	Origin	Insertion	Nerve	Action
Brachioradialis	Lateral supracondylar ridge of humerus	Base of radial styloid process	Radial	Flexes forearm
Extensor carpi radialis longus	Lateral supracondylar ridge of humerus	Dorsum of base of second metacarpal	Radial	Extends and abducts hand
Extensor carpi radialis brevis	Lateral epicondyle of humerus	Posterior base of third metacarpal	Radial	Extends fingers and abducts hands
Extensor digitorum	Lateral epicondyle of humerus	Extensor expansion, base of middle and digital phalanges	Radial	Extends fingers and hand
Extensor digiti minimi	Common extensor tendon and interosseous membrane	Extensor expansion, base of middle and distal phalanges	Radial	Extends little finger
Extensor carpi ulnaris	Lateral epicondyle and posterior surface of ulna	Base of fifth metacarpal	Radial	Extends and adducts hand
Supinator	Lateral epicondyle, radial collateral and annular ligaments	Lateral side of upper part of radius	Radial	Supinates forearm
Abductor pollicis longus	Interosseous membrane, middle third of posterior surfaces of radius and ulna	Lateral surface of base of first metacarpal	Radial	Abducts thumb and hand
Extensor pollicis longus	Interosseous membrane and middle third of posterior surface of ulna	Base of distal phalanx of thumb	Radial	Extends distal phalanx of thumb and abducts hand
Extensor pollicis brevis	Interosseous membrane and posterior surface of middle third of radius	Base of proximal phalanx of thumb	Radial	Extends proximal phalanx of thumb and abducts hand
Extensor indicis	Posterior surface of ulna and interosseous membrane	Extensor expansion of index finger	Radial	Extends index finger

–undergoes thickening, shortening, and fibrosis to produce **Dupuytren's contracture,** a flexion deformity in which the fingers are pulled toward the palm.

C. **Palmar carpal ligament**

–is a thickening of deep antebrachial fascia at the wrist, covering the tendons of the flexor muscles, median nerve, and ulnar artery and nerve, except palmar branches of the median and ulnar nerves.

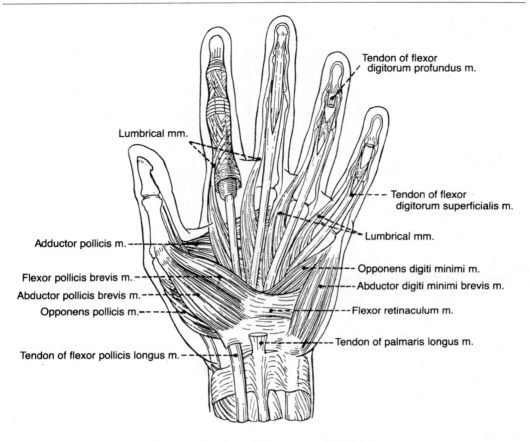

Figure 2-10. Superficial muscles of the hand.

D. Flexor retinaculum (see Figure 2-10)

–serves as an origin for muscles of the thenar eminence.

–forms a **carpal (osteofacial) tunnel** on the anterior aspect of the wrist.

–is attached medially to the triquetrum, the pisiform and the hook of the hamate, and laterally to the tubercles of the scaphoid and trapezium.

–is crossed superficially by the **ulnar nerve, ulnar artery, palmaris longus tendon,** and **palmar cutaneous branch of the median nerve.**

E. Carpal tunnel

–is formed anteriorly by the flexor retinaculum and posteriorly by the carpal bones.

–transmits the **median nerve** and the tendons of **flexor pollicis longus, flexor digitorum profundus,** and **flexor digitorum superficialis muscles.**

F. Fascial spaces of the palm

–are fascial spaces deep to the palmar aponeurosis and divided by a midpalmar (oblique) septum into the **thenar space** and the **midpalmar space.**

1. Thenar space

–is the lateral space that contains the flexor pollicis longus tendon and the other flexor tendons of the index finger.

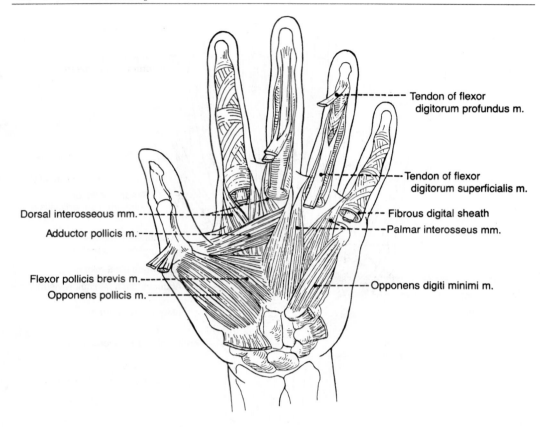

Figure 2-11. Deep muscles of the hand.

2. Midpalmar space

–is the medial space that contains the flexor tendons of the medial three digits.

G. Synovial flexor sheaths

1. Common synovial flexor sheath (ulnar bursa)

–envelops or contains the tendons of both the flexor digitorum superficialis and profundus muscles.

2. Synovial sheath for flexor pollicis longus (radial bursa)

–envelops the tendon of the flexor pollicis longus muscle.

H. Extensor expansion (Figure 2-12)

–is the expansion of the extensor tendon over the metacarpophalangeal joint and is referred to by clinicians as the **extensor hood.**

–provides the insertion of the lumbrical and interosseous muscles as well as the extensor indicis and extensor digiti minimi muscles.

I. Anatomical snuff-box

–is a **triangular interval** bounded medially by the tendon of the extensor pollicis longus muscle and laterally by the tendons of the extensor pollicis brevis and abductor pollicis longus muscles.

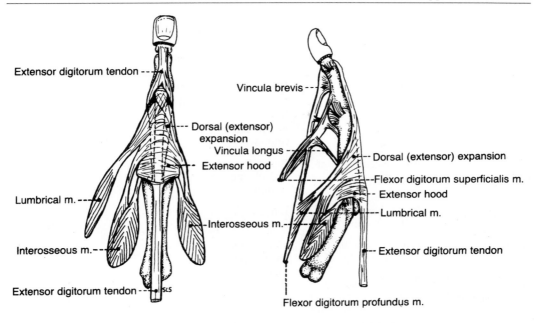

Figure 2-12. Dorsal (extensor) expansion of the middle finger.

–is limited proximally by the styloid process of the radius.
–has a floor formed by the scaphoid and trapezium bones and crossed by the **radial artery.**

J. Fingernails

–are keratinized plates on the dorsum of the tips of the fingers that consist of the proximal hidden part or **root,** the exposed part or **body,** and the distal **free border.** Parts of the nail include:

1. **Nail bed.** The skin underneath the nail is the **nail bed** in which sensory nerve endings and blood vessels are abundant. The **matrix** or proximal part of the nail bed produces hard keratin and is responsible for nail growth.

2. **Other structures.** The root is partially covered by a fold of skin known as the **nail fold.** The narrow band of epidermis prolonged from the proximal nail fold onto the nail is termed the **eponychium.** The half-moon or **lunula** is distal to the eponychium. The **hyponychium** represents the thickened epidermis deep to the distal end of the nail.

III. Vessels of the Hand (see Blood Vessels: IV C–E, G; V D–G; see Figures 2-17 and 2-18)

IV. Nerves of the Hand (see Nerves II: B–D; see Figures 2-17 and 2-18)

Nerves

I. Brachial Plexus (Figure 2-15)

–is formed by the ventral primary rami of the lower four cervical nerves and the first thoracic nerve (C5–T1).

II. **Muscles of the Hand** (Figures 2-13 and 2-14; Table 2-6)

Table 2–6. Muscles of the Hand

Muscle	Origin	Insertion	Nerve	Action
Abductor pollicis brevis	Flexor retinaculum, scaphoid, and trapezium	Lateral side of base of proximal phalanx of thumb	Median	Abducts thumb
Flexor pollicis brevis	Flexor retinaculum and trapezium	Base of proximal phalanx of thumb	Median	Flexes thumb
Opponens pollicis	Flexor retinaculum and trapezium	Lateral side of first metacarpal	Median	Opposes thumb to other digits
Adductor pollicis	Capitate and bases of second and third metacarpals (oblique head); palmar surface of third metacarpal (transverse head)	Medial side of base of proximal phalanx of the thumb	Ulnar	Adducts thumb
Palmaris brevis	Medial side of flexor retinaculum, palmar aponeurosis	Skin of medial side of palm	Ulnar	Wrinkles skin on medial side of palm
Abductor digiti minimi	Pisiform and tendon of flexor carpi ulnaris	Medial side of base of proximal phalanx of little finger	Ulnar	Abducts little finger
Flexor digiti minimi brevis	Flexor retinaculum and hook of hamate	Medial side of base of proximal phalanx of little finger	Ulnar	Flexes proximal phalanx of little finger
Opponens digiti minimi	Flexor retinaculum and hook of hamate	Medial side of fifth metacarpal	Ulnar	Opposes little finger
Lumbricals (4)	Lateral side of tendons of flexor digitorum profundus	Lateral side of extensor expansion	Median (two lateral) and ulnar (two medial)	Flex metacarpophalangeal joints and extend interphalangeal joints
Dorsal interossei (4)	Adjacent sides of metacarpal bones	Lateral sides of bases of proximal phalanges; extensor expansion	Ulnar	Abduct fingers; flex metacarpophalangeal joints; extend interphalangeal joints
Palmar interossei (3)	Medial side of second metacarpal; lateral sides of fourth and fifth metacarpals	Bases of proximal phalanges in same sides as their origins; extensor expansion	Ulnar	Adduct fingers; flex metacarpophalangeal joints; extend interphalangeal joints

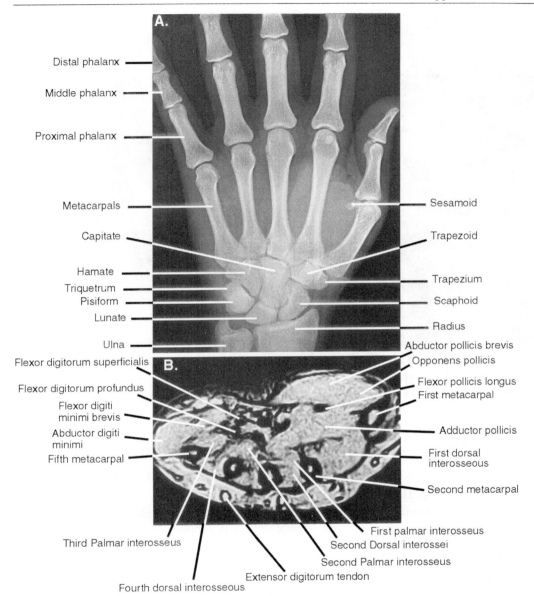

Figure 2-13. Bones and muscles of the hand. (*A*) Radiograph of the wrist and hand. (*B*) Transverse magnetic resonance image (MRI) of the palm of the hand.

–has roots that pass between the scalenus anterior and medius muscles.

–is enclosed with the axillary artery and vein in the **axillary sheath,** which is formed by a prolongation of the prevertebral fascia.

–has the following subdivisions:

A. Branches from the roots

1. Dorsal scapular nerve (C5)

–pierces the scalenus medius muscle to reach the posterior cervical triangle and descends deep to the levator scapulae and the rhomboid minor and major muscles.

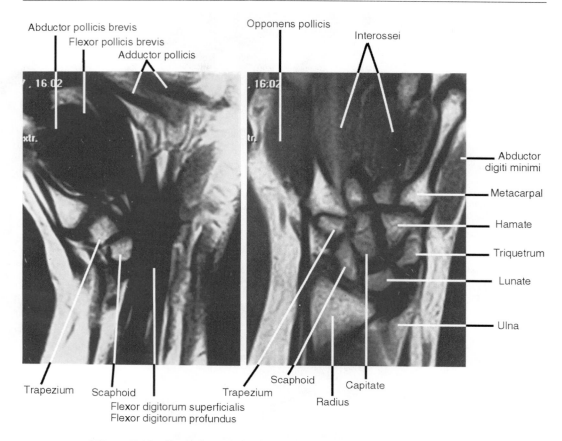

Figure 2-14. Coronal magnetic resonance image (MRI) of the wrist and hand.

–innervates the rhomboids and frequently the levator scapulae muscles.

2. Long thoracic nerve (C5–C7)

–descends behind the brachial plexus and runs on the external surface of the serratus anterior muscle, which it supplies.

–when damaged, causes **winging of the scapula** and makes elevating the arm above a horizontal position impossible.

B. Branches from the upper trunk

1. Suprascapular nerve (C5–C6)

–runs laterally across the posterior cervical triangle.

–passes through the scapular notch under the superior transverse scapular ligament, whereas the suprascapular artery passes over the ligament. [Thus, it can be said that the army **(artery)** runs over the bridge **(ligament),** and the navy **(nerve)** runs under the bridge.]

–supplies the supraspinatus muscle and the shoulder joint and then descends through the notch of the scapular neck to innervate the infraspinatus muscle.

2. Nerve to subclavius (C5)

–descends in front of the brachial plexus and the subclavian artery and behind the clavicle to reach the subclavius muscle.

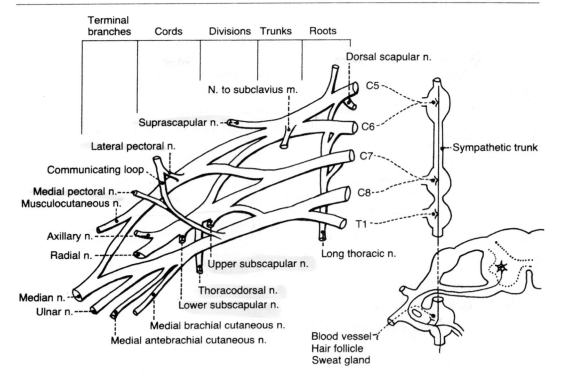

Figure 2-15. Brachial plexus.

–also innervates the sternoclavicular joint.

–usually branches to the **accessory phrenic nerve (C5),** which enters the thorax to join the phrenic nerve.

C. Branches from the lateral cord

1. Lateral pectoral nerve (C5–C7)

–innervates the **pectoralis major muscle** primarily and also supplies the **pectoralis minor muscle** by way of a nerve loop.

–sends a branch over the first part of the axillary artery to the medial pectoral nerve and forms a nerve loop through which the lateral pectoral nerve conveys motor fibers to the pectoralis minor muscle.

–pierces the costocoracoid membrane of the clavipectoral fascia.

–is accompanied by the pectoral branch of the thoracoacromial artery.

2. Musculocutaneous nerve (C5–C7)

–pierces the coracobrachialis muscle, descends between the biceps brachii and brachialis muscles, and innervates these three muscles.

D. Branches from the medial cord

1. Medial pectoral nerve (C8–T1)

–passes forward between the axillary artery and vein and forms a loop in front of the axillary artery with the lateral pectoral nerve.

–enters and supplies the pectoralis minor muscle and reaches the overlying pectoralis major muscle.

2. **Medial brachial cutaneous nerve (C8–T1)**

   –runs along the medial side of the axillary vein.

   –innervates the skin on the medial side of the arm.

   –may communicate with the **intercostobrachial nerve,** which arises as a lateral branch of the second intercostal nerve.

3. **Medial antebrachial cutaneous nerve (C8–T1)**

   –runs between the axillary artery and vein and then runs medial to the brachial artery.

   –innervates the skin on the medial side of the forearm.

4. **Ulnar nerve (C7–T1)**

   –runs down the medial aspect of the arm but does not branch in the brachium.

E. Branches from the medial and lateral cords: median nerve (C5–T1)

–is formed by heads from both the medial and lateral cords.

–runs down the anteromedial aspect of the arm but does not branch in the brachium.

F. Branches from the posterior cord

1. **Upper subscapular nerve (C5–C6)**

   –innervates the upper portion of the subscapularis muscle.

2. **Thoracodorsal nerve (C7–C8)**

   –runs behind the axillary artery and accompanies the thoracodorsal artery to enter the latissimus dorsi muscle.

3. **Lower subscapular nerve (C5–C6)**

   –innervates the lower part of the subscapularis and teres major muscles.

   –runs downward behind the subscapular vessels to the teres major muscle.

4. **Axillary nerve (C5–C6)**

   –innervates the deltoid muscle (by its anterior and posterior branches) and the teres minor muscle (by its posterior branch).

   –gives rise to the **lateral brachial cutaneous nerve.**

   –passes posteriorly through the quadrangular space accompanied by the posterior circumflex humeral artery.

   –winds around the surgical neck of the humerus (may be injured when this part of the bone is fractured).

5. **Radial nerve (C5–T1)**

   –is the largest branch of the brachial plexus and occupies the musculospiral groove on the back of the humerus with the profunda brachii artery.

II. Nerves of the Arm, Forearm, and Hand (Figures 2-16 and 2-17)

A. Musculocutaneous nerve (C5–C7)

–pierces the coracobrachialis muscle and descends between the biceps and brachialis muscles.

–innervates all of the flexor muscles in the anterior compartment of the arm, such as the coracobrachialis, biceps, and brachialis muscles.

–continues into the forearm as the **lateral antebrachial cutaneous nerve.**

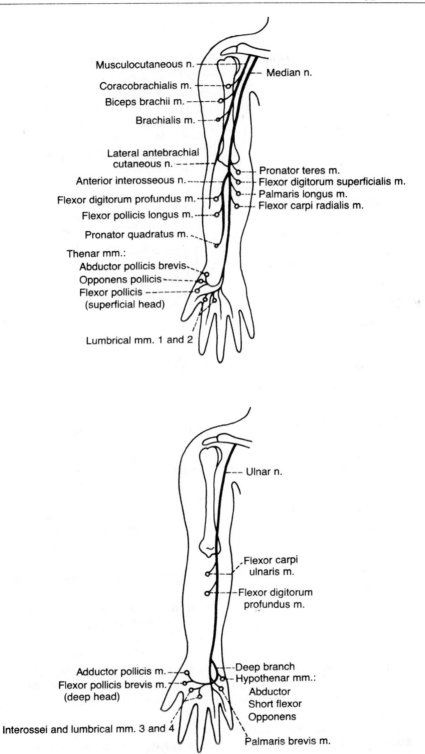

Figure 2-16. Distribution of the musculocutaneous, median, and ulnar nerves.

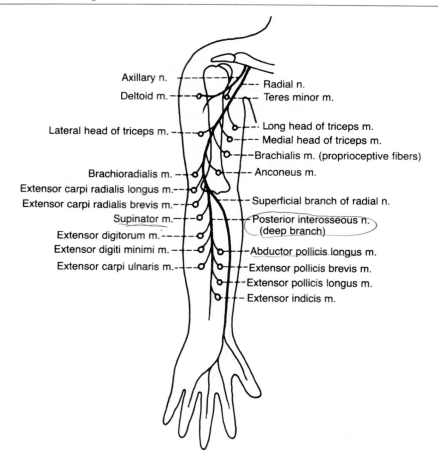

Axillary n.
Radial n.
Deltoid m.
Teres minor m.
Lateral head of triceps m.
Long head of triceps m.
Medial head of triceps m.
Brachialis m. (proprioceptive fibers)
Brachioradialis m.
Anconeus m.
Extensor carpi radialis longus m.
Extensor carpi radialis brevis m.
Superficial branch of radial n.
Supinator m.
Posterior interosseous n. (deep branch)
Extensor digitorum m.
Extensor digiti minimi m.
Abductor pollicis longus m.
Extensor carpi ulnaris m.
Extensor pollicis brevis m.
Extensor pollicis longus m.
Extensor indicis m.

Figure 2-17. Distribution of the axillary and radial nerves.

B. Median nerve (C5–T1)

–runs down the anteromedial aspect of the arm and at the elbow it lies medial to the brachial artery on the brachilis muscle (has no muscular branches in the arm).

–passes through the cubital fossa, deep to the bicipital aponeurosis and medial to the brachial artery.

–enters the forearm between the humeral and ulnar heads of the pronator teres muscle and then passes between the flexor digitorum superficialis and the flexor digitorum profundus muscles.

–in the cubital fossa, gives rise to the **anterior interosseous nerve,** which descends on the interosseous membrane between the flexor digitorum profundus and the flexor pollicis longus, passes behind the pronator quadratus, supplying these three muscles, and then ends in sensory "twigs" to the wrist joint.

–innervates all of the anterior muscles of the forearm except the flexor carpi ulnaris and the ulnar half of the flexor digitorum profundus.

–enters the palm of the hand through the carpal tunnel deep to the flexor retinaculum, gives off a muscular branch **(recurrent branch)** to the thenar muscles, and terminates by dividing into three **common palmar digital nerves,** which then divide into the palmar digital branches.

–innervates also the lateral two lumbricals, the skin of the lateral side of the palm, and the palmar side of the lateral three and one-half fingers, as well as the dorsal side of the index finger, middle finger, and one-half of the ring finger.

C. Radial nerve (C5–T1)

–arises from the posterior cord and the **largest branch** of the brachial plexus.

–descends posteriorly between the long and medial heads of the triceps, after which it passes inferolaterally with the profunda brachii artery in the spiral (radial) groove on the back of the humerus between the medial and lateral heads of the triceps.

–pierces the lateral intermuscular septum to enter the anterior compartment and descends anterior to the lateral epicondyle between the brachialis and brachioradialis muscles to enter the cubital fossa, where it divides into superficial and deep branches.

–gives rise to muscular, articular, and posterior brachial and antebrachial cutaneous branches.

1. Deep branch

–enters the supinator muscle, winds laterally around the radius in the substance of the muscle, and continues as the **posterior interosseous nerve** with the posterior interosseous artery.

–innervates the muscles of the back of the forearm.

2. Superficial branch

–descends in the forearm under cover of the brachioradialis muscle and then passes dorsally around the radius under the tendon of the brachioradialis.

–runs distally to the dorsum of the hand to innervate the skin of the radial side of the hand and the radial two and one-half digits over the proximal phalanx. This nerve does not supply the skin of the distal phalanges.

D. Ulnar nerve (C7–T1)

–arises from the medial cord of the brachial plexus, runs down the medial aspect of the arm, pierces the medial intermuscular septum at the middle of the arm, and descends together with the superior ulnar collateral branch of the brachial artery.

–descends behind the medial epicondyle in a groove, where it is readily palpated and most commonly injured. It may be damaged by a fracture of the medial epicondyle and produce **funny bone** symptoms.

–enters the forearm by passing between the two heads of the flexor carpi ulnaris and descends between and innervates the flexor carpi ulnaris and flexor digitorum profundus muscles.

–enters the hand superficial to the flexor retinaculum and lateral to the pisiform bone, where it is vulnerable to damage from cuts or stab wounds.

–terminates by dividing into superficial and deep branches at the root of the hypothenar eminence.

1. Superficial branch

–innervates the palmaris brevis and the skin over the palmar and dorsal surfaces of the medial one-third of the hand, including the hypothenar eminence.

–terminates in the palm by dividing into **three palmar digital branches,** which supply the skin of the little finger and the medial side of the ring finger.

2. **Deep branch**

–arises at about the level of the pisiform bone and passes between the pisiform and the hook of the hamate, between the origins of the abductor and flexor digiti minimi brevis muscles, and then deep to the opponens digiti minimi.

–curves around the hook of the hamate, and then turns laterally to follow the course of the deep palmar arterial arch across the interossei.

–innervates the hypothenar muscles, the medial two lumbricals, all the interossei, the adductor pollicis, and usually the deep head of the flexor pollicis brevis.

III. Functional Components of the Peripheral Nerves

A. Somatic motor nerves

–includes radial, axillary, median, musculocutaneous, and ulnar nerves.

–contain nerve fibers with cell bodies that are located in the following areas:

1. **Dorsal root ganglia [general somatic afferent (GSA) and general visceral afferent (GVA) fibers]**

2. **Anterior horn of the spinal cord [general somatic efferent (GSE) fibers]**

3. **Sympathetic chain ganglia [sympathetic postganglionic general visceral efferent (GVE) fibers]**

B. Cutaneous nerves

–include medial brachial and medial antebrachial cutaneous nerves.

–contain nerve fibers with cell bodies that are located in the following areas:

1. **Dorsal root ganglia (for GSA and GVA fibers)**

2. **Sympathetic chain ganglia (for sympathetic postganglionic GVE fibers)**

Blood Vessels

I. Branches of the Subclavian Artery (Figure 2-18)

A. Suprascapular artery

–is a branch of the thyrocervical trunk.

–passes over the superior transverse scapular ligament (whereas the suprascapular nerve passes under the ligament).

–anastomoses with the deep branch of the transverse cervical artery **(dorsal scapular artery)** and the circumflex scapular artery around the scapula, providing a collateral circulation.

–supplies the supraspinatus and infraspinatus muscles and the shoulder and acromioclavicular joints.

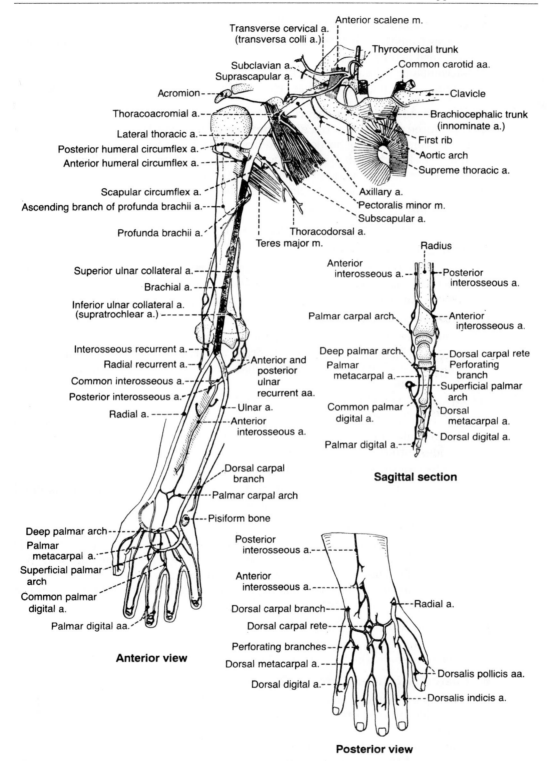

Figure 2-18. Blood supply to the upper limb.

B. Dorsal scapular or descending scapular artery

–arises from the subclavian artery but may be a deep branch of the transverse cervical artery.

–accompanies the dorsal scapular nerve.

–supplies the levator scapulae, rhomboids, and serratus anterior muscles.

II. Axillary Artery (see Figure 2-18)

–is considered to be the **central structure of the axilla.**

–extends from the outer border of the first rib to the inferior border of the teres major muscle, where it becomes the **brachial artery.** The axillary artery is bordered on its medial side by the axillary vein.

–is divided into three parts by the pectoralis minor muscle.

A. Supreme thoracic artery

–supplies the first and second intercostal spaces and adjacent muscles.

B. Thoracoacromial artery

–is a short trunk from the first or second part of the axillary artery and has pectoral, clavicular, acromial, and deltoid branches.

–pierces the costocoracoid membrane (or clavipectoral fascia).

C. Lateral thoracic artery

–runs along the lateral border of the pectoralis minor muscle.

–supplies the pectoralis major, pectoralis minor, and serratus anterior muscles and the axillary lymph nodes, and gives rise to **lateral mammary branches.**

D. Subscapular artery

–is the largest branch of the axillary artery, arises at the lower border of the subscapularis muscle, and descends along the axillary border of the scapula.

–divides into the thoracodorsal and circumflex scapular arteries.

1. Thoracodorsal artery

–accompanies the thoracodorsal nerve and supplies the latissimus dorsi muscle and the lateral thoracic wall.

2. Circumflex scapular artery

–passes posteriorly into the triangular space bounded by the subscapularis muscle and the teres minor muscle above, the teres major muscle below, and the long head of the triceps brachii laterally.

–ramifies in the infraspinous fossa and anastomoses with branches of the dorsal scapular and suprascapular arteries.

E. Anterior humeral circumflex artery

–passes anteriorly around the surgical neck of the humerus.

–anastomoses with the posterior humeral circumflex artery.

F. Posterior humeral circumflex artery

–runs posteriorly with the axillary nerve through the quadrangular space bounded by the teres minor and teres major muscles, the long head of the triceps brachii, and the humerus.

–anastomoses with the anterior humeral circumflex artery and an ascending branch of the profunda brachii artery and also sends a branch to the acromial rete.

III. Brachial Artery (see Figure 2-18)

–extends from the inferior border of the teres major muscle to its bifurcation in the cubital fossa.

–lies on the triceps brachii and then on the brachialis muscles medial to the coracobrachialis and biceps brachii, and is accompanied by the basilic vein in the middle of the arm.

–lies in the center of the cubital fossa, medial to the biceps tendon, lateral to the median nerve, and deep to the bicipital aponeurosis.

–provides muscular branches and terminates by dividing into the radial and ulnar arteries at the level of the radial neck, about 1 cm below the bend of the elbow, in the cubital fossa.

A. Profunda brachii (deep brachial) artery

–descends posteriorly with the radial nerve and gives off an **ascending branch,** which anastomoses with the descending branch of the posterior humeral circumflex artery.

–divides into the **middle collateral artery,** which anastomoses with the interosseous recurrent artery, and the **radial collateral artery,** which follows the radial nerve through the lateral intermuscular septum and ends in front of the lateral epicondyle by anastomosing with the radial recurrent artery of the radial artery.

B. Superior ulnar collateral artery

–pierces the medial intermuscular septum and accompanies the ulnar nerve behind the septum and medial epicondyle.

–anastomoses with the posterior ulnar recurrent branch of the ulnar artery.

C. Inferior ulnar collateral artery

–arises just above the elbow and descends in front of the medial epicondyle.

–anastomoses with the anterior ulnar recurrent branch of the ulnar artery.

IV. Radial Artery (see Figure 2-18; Figure 2-19)

–arises as the smaller lateral branch of the brachial artery in the cubital fossa and descends laterally under cover of the brachioradialis muscle, with the superficial radial nerve on its lateral side, on the supinator and flexor pollicis longus muscles.

–curves over the radial side of the carpal bones beneath the tendons of the abductor pollicis longus muscle, the extensor pollicis longus and brevis muscles, and over the surface of the scaphoid and trapezium bones.

–runs through the anatomical snuff-box, enters the palm by passing between the two heads of the first dorsal interosseous muscle and then between the heads of the adductor pollicis muscle, and divides into the princeps **pollicis artery** and the **deep palmar arch.**

–accounts for the **radial pulse,** which can be felt proximal to the wrist between the tendons of the brachioradialis and flexor carpi radialis muscles. The radial pulse may also be palpated in the anatomical snuff-box between the tendons of the extensor pollicis longus and brevis muscles.

–gives rise to the following branches:

A. Radial recurrent artery

–arises from the radial artery just below its origin and ascends on the supinator and then between the brachioradialis and brachialis muscles.

–anastomoses with the radial collateral branch of the profunda brachii artery.

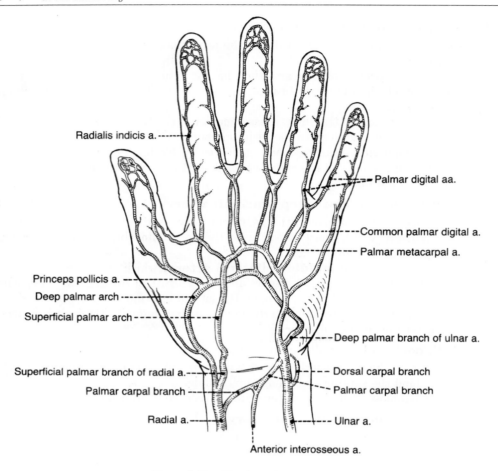

Figure 2-19. Blood supply to the hand.

B. Palmar carpal branch

–joins the palmar carpal branch of the ulnar artery and forms the palmar carpal arch.

C. Superficial palmar branch

–passes through the thenar muscles and anastomoses with the superficial branch of the ulnar artery to complete the superficial palmar arterial arch.

D. Dorsal carpal branch

–joins the dorsal carpal branch of the ulnar artery and the dorsal terminal branch of the anterior interosseous artery to form the **dorsal carpal rete.**

E. Princeps pollicis artery

–descends along the ulnar border of the first metacarpal bone under the flexor pollicis longus tendon.
–divides into two **proper digital arteries** for each side of the thumb.

F. Radialis indicis artery

–also may arise from the deep palmar arch or the princeps pollicis artery.

G. Deep palmar arch

–is formed by the main termination of the radial artery and usually is completed by the deep palmar branch of the ulnar artery.

–passes between the transverse and oblique heads of the adductor pollicis muscle.

–gives rise to three **palmar metacarpal arteries,** which descend on the interossei and join the common palmar digital arteries from the superficial palmar arch.

V. Ulnar Artery (see Figures 2-18 and 2-19)

–is the **larger medial branch of the brachial artery** in the cubital fossa.

–descends behind the ulnar head of the pronator teres muscle and lies between the flexor digitorum superficialis and profundus muscles.

–enters the hand anterior to the flexor retinaculum, lateral to the pisiform bone, and medial to the hook of the hamate bone.

–divides into the superficial palmar arch and the deep palmar branch, which passes between the abductor and flexor digiti minimi brevis muscles and runs medially to join the radial artery to complete the deep palmar arch.

–accounts for the **ulnar pulse,** which is palpable just to the radial side of the insertion of the flexor carpi ulnaris into the pisiform bone.

–gives rise to the following branches:

A. Anterior ulnar recurrent artery

–anastomoses with the inferior ulnar collateral artery.

B. Posterior ulnar recurrent artery

–anastomoses with the superior ulnar collateral artery.

C. Common interosseous artery

–arises from the lateral side of the ulnar artery and divides into the anterior and posterior interosseous arteries.

1. Anterior interosseous artery

–descends with the anterior interosseous nerve in front of the interosseous membrane, located between the flexor digitorum profundus and the flexor pollicis longus muscles.

–perforates the interosseous membrane to anastomose with the posterior interosseous artery and join the dorsal carpal network.

2. Posterior interosseous artery

–gives rise to the interosseous recurrent artery, which anastomoses with a middle collateral branch of the profunda brachii artery.

–descends behind the interosseous membrane in company with the posterior interosseous nerve.

–anastomoses with the dorsal carpal branch of the anterior interosseous artery.

D. Palmar carpal branch

–joins the palmar carpal branch of the radial artery to form the palmar carpal arch.

E. Dorsal carpal branch

–passes around the ulnar side of the wrist and joins the dorsal carpal rete.

F. Superficial palmar arch

–is formed by the main termination of the ulnar artery and usually is completed by the superficial palmar branch of the radial artery.

–lies immediately under the palmar aponeurosis.

–gives rise to three **common palmar digital arteries,** each of which bifurcates into proper palmar digital arteries, which run distally to supply the adjacent sides of the fingers.

G. Deep palmar branch

–accompanies the deep branch of the ulnar nerve through the hypothenar muscles and anastomoses with the radial artery, thereby completing the **deep palmar arch.**

VI. Veins of the Upper Limb (see Figure 2-4)

A. Deep and superficial venous arches

–are formed by a pair of venae comitantes, which accompany each of the deep and superficial palmar arterial arches.

B. Deep veins of the arm and forearm

–follow the course of the arteries, accompanying them as their venae comitantes. (The radial veins receive the dorsal metacarpal veins. The ulnar veins receive tributaries from the deep palmar venous arches. The brachial veins are the vena comitantes of the brachial artery and are joined by the basilic vein to form the axillary vein.)

C. Axillary vein

–begins at the lower border of the teres major muscle as the continuation of the basilic vein and ascends along the medial side of the axillary artery.

–continues as the subclavian vein at the inferior margin of the first rib.

–commonly receives the thoracoepigastric veins directly or indirectly and thus provides a collateral circulation if the inferior vena cava becomes obstructed.

–has tributaries that include the cephalic vein, brachial veins, and veins, which correspond to the branches of the axillary artery, with the exception of the thoracoacromial vein.

Clinical Considerations

I. Breast Cancer Detection and Surgical Treatment

A. Anatomic considerations

–occurs in the upper lateral quadrant (about 60% of cases) and forms a palpable mass in advanced stages.

–enlarges, attaches to Cooper's ligaments, and produces shortening of the ligaments, causing depression or **dimpling** of the overlying skin.

–may also attach to and shorten the lactiferous ducts, resulting in a **retracted** or **inverted nipple.**

–may invade the deep fascia of the pectoralis major muscle, so that contraction of the muscle produces a **sudden upward movement** of the entire breast.

B. Mammography

–is a radiographic examination of the breast to screen for benign and malignant tumors and cysts.

C. Radical mastectomy

–is **extensive surgical removal of the breast and its related structures,** including the pectoralis major and minor muscles, axillary lymph nodes and fascia, and part of the thoracic wall.

–may injure the long thoracic and thoracodorsal nerves.

–may cause postoperative swelling **(edema)** of the upper limb as a result of **lymphatic obstruction** caused by removal of most of the lymphatic channels that drain the arm, or by venous obstruction caused by thrombosis of the axillary vein.

D. Modified radical mastectomy

–involves **excision of the entire breast and axillary lymph nodes,** with preservation of the pectoralis major and minor muscles. (The pectoralis minor muscle is usually retracted or severed near its insertion into the coracoid process.)

E. Lumpectomy (tylectomy)

–is surgical excision of only the palpable mass in carcinoma of the breast.

II. Fractures and Syndromes

A. Fracture of the clavicle

–results in upward displacement of the proximal fragment, owing to the pull of the sternocleidomastoid muscle, and downward displacement of the distal fragment, owing to the pull of the deltoid muscle and gravity.

–may be caused by the obstetrician in breech (buttocks) presentation or may occur when the infant presses against the maternal pubic symphysis during its passage through the birth canal.

–may cause injury to the brachial plexus (lower trunk) and fatal hemorrhage from the subclavian vein.

–is also responsible for thrombosis of the subclavian vein, leading to pulmonary embolism.

B. Colles' fracture of the wrist

–is a fracture of the lower end of the radius in which the distal fragment is displaced (tilted) posteriorly, producing a characteristic hump described as **silver fork deformity.**

–is called a reverse Colles' fracture **(Smith's fracture)** if the distal fragment is displaced anteriorly.

C. Inferior dislocation of the humerus

–is not uncommon because the inferior aspect of the shoulder joint is not supported by muscles.

–may damage the axillary nerve and the posterior humeral circumflex vessels.

D. Referred pain to the shoulder

–most probably indicates involvement of the phrenic nerve (or diaphragm). The supraclavicular nerve (C3–C4), which supplies sensory fibers over the shoulder, has the same origin as the phrenic nerve (C3–C5), which supplies the diaphragm.

E. Carpal tunnel syndrome

–is caused by **compression of the median nerve** due to the reduced size of the osseofibrous carpal tunnel, resulting from inflammation of the flexor retinaculum, anterior dislocations of the lunate bone, arthritic changes, or inflammation of the tendon and its sheath by fibers of the flexor retinaculum.

–leads to **pain** and **paresthesia** (tingling, burning, and numbness) in the hand in the area of the median nerve.

–may also cause **atrophy of the thenar muscles** in cases of severe compression.

F. Dupuytren's contracture

–is a **disease of the palmar fascia** resulting in thickening and contracture of fibrous bands on the palmar surface of the hand and fingers.

III. Lesions of Peripheral Nerves

A. Upper trunk injury (Erb-Duchenne paralysis or Erb palsy)

–is caused by a birth injury during a breech delivery or a violent displacement of the head from the shoulder such as might result from a fall from a motorcycle or horse.

–results in a loss of abduction, flexion and lateral rotation of the arm, producing a **waiter's tip hand,** in which the arm tends to lie in medial rotation due to paralysis of lateral rotator muscles.

B. Lower trunk injury (Klumpke's paralysis)

–may be caused during a difficult breech delivery **(birth palsy or obstetric paralysis),** by a cervical rib **(cervical rib syndrome),** or by abnormal insertion or spasm of the anterior and middle scalene muscles **(scalene syndrome).**

–results in a **claw hand.**

C. Injury to the posterior cord

–is caused by the pressure of the crosspiece of a crutch, resulting in paralysis of the arm called **crutch palsy.**

–results in loss in function of the extensors of the arm, forearm, and hand.

–produces a **wrist drop.**

D. Injury to the long thoracic nerve

–is caused by a stab wound or during thoracic surgery.

–results in paralysis of the serratus anterior muscle and inability to elevate the arm above the horizontal.

–produces a **winged scapula** in which the vertebral (medial) border of the scapula protrudes away from the thorax.

E. Injury to the musculocutaneous nerve

–results in weakness of supination (biceps) and forearm flexion (brachialis and biceps).

F. Injury to the axillary nerve

–is caused by a fracture of the surgical neck of the humerus or inferior dislocation of the humerus.

–results in weakness of lateral rotation and abduction of the arm (the supraspinatus can abduct the arm but not to a horizontal level).

G. Injury to the radial nerve

–is caused by a **fracture of the midshaft of the humerus.**

–results in loss of function in the extensors of the forearm, hand, metacarpals, and phalanges.

–results in loss of wrist extension, leading to **wrist drop,** and produces a weakness of abduction and adduction of the hand.

H. Injury to the ulnar nerve

–is caused by a fracture of the medial epicondyle, and results in a **claw hand,** in which the ring and little fingers are hyperextended at the metacarpophalangeal joints and flexed at the interphalangeal joints.

–results in loss of abduction and adduction of the fingers and flexion of the metacarpophalangeal joints, owing to paralysis of the palmar and dorsal interossei muscles and the medial two lumbricals.

–produces a wasted hypothenar eminence and palm and also leads to loss of adduction of the thumb, owing to paralysis of the adductor pollicis muscle.

I. Injury to the median nerve

–may be caused by a supracondylar fracture of the humerus or a compression in the carpal tunnel.

–results in loss of pronation, opposition of the thumb, flexion of the lateral two interphalangeal joints, and impairment of the medial two interphalangeal joints.

–produces a characteristic flattening of the thenar eminence, often referred to as **ape hand.**

Summary of Muscle Actions of the Upper Limb

Movement of the Scapula
Elevation—trapezius (upper part), levator scapulae
Depression—trapezius (lower part), serratus, anterior, pectoralis minor
Protrusion (forward or lateral movement; abduction)—serratus anterior
Retraction (backward or medial movement; adduction)—trapezius, rhomboids
Anterior or inferior rotation of the glenoid fossa—rhomboid major
Posterior or superior rotation of the glenoid fossa—serratus anterior, trapezius

Movement at the Shoulder Joint (Ball-and-Socket Joint)
Adduction—pectoralis major, latissimus dorsi, deltoid (posterior part)
Abduction—deltoid, supraspinatus
Flexion—pectoralis major (clavicular part), deltoid (anterior part), coracobrachialis, biceps
Extension—latissimus dorsi, deltoid (posterior part)
Medial rotation—subscapularis, pectoralis major, deltoid (anterior part), latissimus dorsi, teres major
Lateral rotation—infraspinatus, teres minor, deltoid (posterior part)

Movement at the Elbow Joint (Hinge Joint)
Flexion—brachialis, biceps, brachioradialis, pronator teres
Extension—triceps, anconeus

Movement at the Radioulnar Joints (Pivot Joints)
Pronation—pronator quadratus, pronator teres
Supination—supinator, biceps brachii

Movement at the Wrist (Radiocarpal) Joint (Ellipsoidal Joint)
Adduction—flexor carpi ulnaris, extensor carpi ulnaris
Abduction—flexor carpi radialis, extensor carpi radialis longus and brevis
Flexion—flexor carpi radialis, flexor carpi ulnaris, palmaris longus, abductor pollicis
  longus
Extension—extensor carpi radialis longus and brevis, extensor carpi ulnaris

Movement at the Metacarpophalangeal Joint (Condyloid Joint)
Adduction—palmar interossei
Abduction—dorsal interossei
Flexion—lumbricals and interossei
Extension—extensor digitorum

Movement at the Interphalangeal Joint (Hinge Joint)
Flexion—flexor digitorum superficialis (proximal interphalangeal joint), flexor digitorum profundus (distal interphalangeal joint)
Extension—lumbricals and interossei (when metacarpophalangeal joint is extended by
  extensor digitorum)
Extension—extensor digitorum (when metacarpophalangeal joint is flexed by lumbricals
  and interossei)

Summary of Muscle Innervations of the Upper Limb

Muscles of the Anterior Compartment of the Arm: Musculocutaneous Nerve
Biceps brachii
Coracobrachialis
Brachialis

Muscles of the Posterior Compartment of the Arm: Radial Nerve
Triceps
Anconeus

Muscles of the Posterior Compartment of the Forearm: Radial Nerve
Superficial layer—brachioradialis; extensor carpi radialis longus; extensor carpi radialis
  brevis; extensor carpi ulnaris; extensor digitorum communis; extensor digiti minimi
Deep layer—supinator; abductor pollicis longus; extensor pollicis longus; extensor pollicis brevis; extensor indicis

Muscles of the Anterior Compartment of the Forearm: Median Nerve
Superficial layer—pronator teres; flexor carpi radialis; palmaris longus; flexor carpi
  ulnaris (ulnar nerve)*
Middle layer—flexor digitorum superficialis
Deep layer—flexor digitorum profundus (median nerve and ulnar nerve)*; flexor pollicis
  longus; pronator quadratus

Thenar Muscles: Median Nerve
   Abductor pollicis brevis
   Opponens pollicis
   Flexor pollicis brevis (median and ulnar nerves)*

Adductor Pollicis Muscle: Ulnar Nerve

Hypothenar Muscles: Ulnar Nerve
   Abductor digiti minimi
   Opponens digiti minimi
   Flexor digiti minimi

Interossei (Dorsal and Palmar) Muscles: Ulnar Nerve

Lumbrical Muscles (Medial Two): Ulnar Nerve

Lumbrical Muscles (Lateral Two): Median Nerve

---

*Indicates exception or dual innervation supply to the hand.

Review Test

Directions: Each of the numbered items or incomplete statements in this section is followed by answers or by completions of the statement. Select the **one** lettered answer or completion that is **best** in each case.

1. A 21-year-old patient has a lesion of the upper trunk of the brachial plexus (Erb-Duchenne paralysis). Which of the following is the most likely diagnosis?

(A) Paralysis of the rhomboid major
(B) Inability to elevate the arm above the horizontal
(C) Arm tending to lie in medial rotation
(D) Loss of sensation on the medial side of the arm
(E) Damage to nerve fibers from dorsal primary rami of C5 and C6

2. If the thoracoacromial trunk were ligated, which of the following arterial branches would maintain blood flow?

(A) Acromial
(B) Pectoral
(C) Clavicular
(D) Deltoid
(E) Superior thoracic

3. The defect known as winged scapula is caused by damage to a nerve that arises from which of the following structures of the brachial plexus?

(A) Medial cord
(B) Posterior cord
(C) Lower trunk
(D) Roots
(E) Upper trunk

4. Which of the following muscles is able to do the following: (1) flex the metacarpophalangeal joint and extend the interphalangeal joint of the ring finger, and (2) adduct the ring finger?

(A) Flexor digitorum profundus
(B) Extensor digitorum
(C) Lumbrical
(D) Dorsal interosseous
(E) Palmar interosseous

5. Paralysis of the pectoralis minor muscle may be associated with which of the following conditions?

(A) Fracture of the clavicle
(B) Injury to the posterior cord of the brachial plexus
(C) Fracture of the coracoid process
(D) Inability to elevate the shoulder
(E) Defects in the posterior wall of the axilla

6. A 22-year-old patient with a lesion of the intercostobrachial nerve experiences which of the following?

(A) Inability to move the ribs
(B) Loss of tactile sensation on the lateral aspect of the arm
(C) Absence of sweating on the posterior aspect of the arm
(D) Loss of sensory fibers from the second intercostal nerve
(E) Damage to the sympathetic preganglionic fibers

7. A patient with a severely damaged radial nerve in the spiral groove of the humerus eventually experiences which of the following?

(A) Loss of wrist extension, leading to wrist drop
(B) Weakness in pronating the forearm
(C) Sensory loss over the ventral aspect of the base of the thumb
(D) Inability to oppose the thumb
(E) Inability to abduct the fingers

8. A patient is unable to flex the proximal interphalangeal joints as a result of paralysis of which of the following muscles?

(A) Palmar interossei
(B) Flexor digitorum profundus
(C) Dorsal interossei
(D) Flexor digitorum superficialis
(E) Lumbricals

9. A patient is incapable of adducting the arm because of paralysis of which of the following muscles?

(A) Teres minor
(B) Supraspinatus
(C) Latissimus dorsi
(D) Infraspinatus
(E) Serratus anterior

10. If the most medial structure of the proximal portion of the cubital fossa is severed by a knife, which of the following structures most likely suffers damage?

(A) Biceps brachii tendon
(B) Radial nerve
(C) Brachial artery
(D) Radial recurrent artery
(E) Median nerve

11. A bullet strikes a murder suspect, who is involved in a gun fight with a police officer, in the arm, injuring the median nerve. Which of the following signs is most likely to be present?

(A) Waiter's tip hand
(B) Claw hand
(C) Wrist drop
(D) Ape hand
(E) Flattening of the hypothenar eminence

12. An automobile body shop worker experiences a crush injury to his middle finger. The functions of which groups of muscles are most likely to be impaired?

(A) Extensor digitorum, one lumbrical, one dorsal interosseous, and one palmar interosseous
(B) Flexor digitorum profundus, one lumbrical, one palmar interosseous, and two dorsal interosseous
(C) Extensor digitorum, one lumbrical, and two dorsal interosseous
(D) Extensor indicis, one lumbrical, and one dorsal interosseous
(E) Extensor digitorum, one lumbrical, and one palmar interosseous

13. A 27-year-old patient is given radiopaque dye in preparation for an arteriogram of the radial artery that

(A) enters the hand through the carpal tunnel
(B) accompanies the posterior interosseous nerve in the forearm
(C) is the principal source of blood to the superficial palmar arterial arch
(D) has the princeps pollicis artery as one of its branches
(E) runs between the flexor digitorum superficialis and profundus muscles

14. Which of the following groups of nerves is intimately related to a portion of the humerus and can most likely be affected by fractures of the humerus?

(A) Axillary, musculocutaneous, radial
(B) Axillary, median, ulnar
(C) Axillary, radial, ulnar
(D) Axillary, median, musculocutaneous
(E) Median, radial, ulnar

15. A man injures his wrist on broken glass. Which of the following structures entering the palm superficial to the flexor retinaculum may be damaged?

(A) Ulnar nerve and median nerve
(B) Median nerve and flexor digitorum profundus
(C) Median nerve and flexor pollicis longus
(D) Ulnar artery and ulnar nerve
(E) Ulnar nerve and flexor digitorum superficialis

16. Fracture of the first metacarpal bone may injure which of the following intrinsic muscles of the thumb?

(A) Abductor pollicis brevis
(B) Flexor pollicis brevis (superficial head)
(C) Opponens pollicis
(D) Adductor pollicis
(E) Flexor pollicis brevis (deep head)

17. A lesion of the median nerve produces a paralysis of which of the following muscles?

(A) Palmar interossei and adductor pollicis
(B) Dorsal interossei and lateral two lumbricals
(C) Lateral two lumbricals and opponens pollicis
(D) Abductor pollicis brevis and palmar interossei
(E) Medial two and lateral two lumbricals

18. An infection in the ulnar bursa could result in necrosis of which of the following tendons?

(A) Tendon of the flexor carpi ulnaris
(B) Tendon of the flexor pollicis longus
(C) Tendon of the flexor digitorum profundus
(D) Tendon of the flexor carpi radialis
(E) Tendon of the palmaris longus

19. Abductors of the arm are paralyzed resulting from a lesion of which of the following nerves?

(A) Suprascapular and axillary
(B) Thoracodorsal and upper subscapular
(C) Axillary and musculocutaneous
(D) Radial and lower subscapular
(E) Suprascapular and dorsal scapular

20. If the brachial artery is ligated at its origin, the profunda brachii artery would receive blood from which of the following arteries?

(A) Lateral thoracic
(B) Subscapular
(C) Posterior humeral circumflex
(D) Superior ulnar collateral
(E) Radial recurrent

21. A woman is unable to move the metacarpophalangeal joint of her ring finger. Which of the following pairs of nerves are damaged?

(A) Median and ulnar
(B) Radial and median
(C) Musculocutaneous and ulnar
(D) Ulnar and radial
(E) Radial and axillary

22. The muscles that form the floor of the cubital fossa are torn. Which of the following groups of muscles has lost function?

(A) Brachioradialis and supinator
(B) Brachialis and supinator
(C) Pronator teres and supinator
(D) Supinator and pronator quadratus
(E) Brachialis and pronator teres

23. The cell bodies of nerve fibers in the medial brachial cutaneous nerve are damaged. Which of the following nervous structures are involved in structural and functional changes?

(A) Dorsal root ganglia and anterior horn of the spinal cord
(B) Anterior and lateral horns of the spinal cord
(C) Sympathetic chain ganglia and dorsal root ganglia
(D) Lateral horn of the spinal cord and sympathetic chain ganglia
(E) Dorsal root ganglia and lateral horn of the spinal cord

24. Inability to supinate the forearm could result from an injury to which of the following nerves?

(A) Suprascapular and axillary
(B) Musculocutaneous and median
(C) Axillary and radial
(D) Radial and musculocutaneous
(E) Median and ulnar

25. A patient complains of sensory loss over the anterior and posterior surfaces of the medial third of the hand and the medial one and one-half fingers. Which of the following nerves is injured?

(A) Axillary
(B) Radial
(C) Median
(D) Ulnar
(E) Musculocutaneous

26. Injury to the anterior interosseous nerve could result in paralysis of which of the following muscles?

(A) Flexor pollicis longus and brevis
(B) Flexor pollicis longus and opponens pollis
(C) Flexor digitorum profundus and pronator quadratus
(D) Flexor digitorum profundus and superficialis
(E) Flexor pollicis brevis and pronator quadratus

27. Nerve damage that impairs flexion of the distal interphalangeal joint of the index finger also produces which of the following conditions?

(A) Similar paralysis of the little finger
(B) Atrophy of the hypothenar eminence
(C) Loss of sensation over the distal part of the second digit
(D) Complete paralysis of the thumb
(E) Loss of supination

28. Damage to the ulnar nerve at the elbow most likely results in paralysis of which of the following muscles?

(A) Flexor digitorum superficialis
(B) Opponens pollicis
(C) Two medial lumbricals
(D) Pronator teres
(E) Supinator

29. In a patient with carpal tunnel syndrome, which of the following conditions most likely occurs?

(A) Inability to adduct the middle finger
(B) Inability to flex the distal interphalangeal joint of the ring finger
(C) Flattened thenar eminence
(D) Loss of skin sensation of the medial one and one-half fingers
(E) Atrophied adductor pollicis muscle

30. A man is unable to hold typing paper between his index and middle fingers because of an injury to which of the following nerves?

(A) Radial nerve
(B) Median nerve
(C) Ulnar nerve
(D) Musculocutaneous nerve
(E) Axillary nerve

31. The victim of an automobile accident has a destructive injury of the proximal row of carpal bones. Which of the following bones is most likely damaged?

(A) Capitate
(B) Hamate
(C) Trapezium
(D) Triquetrum
(E) Trapezoid

32. A patient has a torn rotator cuff of the shoulder joint as the result of an automobile accident. Which of the following muscle tendons is intact and has normal function?

(A) Supraspinatus
(B) Subscapularis
(C) Teres major
(D) Teres minor
(E) Infraspinatus

33. Occlusion of the radial artery just distal to its origin is most likely to cause which of the following conditions?

(A) A marked decrease in the blood flow in the superficial palmar arterial arch
(B) Decreased pulsation in the artery passing superficial to the flexor retinaculum
(C) Ischemia of the entire extensor muscles of the forearm
(D) A marked decrease in the blood flow in the princeps pollicis artery
(E) A low blood pressure in the anterior interosseous artery

34. A patient bleeding from the shoulder secondary to a knife wound is in fair condition because of the vascular anastomosis around the shoulder. Which of the following arteries is most likely a direct branch of the subclavian artery and involved in the anastomosis?

(A) Dorsal scapular artery
(B) Thoracoacromial artery
(C) Subscapular artery
(D) Transverse cervical artery
(E) Suprascapular artery

35. During a breast examination of a 56-year-old woman, the physician found evidence of breast cancer. Which of the following statements about breast cancer and its diagnosis is correct?

(A) Elevated nipple is a common presenting sign
(B) Severe pain due to compression of the medial brachial cutaneous nerve frequently is present
(C) Shortening of the clavipectoral fascia leads to breast asymmetry
(D) Dimpling of the overlying skin is not uncommon
(E) Mammography is a poor screening tool for breast cancer

36. If the musculocutaneous nerve is severed, which of the following is most likely to occur?

(A) Lack of sweating on the lateral side of the arm
(B) Chromatolysis of neuron cell bodies in the lateral horn of the spinal cord
(C) Paralysis of brachioradialis muscle
(D) Loss of tactile sensation on the hand
(E) Degeneration of cell bodies in the anterior horn of the spinal cord

37. A lesion of the lateral cord of the brachial plexus most likely leads to paralysis of which of the following muscles?

(A) Subscapularis
(B) Teres major
(C) Latissimus dorsi
(D) Teres minor
(E) Pectoralis major

38. If a 24-year-old carpenter suffers a crush injury of his entire little finger, which of the following muscles is most likely to be spared?

(A) Flexor digitorum profundus
(B) Extensor digitorum
(C) Palmar interossei
(D) Dorsal interossei
(E) Lumbricals

39. Which of the following conditions is most likely to cause a loss of the axillary nerve function?

(A) Injury to the lateral cord of the brachial plexus
(B) Fracture of the anatomical neck of the humerus
(C) Knife wound on the teres major muscle
(D) Inferior dislocation of the head of the humerus
(E) A tumor in the triangular space in the shoulder region

40. Lymph from the breast drains primarily into which of the following nodes?

(A) Apical nodes
(B) Anterior (pectoral) nodes
(C) Parasternal (internal thoracic) nodes
(D) Supraclavicular nodes
(E) Nodes of the anterior abdominal wall

41. If the musculocutaneous nerve is severed, which of the following types of axons is most likely spared?

(A) Postganglionic sympathetic axons
(B) Somatic afferent axons
(C) Preganglionic sympathetic axons
(D) Somatic efferent axons
(E) Visceral afferent axons

42. A construction worker suffers a destructive injury of the structures related to the anatomical snuff-box. Which of the following structures would most likely be damaged?

(A) Triquetral bone
(B) Trapezoid bone
(C) Extensor indicis tendon
(D) Abductor pollicis brevis tendon
(E) Radial artery

43. A rock climber falls on his shoulder, resulting in the chipping off of a lesser tubercle of the humerus. Which of the following structures would most likely have structural and functional damage?

(A) Supraspinatus muscle
(B) Infraspinatus muscle
(C) Subscapularis muscle
(D) Teres minor muscle
(E) Coracohumeral ligament

Questions 44–47

A patient with a fracture of the clavicle at the junction of the inner and middle third of the bone exhibits overriding of the medial and lateral fragments. The arm is rotated medially.

44. The lateral portion of the fractured clavicle is displaced downward by which of the following?

(A) Deltoid and trapezius muscles
(B) Pectoralis major and deltoid muscles
(C) Pectoralis minor muscle and gravity
(D) Trapezius and pectoralis minor muscles
(E) Deltoid muscle and gravity

45. Which of the following muscles causes upward displacement of the medial fragment?

(A) Pectoralis major
(B) Deltoid
(C) Trapezius
(D) Sternocleidomastoid
(E) Scalenus anterior

46. Which of the following conditions is most likely to occur secondary to the fractured clavicle?

(A) A fatal hemorrhage from the brachiocephalic vein
(B) Thrombosis of the subclavian vein, causing a pulmonary embolism
(C) Thrombosis of the subclavian artery, causing an embolism in the ascending aorta
(D) Damage to the upper trunk of the brachial plexus
(E) Damage to the long thoracic nerve, causing the winged scapula

47. The woman is unable to rotate her arm laterally. Which of the following muscles is most likely paralyzed?

(A) Pectoralis major
(B) Subscapularis
(C) Teres major
(D) Latissimus dorsi
(E) Teres minor

Questions 48–50

A 21-year-old man suffers an injury of the right arm in an automobile accident. Radiographic examination reveals a fracture of the medial epicondyle of the humerus.

48. Which of the following nerves is most likely injured as a result of this accident?

(A) Axillary
(B) Musculocutaneous
(C) Radial
(D) Median
(E) Ulnar

49. Which of the following muscles is most likely paralyzed as a result of this accident?

(A) Extensor pollicis brevis
(B) Abductor pollicis longus
(C) Abductor pollicis brevis
(D) Adductor pollicis
(E) Opponens pollicis

50. After this injury, the patient is unable to

(A) flex his proximal interphalangeal joint of the ring finger
(B) flex his distal interphalangel joint of the index finger
(C) feel sensation on his middle finger
(D) abduct his thumb
(E) adduct his index finger

Questions 51–53

A 10-year-old boy falls off his bike and fractures the surgical neck of his humerus.

51. Which of the following nerves is most likely injured as a result of this accident?

(A) Musculocutaneous
(B) Axillary
(C) Radial
(D) Median
(E) Ulnar

52. The damaged nerve leads to degenerative changes in neuronal cells. Which of the following structures would most likely be involved in cellular alteration?

(A) Anterior, lateral, and posterior horns of the spinal cord
(B) Anterior horn, lateral horn, and dorsal root ganglia
(C) Lateral horn, dorsal root ganglia, and sympathetic chain ganglia
(D) Anterior horn, dorsal root ganglia, and sympathetic chain ganglia
(E) Posterior horn, sympathetic chain ganglia, and enteric ganglia

53. This accident most likely leads to damage of which of the following arteries?

(A) Axillary
(B) Deep brachial
(C) Posterior humeral circumflex
(D) Superior ulnar collateral
(E) Scapular circumflex

Questions 54–55

In an attempt to obtain a blood sample from an individual's median cubital vein, a registered nurse inadvertently procures arterial blood.

54. The blood most likely comes from which of the following arteries?

(A) Brachial
(B) Radial
(C) Ulnar
(D) Common interosseous
(E) Superior ulnar collateral

55. During the procedure, the needle hits a nerve medial to the artery. Which of the following nerves is most likely damaged?

(A) Radial
(B) Median
(C) Ulnar
(D) Lateral antebrachial
(E) Medial antebrachial

Questions 56–60

A 17-year-old boy suffers a fracture of the shaft of the humerus as the result of an automobile accident.

56. Which of the following nerves is most likely damaged?

(A) Axillary nerve
(B) Radial nerve
(C) Musculocutaneous nerve
(D) Median nerve
(E) Ulnar nerve

57. As a result of this fracture, the cell bodies in which of the following structures undergo degenerative changes?

(A) Anterior and lateral horns of the spinal cord
(B) Sympathetic chain ganglia and lateral horn
(C) Lateral horn and dorsal root ganglia
(D) Anterior horn and sympathetic chain ganglia
(E) Dorsal root ganglia and dorsal horns

58. Following this accident, the patient has no cutaneous sensation in which of the following areas?

(A) Medial aspect of the arm
(B) Lateral aspect of the forearm
(C) Palmar aspect of the second and third digits
(D) Area of the anatomical snuff-box
(E) Medial one and half fingers

59. Which of the following arteries may be damaged?

(A) Brachial artery
(B) Posterior humeral circumflex artery
(C) Profunda brachii artery
(D) Radial artery
(E) Radial recurrent artery

60. After this accident, supination is still possible through contraction of which of the following muscles?

(A) Supinator
(B) Pronator teres
(C) Brachioradialis
(D) Biceps brachii
(E) Supraspinatus

Questions 61–62

A physician examines a radiograph of the shoulder region in an 11-year-old boy.

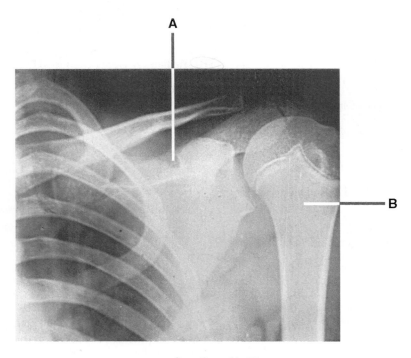

Questions 61–62.

61. If the structure indicated by the letter A is calcified, which of the following muscles is most likely paralyzed?

(A) Deltoid
(B) Teres major
(C) Teres minor
(D) Infraspinatus
(E) Subclapularis

62. If the structure indicated by the letter B is fractured, which of the structures is most likely injured?

(A) Musculocutaneous nerve
(B) Radial nerve
(C) Deep brachial artery
(D) Posterior humeral circumflex artery
(E) Scapular circumflex artery

Questions 63–65

Choose the appropriate lettered site or structure in this radiograph of the elbow joint and its associated structures to match the following descriptions.

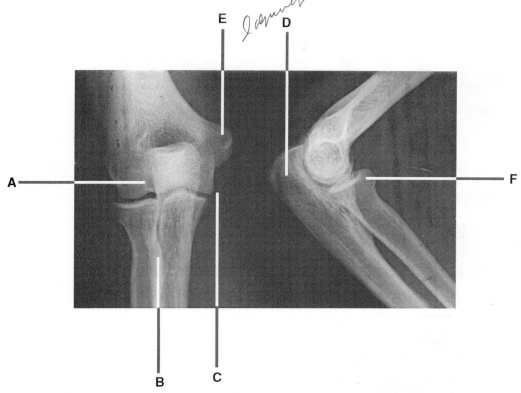

Questions 63–65.

63. Destruction of this area would most likely cause weakness of supination and flexion of the forearm.

64. Destruction of this area would most likely cause weakness of pronation of the forearm and flexion of the wrist joints.

65. A lesion of the radial nerve would most likely cause paralysis of muscles that are attached to this area.

Questions 66–67

Choose the appropriate lettered site or structure in this radiograph of the wrist and hand.

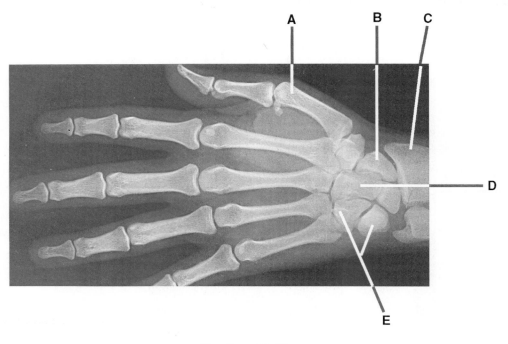

Questions 66–67.

66. Destruction of a structure indicated by the letter E most likely causes weakness of which of the following muscles?

(A) Flexor carpi radialis
(B) Palmaris longus
(C) Flexor carpi ulnaris
(D) Brachioradialis
(E) Flexor digitorum superficialis

67. If the floor of the anatomical snuff box and origin of the abductor pollicis brevis are damaged, which of the following bones is most likely to be involved?

(A) A
(B) B
(C) C
(D) D
(E) E

Questions 68–70

Choose the appropriate lettered site or structure in this transverse magnetic resonance imaging (MRI) scan through the middle of the palm of a woman's right hand that matches the following descriptions.

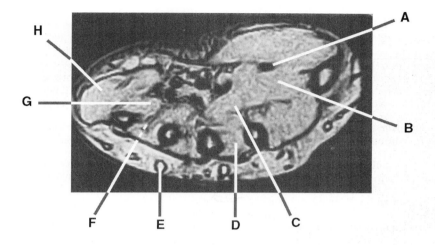

Questions 68–70.

68. A patient is unable to abduct her middle finger due to paralysis of this structure.

D dorsal int

69. A lesion of the median nerve causes paralysis of this structure.

A

70. A patient is unable to adduct her little finger because of paralysis of this structure.

6 palm interosseus

Answers and Explanations

1-C. A lesion of the upper trunk of the brachial plexus results in a condition called "waiter's tip hand" in which the arm tends to lie in medial rotation due to paralysis of lateral rotators and abductors of the arm. The long thoracic nerve, which arises from the root (C5–C7) of the brachial plexus, innervates the serratus anterior muscle that can elevate the arm above the horizontal. The dorsal scapular nerve, which arises from the root (C5), innervates the rhomboid major. The medial side of the arm receives cutaneous innervation from the medial brachial cutaneous nerve of the medial cord. Nerve fibers from dorsal primary rami of C5 and C6 supply the deep muscles of the back.

2-E. The superior thoracic artery is a direct branch of the axillary artery. The thoracoacromial trunk has four branches: the pectoral, clavicular, acromial, and deltoid branches.

3-D. Winged scapula is caused by paralysis of the serratus anterior muscle that results from damage to the long thoracic nerve that arises from the roots of the brachial plexus (C5–C7).

4-E. The dorsal and palmar interosseous and lumbrical muscles can flex the metacarpophalangeal joints and extend the interphalangeal joints. The palmar interosseous muscles adduct the fingers, and the dorsal interosseous muscles abduct the fingers.

5-C. The pectoralis minor originates from the second to the fifth ribs, inserts on the coracoid process, and is innervated by the medial and lateral pectoral nerves which arise from the medial and lateral cords of the brachial plexus. It depresses the shoulder and forms the anterior wall of the axilla. The clavicle provides no attachment for the pectoralis minor.

6-D. The intercostobrachial nerve arises from the lateral cutaneous branch of the second intercostal nerve and pierces the intercostal and serratus anterior muscles. It may communicate with the medial brachial cutaneous nerve, and it supplies skin on the medial side of the arm. It contains no skeletal motor fibers but does contain sympathetic postganglionic fibers, which supply sweat glands.

7-A. Injury to the radial nerve results in loss of wrist extension, leading to wrist drop. The median nerve innervates the pronator teres, pronator quadratus, and opponens pollicis muscles, as well as the skin over the ventral aspect of the thumb. The ulnar nerve innervates the dorsal interosseous muscles, which act to abduct the fingers.

8-D. The flexor digitorum superficialis muscle flexes the proximal interphalangeal joints. The flexor digitorum profundus muscle flexes the distal interphalangeal joints. The palmar and dorsal interossei and lumbricals can flex metacarpophalangeal joints and extend the interphalangeal joints. The palmar interossei adduct the fingers, and the dorsal interossei abduct the fingers.

9-C. The latissimus dorsi adducts the arm, and the supraspinatus muscle abducts the arm. The infraspinatus and the teres minor rotate the arm laterally. The serratus anterior rotates the glenoid cavity of the scapula upward, abducts the arm, and elevates it above a horizontal position.

10-E. The contents of the cubital fossa from medial to lateral side are the median nerve, the brachial artery, the biceps brachii tendon, and the radial nerve. So the median nerve is damaged. The radial recurrent artery ascends medial to the radial nerve.

11-D. Injury to the median nerve produces the ape hand (a hand with the thumb permanently extended). Injury to the radial nerve results in loss of wrist extension, leading to wrist drop. Damage to the upper trunk of the brachial plexus produces waiter's tip hand. A claw hand results from damage to the ulnar nerve.

12-C. The extensor digitorum, flexor digitorum profundus and superficialis, one lumbrical muscle, and two dorsal interosseous muscles are attached to the middle digit, but no palmar interosseous muscles and extensor indicis are attached.

13-D. The radial artery descends laterally beneath the brachioradialis with the superficial radial nerve, passes through the anatomical snuff-box, enters the palm by passing between the two heads of the first dorsal interosseous muscle, and divides into the princeps pollicis artery and the deep palmar arch. The median nerve runs between the flexor digitorum superficialis and profundus in the forearm and enters the hand through the carpal tunnel. The posterior interosseous nerve accompanies the posterior interosseous artery, which is a branch of the common interosseous artery of the ulnar artery, the principal source of blood to the superficial palmar arch.

14-C. To be injured in a fracture, the nerve must lie close to, or contact, the bone. The axillary nerve passes posteriorly around the surgical neck of the humerus, the radial nerve lies in the radial groove of the middle of the shaft of the humerus, and the ulnar nerve passes behind the medial epicondyle.

15-D. Structures entering the palm superficial to the flexor retinaculum include the ulnar nerve, ulnar artery, palmaris longus tendon, and palmar cutaneous branch of the median nerve. The median nerve, the flexor pollicis longus, and the flexor digitorum superficialis and profundus run deep to the flexor retinaculum.

16-C. The opponens pollicis inserts on the first metacarpal. All other short muscles of the thumb, including the abductor pollicis brevis, the flexor pollicis brevis, and the adductor pollicis muscles, insert on the proximal phalanges.

17-C. The median nerve innervates the abductor pollicis brevis, opponens pollicis, and two lateral lumbricals. The ulnar nerve innervates all interossei (palmar and dorsal), the adductor pollicis, and the two medial lumbricals.

18-C. The ulnar bursa, or common synovial flexor sheath, contains the tendons of both the flexor digitorum superficialis and profundus muscles. The radial bursa envelops the tendon of the flexor pollicis longus.

19-A. The abductors of the arm are the deltoid and supraspinatus muscles, which are innervated by the axillary and suprascapular nerves, respectively. The thoracodoral nerve supplies the latissimus dorsi, which can adduct, extend, and rotate the arm medially. The upper and lower subscapular nerves supply the subscapularis, and the lower subscapular nerve also supplies the teres major; both of these sturctures can adduct and rotate the arm medially. The musculocutaneous nerve supplies the flexors of the arm, and the radial nerve supplies the extensors of the arm. The dorsal scapular nerve supplies the levator scapulae and rhomboid muscles; these muscles elevate and adduct the scapula, respectively.

20-C. The posterior humeral circumflex artery anastomoses with an ascending branch of the profunda brachii artery, whereas the lateral thoracic and subscapular arteries do not. The superior ulnar collateral and radial recurrent arteries arise inferior to the origin of the profunda brachii artery.

21-D. The metacarpophalangeal joint of the ring finger is flexed by the lumbrical, palmar, and dorsal interosseous muscles, which are innervated by the ulnar nerve. The extensor digitorum, which is innervated by the radial nerve, extends this joint. The musculocutaneous and axillary nerves do not supply muscles of the hand. The median nerve supplies the lateral two lumbricals, which can flex metacarpophalangeal joints of the index and middle fingers.

22-B. The brachialis and supinator muscles form the floor of the cubital fossa. The brachioradialis and pronator teres muscles form the lateral and medial boundaries, respectively. The pronator quadratus is attached to the distal ends of the radius and the ulna.

23-C. The medial brachial cutaneous nerve contains sensory fibers that have cell bodies in the dorsal root ganglia. It also contains sympathetic postganglionic fibers that have cell bodies in the sympathetic chain ganglia. The anterior horn contains cell bodies of skeletal motor fibers, and the lateral horn contains cell bodies of sympathetic preganglionic fibers.

24-D. The supinator and biceps brachii muscles, which are innervated by the radial and musculocutaneous nerves, respectively, produce supination of the forearm.

25-D. The ulnar nerve supplies sensory fibers to the skin over the palmar and dorsal surfaces of the medial third of the hand and the medial one and one-half fingers. The median nerve innervates the skin of the lateral side of the palm; the palmar side of the lateral three and one-half fingers; and the dorsal side of the index finger, the middle finger, and one-half of the ring finger. The radial nerve innervates the skin of the radial side of the hand and the radial two and one-half digits over the proximal phalanx.

26-C. The anterior interosseous nerve is a branch of the median nerve and supplies the flexor pollicis longus, half of the flexor digitorum profundus, and the pronator quadratus. The median nerve supplies the pronator teres, flexor digitorum superficialis, palmaris longus, and flexor carpi radialis muscles. A muscular branch (the recurrent branch) of the median nerve innervates the thenar muscles.

27-C. The flexor digitorum profundus muscle, which is innervated by the median nerve, leads to flexion of the distal interphalangeal joints of the index and middle fingers. The same muscle produces flexion of the ring and little fingers but receives innervation from the ulnar nerve. The median nerve innervates the skin over the distal part of the second digit, the pronator teres, and the thenar muscles. The radial nerve innervates the supinator, abductor pollicis and longus, and extensor pollicis longus and brevis muscles. The ulnar nerve innervates the adductor pollicis. The musculocutaneous nerve supplies the biceps brachii that can supinate the arm.

28-C. The ulnar nerve innervates the two medial lumbricals. However, the median nerve innervates the two lateral lumbricals, the flexor digitorum superficialis, the opponens pollicis, and the pronator teres muscles.

29-C. The carpal tunnel contains the median nerve and the tendons of flexor pollicis longus, flexor digitorum profundus, and flexor digitorum superficialis muscles. Carpal tunnel syndrome results from injury to the median nerve, which supplies the thenar muscle. So injury to this nerve causes the flattened thenar eminence. The middle finger has no attachment for the adductors. The flexor digitorum profundus muscle, which is innervated by the ulnar nerve, allows flexion of the distal interphalangeal joint of the ring finger. The ulnar nerve supplies the skin over the medial one and one-half fingers and adductor pollicis muscle.

30-C. To hold typing paper, the index finger is adducted by the palmar interosseous muscle, and the middle finger is abducted by the dorsal interosseous muscle. Both muscles are innervated by the ulnar nerve.

31-D. The proximal row of carpal bones consists of the scaphoid, lunate, triquetrum, and pisiform bones, whereas the distal row consists of trapezium, trapezoid, capitate and hamate bones.

32-C. The rotator cuff consists of the tendons of the supraspinatus, infraspinatus, subscapularis, and teres minor muscles. It stabilizes the shoulder joint by holding the head of the humerus in the glenoid cavity during movement. The teres major inserts on the medial lip of the intertubercular groove of the humerus.

33-D. The radial artery gives off the princeps pollicis artery and the deep palmar arterial arch. So ligation of the radial artery results in a decreased blood flow, blood pressure, and pulsation in its branches. The superficial palmar arterial arch is formed primarily by the ulnar artery. The extensor compartment of the forearm receives blood from the posterior interosseous artery, which arises from the common interosseous branch of the ulnar artery. However, the radial and radial recurrent arteries supply the brachioradialis and the extensor carpi radialis longus and brevis.

34-A. The dorsal scapular artery usually arises directly from the third part of the subclavian artery and replaces the deep (descending) branch of the transverse cervical artery. The suprascapular artery is a branch of the thyrocervical trunk of the subclavian artery.

35-D. Breast cancer may cause dimpling of the overlying skin due to shortening of the suspensory (Cooper's) ligaments, inverted or retracted nipple by pulling on the lactiferous ducts, and severe pain (in late-stage) due to compression of sensory nerves that arise from the second to sixth intercostal nerves. The majority of mammary gland tissue is located in the superficial fascia, except the axillary tail, which invades the deep fascia in the axilla.

36-E. The musculocutaneous nerve contains general somatic motor fibers that have cell bodies in the anterior horn of the spinal cord and supply the flexor of the arm. It also contains sympathetic postganglionic fibers that supply blood vessels and have cell bodies in the sympathetic chain ganglia.

37-E. The pectoralis major is innervated by the lateral and medial pectoral nerves originated from the lateral and medial cords of the brachial plexus, respectively. The subscapularis, teres major, latissimus dorsi, and teres minor muscles are innervated by nerves originating from the posterior cord of the brachial plexus.

38-D. The dorsal interossei are abductors of the fingers. The little finger has no attachment for the dorsal interosseous muscle because it has its own abductor.

39-D. The axillary nerve arises from the posterior cord of the brachial plexus, passes posteriorly through the quadrangular space accompanied by the posterior humeral circumflex vessels around the surgical neck of the humerus, and supplies the deltoid and teres minor muscles. Thus, it is damaged by fracture of the surgical neck, inferior dislocation of the head of the humerus, or a tumor in the quadrangular space.

40-B. Lymph from the breast drains mainly (75%) to the axillary nodes, more specifically to the pectoral (anterior) nodes.

41-C. The musculocutaneous nerve contains postganglionic sympathetic axons that innervate blood vessels, hair follicles, and sweat glands; afferent axons that innervate cutaneous tissues; and somatic efferent fibers that innervate skeletal muscles.

42-E. The tendons of the extensor pollicis longus, extensor pollicis brevis and abductor pollicis longus muscles form the boundaries of the anatomical snuff-box. The scaphoid and trapezium bones form its floor, and the radial artery crosses it.

43-C. The subscapularis muscle inserts on the lesser tubercle of the humerus. The supraspinatus, infraspinatus, and teres minor muscles insert on the greater tubercle of the humerus. The coracohumeral ligament attaches to the greater tubercle.

44-E. The lateral fragment of the clavicle is displaced downward by the pull of the deltoid muscle and gravity. The medial fragment is displaced upward by the pull of the sternocleidomastoid muscle.

45-D. The sternocleidomastoid muscle is attached to the superior border of the medial third of the clavicle, and the medial fragment of a fractured clavicle is displaced upward by the pull of the muscle.

46-B. The fractured clavicle may damage the subclavian vein, resulting in a pulmonary embolism; cause thrombosis of the subclavian artery, resulting in embolism of the brachial artery; or damage the lower trunk of the brachial plexus.

47-E. The pectoralis major, subscapularis, teres major, and latissimus dorsi muscles can rotate the arm medially. The teres minor muscle rotates the arm laterally.

48-E. The ulnar nerve runs down the medial aspect of the arm and behind the medial epicondyle in a groove, where it is vulnerable to damage by fracture of the medial epicondyle. Other nerves are not in contact with the medial epicondyle.

49-D. Uninjured, the ulnar nerve innervates the adductor pollicis muscle. The radial nerve innervates the abductor pollicis long and extensor pollicis brevis muscles, whereas the median nerve innervates the abductor pollicis brevis and opponens pollicis muscles.

50-E. The fingers are abducted by the dorsal interosseous muscles, whereas adduction of the fingers is performed by the palmar interosseous muscles. The palmar and dorsal interosseous muscles are innervated by the ulnar nerve. The proximal interphalangeal joints are flexed by the flexor digitorum superficialis, which is innervated by the median nerve. However, the distal interphalangeal joints are flexed by the flexor digitorum profundus, which is innervated by the median nerve (except the medial half of the muscle, which is innervated by the ulnar nerve).

51-B. The axillary nerve runs posteriorly around the surgical neck of the humerus and is vulnerable to injury such as fracture of the surgical neck of the humerus or inferior dislocation of the humerus. Other nerves are not in contact with the surgical neck of the humerus.

52-D. The (injured) axillary nerve contains general somatic efferent (GSE), general somatic afferent (GSA), and sympathetic postganglionic general visceral efferent (GVE) fibers, whose cell bodies are located in the anterior horn of the spinal cord, dorsal root ganglia, and sympathetic chain ganglia, respectively.

53-C. The posterior humeral circumfex artery accompanies the (injured) axillary nerve around the surgical neck of the humerus.

54-A. The median cubital vein lies superficial to the bicipital aponeurosis and thus separates it from the brachial artery, which can be punctured during intravenous injections and blood transfusions.

55-B. The bicipital aponeurosis lies on the brachial artery and the median nerve. The V-shaped cubital fossa contains (from medial to lateral) the median nerve, brachial artery, biceps tendon, and radial nerve.

56-B. The radial nerve runs in the radial groove on the back of the shaft of the humerus with the profunda brachii artery.

57-D. The (damaged) radial nerve contains axons that have cell bodies in the dorsal root ganglia for general somatic afferent (GSA) and general visceral afferent (GVA) fibers, sympathetic chain ganglia for general visceral efferent (GVE) fibers, and anterior horn of the spinal cord for general somatic efferent (GSE) fibers.

58-D. The superficial branch of the radial nerve runs distally to the dorsum of the hand to innvervate the radial side of the hand, including the area of the anatomical snuff-box and the radial two and one-half digits over the proximal phalanx. The medial aspect of the arm is innervated by the medial brachial cutaneous nerve, the lateral aspect of the forearm by the lateral antebrachial cutaneous nerve of the musculocutaneous nerve, the palmar aspect of the second and third digits by the median nerve, and the medial one and one-half fingers by the ulnar nerve.

59-C. The radial nerve accompanies the profunda brachii artery in the radial groove on the posterior aspect of the shaft of the humerus. The posterior humeral circumflex artery accompanies the axillary nerve around the surgical neck of the humerus. Other arteries are not associated with the radial groove of the humerus.

60-D. A lesion of the radial nerve causes paralysis of the supinator. The biceps brachii muscle is a flexor of the elbow and also a strong supinator. Other muscles cannot supinate the forearm.

61-D. The suprascapular notch transmits the suprascapular nerve below the superior transverse ligament, whereas the suprascapular artery and vein run over the ligament. The suprascapular nerve supplies the supraspinatus and infraspinatus muscles. The axillary nerve innervates the deltoid and teres minor muscles. The subscapular nerves innervate the teres major and subscapularis muscles.

62-D. Fracture of the surgical neck of the humerus occurs commonly and would damage the axillary nerve and the posterior humeral circumflex artery.

63-B. The radial tuberosity is the site for tendinous attachment of the biceps brachii muscle, which supinates and flexes the forearm. When the tuberosity is destroyed, the biceps brachii is paralyzed.

64-E. The medial epicondyle is the site of origin for the common flexor tendon and pronator teres. The common flexors include the flexor carpi radialis and ulnaris and palmaris longus muscles, which can flex the elbow and wrist joints. So destruction of this area causes weakness of pronation, because the pronator teres is paralyzed but the pronator quadratus is normal. Similarly, destruction of this area causes paralysis of the flexors of the wrist. However, it can be weakly flexed by the flexor pollicis longus, flexor digitorum superficialis, and profundum muscles.

65-D. The olecranon is the site for insertion of the triceps brachii, which is innervated by the radial nerve. When the olecranon is destroyed, the triceps brachii is paralyzed.

66-C. The hook of hamate and the pisiform provide insertion for the flexor carpi ulnaris.

67-B. The scaphoid forms the floor of the anatomical snuff box and provides a site for origin of the abductor pollicis brevis.

68-D. This is the second dorsal interosseous muscle, which abducts the middle finger.

69-A. This is the flexor pollicis longus, which is innervated by the median nerve.

70-G. This is the third palmar interosseous muscle, which adducts the little finger.

3
Lower Limb

Bones and Joints

I. Coxal (Hip) Bone (Figures 3-1 and 3-2)
   –is formed by the fusion of the **ilium, ischium,** and **pubis** on each side of the pelvis.
   –articulates with the sacrum at the sacroiliac joint to form the **pelvic girdle.**

A. Ilium
   –forms the lateral part of the hip bone and consists of the **body,** which joins the pubis and ischium to form the acetabulum and the **ala** or wing.
   –also comprises the anterior–superior iliac spine, anterior–inferior iliac spine, posterior iliac spine, **greater sciatic notch, iliac fossa,** and gluteal lines.

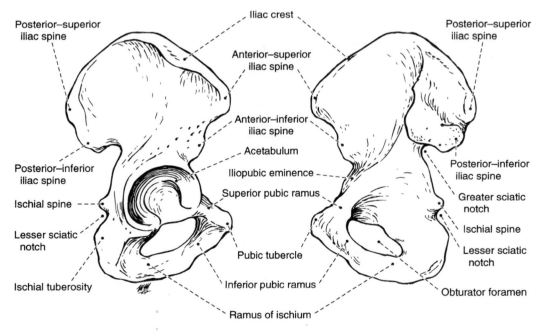

Figure 3–1. Coxal (hip) bone (lateral view).

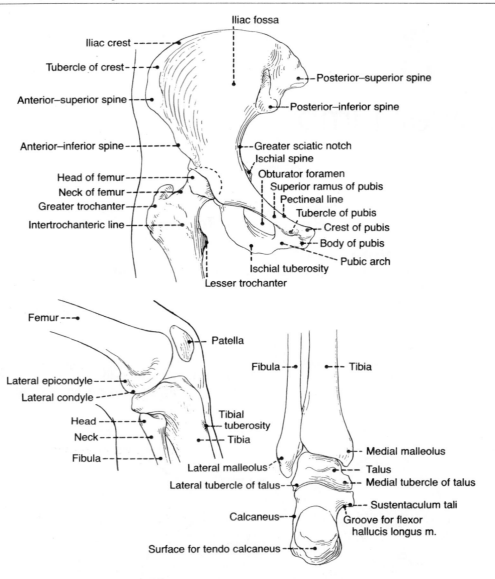

Figure 3–2. Bones of the lower limb.

B. Pubis

–forms the anterior part of the acetabulum and the anteromedial part of the hip bone.

–comprises the following structures: the **body,** which articulates at the symphysis pubis; the **superior ramus,** which enters the formation of the acetabulum; the **inferior ramus,** which joins the ramus of the ischium; the obturator foramen, which is formed by fusion of the ischium and pubis; and the crest of the pubis, pubic tubercle, and pectineal line (or pecten pubis).

C. Ischium

–forms the posteroinferior part of the acetabulum and the lower posterior part of the hip bone.

–consists of the following structures: the **body,** which joins the ilium and superior ramus of the pubis to form the acetabulum; and the **ramus,** which joins the inferior pubic ramus to form the ischiopubic ramus.

–has the **ischial spine, ischial tuberosity,** and lesser sciatic notch.

D. Acetabulum

–is a cup-shaped cavity on the lateral side of the hip bone in which the head of the femur fits.

–includes the **acetabular notch,** which is bridged by the transverse acetabular ligament.

–is formed by the **ilium** superiorly, the **ischium** posteroinferiorly, and the **pubis** anteromedially.

II. Bones of the Thigh and Leg (Figure 3-3; see Figure 3-2)

A. Femur

–is the longest and strongest bone of the body.

1. Head

–forms about two-thirds of a sphere and is directed medially, upward, and slightly forward to fit into the acetabulum.

–has a depression in its articular surface, the **fovea capitis femoris,** to which the ligamentum capitis femoris is attached.

2. Neck

–connects the head to the body (shaft), forms an angle of about 125° with the shaft, and is a **common site of fractures.**

–is separated from the shaft in front by the **intertrochanteric line,** to which the iliofemoral ligament is attached.

3. Greater trochanter

–projects upward from the junction of the neck with the shaft.

–provides an insertion for the gluteus medius and minimus, piriformis, and obturator internus muscles.

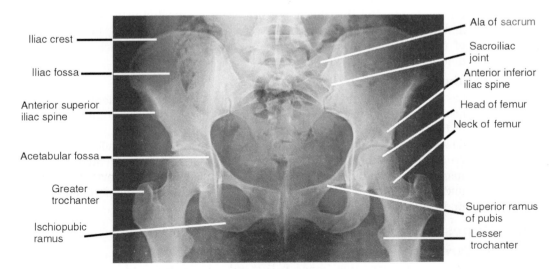

Figure 3–3. Radiograph of the hip, thigh, and pelvis.

–receives the obturator externus tendon on the medial aspect of the **trochanteric fossa.**

4. Lesser trochanter

–lies in the angle between the neck and the shaft.
–projects at the inferior end of the **intertrochanteric crest.**
–provides an insertion for the iliopsoas tendon.

5. Linea aspera

–is the rough line or ridge on the body (shaft) of the femur.
–exhibits lateral and medial lips that provide attachments for many muscles and the three intermuscular septa.

6. Pectineal line

–runs from the lesser trochanter to the medial lip of the linea aspera.
–provides an insertion for the pectineus muscle.

7. Adductor tubercle

–is a small prominence at the uppermost part of the medial femoral condyle.
–provides an insertion for the adductor magnus muscle.

B. Patella

–is the **largest sesamoid bone** located within the tendon of the quadriceps, which articulates with the femur but not with the tibia.
–attaches to the tibial tuberosity by a continuation of the quadriceps tendon called the **patellar ligament.**
–functions to obviate wear and attrition on the quadriceps tendon as it passes across the trochlear groove and to increase the angle of pull of the quadriceps femoris, thereby magnifying its power.

C. Tibia

–is the weight-bearing medial bone of the leg.
–has the **tibial tuberosity,** into which the patellar ligament inserts.
–has medial and lateral condyles that articulate with the condyles of the femur.
–has a projection called the **medial malleolus** with a **malleolar groove** for the tendons of the tibialis posterior and flexor digitorum longus muscles and another **groove** (posterolateral to the malleolus groove) for the tendon of the flexor hallucis longus muscle. It also provides attachment for the deltoid ligament.

D. Fibula

–has little or no function in weightbearing but provides attachment for muscles.
–has a **head** (apex) that provides attachment for the fibular collateral ligament of the knee joint.
–has a projection called the **lateral malleolus** that articulates with the trochlea of the talus, lies more inferior and posterior than the medial malleolus, and provides attachment for the anterior talofibular, posterior talofibular, and calcaneofibular ligaments. It also has the **sulcus** for the peroneus longus and brevis muscle tendons.

III. Bones of the Ankle and Foot (Figure 3-4; see Figures 3-7 and 3-12)

A. Tarsus

–consists of seven tarsal bones: **talus, calcaneus, navicular bone, cuboid bone,** and **three cuneiform bones.**

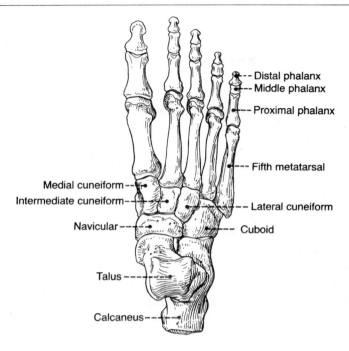

Figure 3–4. Bones of the foot.

1. Talus
–transmits the weight of the body from the tibia to the foot and is the only tarsal bone without muscle attachments.
–has a **neck** with a deep groove, the **sulcus tali,** for the **interosseous ligaments** between the talus and the calcaneus.
–has a **body** with a **groove** on its posterior surface for the **flexor hallucis longus tendon.**
–has a **head,** which serves as **keystone** of the **medial longitudinal arch** of the foot.

2. Calcaneus
–is the largest and strongest bone of the foot and lies below the talus.
–forms the **heel** of the foot and articulates with the talus superiorly and the cuboid anteriorly.
–has a shelf-like medial projection called the **sustentaculum tali**, which **supports** the **head** of the **talus** (with the spring ligament) and has a **groove** on its inferior surface for the **flexor hallucis longus tendon.**

3. Navicular bone
–is a boat-shaped tarsal bone lying between the head of the talus and the three cuneiform bones.

4. Cuboid bone
–is the most laterally placed tarsal bone and has a notch and **groove** for the **peroneus longus muscle tendon.**
–serves as the **keystone** of the **lateral longitudinal arch** of the foot.

5. Cuneiform bones

  –are wedge-shaped bones that are related to the transverse arch.

  –articulate with the navicular bone posteriorly and with three metatarsals anteriorly.

B. Metatarsus

  –consists of **five metatarsals** and has prominent medial and lateral sesamoid bones on the first metatarsal.

C. Phalanges

  –consists of 14 structures (phalanges) [two in the first digit and three in each of the others].

Joints and Ligaments

I. Hip (Coxal) Joint (see Figures 3-2 and 3-3)

  –is a **multiaxial ball-and-socket synovial joint** between the acetabulum of the hip bone and the head of the femur, and allows abduction and adduction, flexion and extension, and circumduction and rotation.

  –is stabilized by the acetabular labrum, the fibrous capsule, and capsular ligaments such as the iliofemoral, ischiofemoral, and pubofemoral ligaments.

  –has a cavity that is deepened by the fibrocartilaginous **acetabular labrum** and is completed below by the **transverse acetabular ligament,** which bridges and converts the **acetabular notch** into a foramen for passage of **nutrient vessels** and nerves.

  –receives blood from branches of the medial and lateral femoral circumflex, superior and inferior gluteal, and obturator arteries. The posterior branch of the obturator artery gives rise to the artery of the ligamentum capitis femoris (ligamentum teres femoris).

  –is innervated by branches of the femoral, obturator, sciatic, and superior gluteal nerves and by the nerve to the quadratus femoris.

A. Structures

1. Acetabular labrum

  –is a complete fibrocartilage rim that deepens the articular socket for the head of the femur and consequently stabilizes the hip joint.

2. Fibrous capsule

  –is attached proximally to the margin of the acetabulum and to the transverse acetabular ligament.

  –is attached distally to the neck of the femur as follows: anteriorly to the intertrochanteric line and the root of the greater trochanter and posteriorly to the intertrochanteric crest.

  –encloses part of the head and most of the neck of the femur.

  –is reinforced anteriorly by the **iliofemoral** ligament, posteriorly by the **ischiofemoral** ligament, and inferiorly by the **pubofemoral** ligament.

B. Ligaments

1. Iliofemoral ligament

  –is the largest and most important ligament that reinforces the fibrous capsule anteriorly and is in the form of an inverted Y.

–is attached proximally to the anterior–inferior iliac spine and the acetabular rim and distally to the intertrochanteric line and the front of the greater trochanter of the femur.

–resists hyperextension and lateral rotation at the hip joint during standing.

2. **Ischiofemoral ligament**

    –reinforces the fibrous capsule posteriorly, extends from the ischial portion of the **acetabular rim** to the neck of the femur medial to the base of the greater trochanter, and limits extension and medial rotation of the thigh.

3. **Pubofemoral ligament**

    –reinforces the fibrous capsule inferiorly, extends from the pubic portion of the acetabular rim and the superior pubic ramus to the lower part of the femoral neck, and limits extension and abduction.

4. **Ligamentum teres capitis femoris (round ligament of head of femur)**

    –arises from the floor of the acetabular fossa (more specifically, from the margins of the acetabular notch and from the transverse acetabular ligament) and attaches to the **fovea capitis femoris.**

    –provides a pathway for the artery of the ligamentum capitis femoris (foveolar artery) from the obturator artery, which is of variable size but represents a significant portion of the blood supply to the femoral head during childhood.

5. **Transverse acetabular ligament**

    –is a fibrous band that bridges the acetabular notch and converts it into a foramen.

II. **Knee Joint** (Figures 3-5 and 3-6; see Figure 3-2)

–is the largest and most complicated joint. Although structurally it resembles a hinge joint, it is a **condylar-type of synovial joint** between two condyles of the femur and tibia. In addition, it includes a **saddle joint** between the femur and the patella.

–is encompassed by a **fibrous capsule** that is rather thin, weak, and incomplete, but it is attached to the margins of the femoral and tibial condyles, to the patella and patellar ligament, and surrounds the lateral and posterior aspects of the joint.

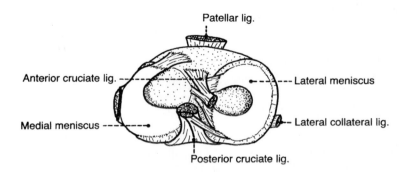

Patellar lig.

Anterior cruciate lig.

Lateral meniscus

Medial meniscus

Lateral collateral lig.

Posterior cruciate lig.

Figure 3–5. Ligaments of the knee.

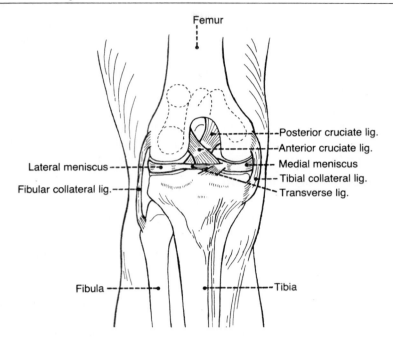

Figure 3–6. Ligaments of the knee joint (anterior view).

–permits flexion, extension, and some gliding and rotation in the flexed position of the knee; full extension is accompanied by medial rotation of the femur on the tibia, pulling all ligaments taut.

–is stabilized laterally by the biceps and gastrocnemius (lateral head) tendons, the **iliotibial tract,** and the fibular collateral ligaments.

–is stabilized medially by the sartorius, gracilis, gastrocnemius (medial head), semitendinosus, and semimembranosus muscles, and the tibial collateral ligament.

–receives blood from the genicular branches (superior medial and lateral, inferior medial and lateral, and middle) of the popliteal artery, a descending branch of the lateral femoral circumflex artery, an articular branch of the descending genicular artery, and the anterior tibial recurrent artery.

–is innervated by branches of the sciatic, femoral, and obturator nerves.

–is supported by various ligaments and menisci.

A. Ligaments

1. Intracapsular ligaments

a. Anterior cruciate ligament

–lies inside the knee joint capsule but outside the synovial cavity of the joint.

–arises from the anterior intercondylar area of the tibia and passes upward, backward, and laterally to insert into the medial surface of the lateral femoral condyle.

–is slightly shorter than the posterior cruciate ligament.

–**prevents posterior displacement** (backward slipping) **of the femur on the tibia** (or anterior displacement of the tibia on the femur) and limits hyperextension of the knee joint.

–is lax when the knee is flexed and becomes taut when the knee is fully extended.

–may be torn when the knee is hyperextended.

b. Posterior cruciate ligament

–lies outside the synovial cavity but within the fibrous joint capsule.

–arises from the posterior intercondylar area of the tibia and passes upward, forward, and medially to insert into the lateral surface of the medial femoral condyle.

–is shorter and stronger than the anterior cruciate ligament.

–**prevents anterior displacement of the femur on the tibia** (or posterior displacement of the tibia on the femur).

–is lax when the knee is flexed and becomes taut when the knee is extended.

c. Medial meniscus

–lies outside the synovial cavity but within the joint capsule.

–is **C-shaped** (i.e., forms a semicircle) and is attached to the medial collateral ligament and interarticular area of the tibia.

–acts as a cushion or shock absorber and lubricates the articular surfaces by distributing synovial fluid in windshield-wiper fashion.

–is **more frequently torn** in injuries than the lateral meniscus.

d. Lateral meniscus

–lies outside the synovial cavity but within the joint capsule.

–is nearly **circular**, acts as a cushion, and facilitates lubrication.

–is separated laterally from the fibular (or lateral) collateral ligament by the tendon of the popliteal muscle and aids in forming a more stable base for the articulation of the femoral condyle.

e. Transverse ligament

–binds the anterior horns (ends) of the lateral and medial semilunar cartilages (menisci).

2. Extracapsular ligaments

a. Medial (tibial) collateral ligament

–is a broad band that extends from the medial femoral epicondyle to the medial tibial condyle.

–is **firmly attached to the medial meniscus** and its attachment is of clinical significance because injury to the ligament results in concomitant damage to the medial meniscus.

–prevents medial displacement of the two long bones and thus abduction of the leg at the knee.

–becomes taut on extension and thus limits extension and abduction of the leg.

b. Lateral (fibular) collateral ligament

–is a rounded cord that is separated from the lateral meniscus by the tendon of the popliteus muscle and also from the capsule of the joint.

–extends between the lateral femoral epicondyle and the head of the fibula.

–becomes taut on extension and limits extension and adduction of the leg.

c. Patellar ligament

–is a strong flattened fibrous band that is the continuation of the **quadriceps femoris tendon.**

–extends from the apex of the patella to the tuberosity of the tibia.

d. Arcuate popliteal ligament

–arises from the head of the fibula, arches superiorly and medially over the tendon of the popliteus muscle on the back of the knee joint, and fuses with the articular capsule.

e. Oblique popliteal ligament

–is an oblique expansion of the **semimembranosus tendon** and passes upward obliquely across the posterior surface of the knee joint from the medial condyle of the tibia.

–resists hyperextension of the leg and lateral rotation during the final phase of extension.

B. Bursae

1. Suprapatellar bursa

–lies deep to the quadriceps femoris muscle and is the major bursa communicating with the knee joint cavity (the semimembranosus bursa also may communicate with it).

2. Prepatellar bursa

–lies over the superficial surface of the patella.

3. Infrapatellar bursa

–consists of a **subcutaneous infrapatellar bursa** over the patellar ligament and a **deep infrapatellar bursa** deep to the patellar ligament.

4. Anserine bursa (known as the **pes anserinus** [goose's foot])

–lies between the tibial collateral ligament and the tendons of the sartorius, gracilis, and semitendinosus muscles.

III. Tibiofibular Joints

A. Proximal tibiofibular joint

–is a plane-type synovial joint between the head of the fibula and the tibia, which allows a little gliding movement.

B. Distal tibiofibular joint

–is a fibrous joint between the tibia and the fibula.

IV. Ankle (Talocrural) Joint (Figure 3-7; see Figure 3-2)

–is a **hinge-type (ginglymus) synovial joint** between superiorly the tibia and fibula and inferiorly the trochlea of the talus, permitting dorsiflexion and plantar flexion.

A. Articular capsule

–is a thin fibrous capsule that lies both anteriorly and posteriorly, allowing movement.

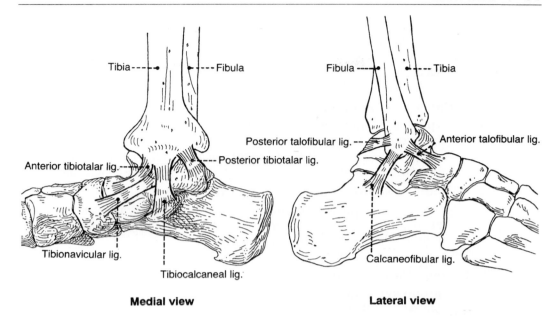

Figure 3–7. Ligaments of the ankle joint.

–is reinforced medially by the medial (or deltoid) ligament and laterally by the lateral ligament, which prevents anterior and posterior slipping of the tibia and fibula on the talus.

B. Ligaments

1. Medial (deltoid) ligament

–has four parts: the tibionavicular, tibiocalcaneal, anterior tibiotalar, and posterior tibiotalar ligaments.
–extends from the medial malleolus to the navicular bone, calcaneus, and talus.
–prevents overeversion of the foot and helps maintain the medial longitudinal arch.

2. Lateral ligament

–consists of the anterior talofibular, posterior talofibular, and calcaneofibular (cord-like) ligaments.
–resists inversion of the foot and may be torn during an **ankle sprain** (inversion injury).

V. Tarsal Joints

A. Intertarsal joints

1. Talocalcaneal (subtalar) joint

–is a plane synovial joint (part of the talocalcaneonavicular joint), formed between the talus and calcaneus bones.
–allows inversion and eversion of the foot.

2. Talocalcaneonavicular joint

–is a ball-and-socket joint (part of the transverse tarsal joint), formed between the head of the talus (ball) and the calcaneus and navicular bones (socket).

–is supported by the **spring** (plantar calcaneonavicular) ligament.

3. Calcaneocuboid joint

–is part of the transverse tarsal joint and resembles a saddle joint between the calcaneus and the cuboid bones.

–is supported by the **short plantar** (plantar calcaneocuboid) and **long plantar** ligaments and by the tendon of the peroneus longus muscle.

4. Transverse tarsal (midtarsal) joint

–is a collective term for the **talonavicular part** of the talocalcaneonavicular joint and the calcaneocuboid joint. The two joints are separated anatomically but act together functionally.

–is important in inversion and eversion of the foot.

B. Tarsometatarsal joints

–are **plane synovial joints** that strengthen the transverse arch.

–are united by articular capsules and are reinforced by the plantar, dorsal, and interosseous ligaments.

C. Metatarsophalangeal joints

–are **ellipsoid (condyloid) synovial joints** that are joined by articular capsules and are reinforced by the plantar and collateral ligaments.

D. Interphalangeal joints

–are **hinge-type (ginglymus) synovial joints** that are enclosed by articular capsules and are reinforced by the plantar and collateral ligaments.

Cutaneous Nerves, Superficial Veins, and Lymphatics

I. Cutaneous Nerves (Figure 3-8)

A. Lateral femoral cutaneous nerve

–arises from the lumbar plexus (L2–L3), emerges from the lateral border of the psoas major, crosses the iliacus, and passes under the inguinal ligament near the anterior–superior iliac spine.

–innervates the **skin on the anterior and lateral aspects of the thigh** as far as the knee.

B. Clunial (buttock) nerves

–innervate the **skin of the gluteal region.**

–consist of **superior** (lateral branches of the dorsal rami of the upper three lumbar nerves), **middle** (lateral branches of the dorsal rami of the upper three sacral nerves), and **inferior** (gluteal branches of the posterior femoral cutaneous nerve) nerves.

C. Posterior femoral cutaneous nerve

–arises from the **sacral plexus** (S1–S3), passes through the greater sciatic foramen below the piriformis muscle, runs deep to the gluteus maximus muscle, and emerges from the inferior border of this muscle.

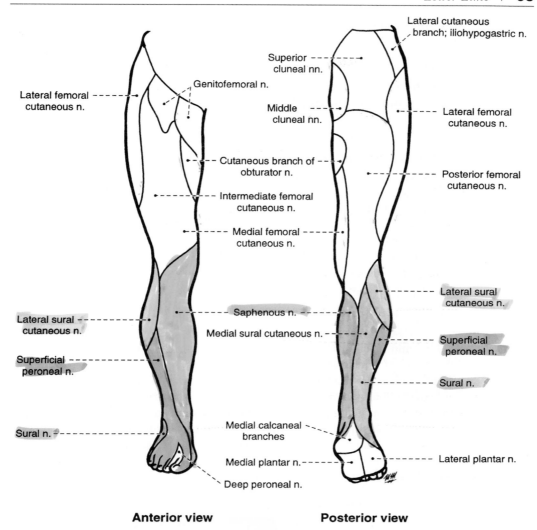

Figure 3–8. Cutaneous nerves of the lower limb.

–descends in the posterior midline of the thigh deep to the fascia lata and pierces the fascia lata near the popliteal fossa.

–innervates the **skin of the buttock, thigh,** and **calf.**

D. Saphenous nerve

–arises from the **femoral nerve** in the **femoral triangle** and descends with the femoral vessels through the femoral triangle and the adductor canal.

–pierces the fascial covering of the adductor canal at its distal end in company with the saphenous branch of the descending genicular artery.

–becomes cutaneous between the sartorius and the gracilis and descends behind the condyles of the femur and tibia and medial aspect of the leg in company with the great saphenous vein.

–**innervates the skin on the medial side of the leg and foot.**

–is **vulnerable to injury** (proximal portion) during surgery to repair varicose veins.

E. Lateral sural cutaneous nerve

–arises from the **common peroneal nerve** in the **popliteal fossa** and may have a **communicating branch** that joins the medial sural cutaneous nerve.

–innervates the **skin on the posterolateral side of the leg.**

F. Medial sural cutaneous nerve

–arises from the tibial nerve in the popliteal fossa and may join the lateral sural nerve or its communicating branch to form the **sural nerve.**

–innervates the **back of the leg** and the **lateral side of the heel and foot.**

G. Sural nerve

–is formed by the union of the medial sural and lateral sural nerves (or the communicating branch of the lateral sural nerve).

–innervates the **back of the leg** and the **lateral side of the heel and foot.**

H. Superficial peroneal nerve

–passes distally between the peroneus muscles and the extensor digitorum longus and pierces the deep fascia in the lower third of the leg to innervate the **skin of the lower part of the leg.**

–divides into a **medial dorsal cutaneous nerve,** which supplies the medial side of the foot and ankle, the medial sides of the great toe, and the adjacent sides of the second and third toes, and an **intermediate dorsal cutaneous nerve,** which supplies the skin of the lateral side of the foot and ankle and the adjacent sides of the third, fourth, and little toes.

II. Superficial Veins

A. Great saphenous vein

–begins at the medial end of the **dorsal venous arch** of the foot.

–ascends in front of the medial malleolus and along the medial aspect of the tibia along with the saphenous nerve, passes behind the medial condyles of the tibia and femur, and then ascends along the medial side of the femur.

–passes through the **saphenous opening (fossa ovalis)** in the fascia lata and pierces the femoral sheath to join the femoral vein.

–receives the external pudendal, superficial epigastric, superficial circumflex ilia, lateral femoral cutaneous, and accessory saphenous veins.

–is a suitable vessel for use in coronary arterial bypass surgery and for venipuncture.

B. Small (short) saphenous vein

–begins at the lateral end of the **dorsal venous arch** and passes upward along the lateral side of the foot with the sural nerve, behind the lateral malleolus.

–passes to the popliteal fossa, where it perforates the deep fascia and terminates in the **popliteal vein.**

III. Lymphatics

A. Vessels

1. Superficial lymph vessels

–are divided into a **medial group,** which follows the great saphenous vein, and a **lateral group,** which follows the small saphenous vein.

2. Deep lymph vessels

–consist of the **anterior tibial, posterior tibial,** and **peroneal vessels,** which follow the course of the corresponding blood vessels and enter the **popliteal lymph nodes.**

B. Lymph nodes

1. Superficial inguinal group of lymph nodes

–is located subcutaneously near the **saphenofemoral junction** and drains the superficial thigh region.

–receives lymph from the anterolateral abdominal wall below the umbilicus, gluteal region, lower parts of the vagina and anus, and external genitalia except the glans, and drains into the **external iliac nodes.**

2. Deep inguinal group of lymph nodes

–lies deep to the fascia lata on the medial side of the femoral vein.

–receives lymph from deep lymph vessels (i.e., efferents of the popliteal nodes) that accompany the femoral vessels and from the glans penis or glans clitoris, and drains into the external iliac nodes through the femoral canal.

Gluteal Region and Posterior Thigh

I. Fibrous Structures

A. Sacrotuberous ligament

–extends from the ischial tuberosity to the posterior iliac spines, lower sacrum, and coccyx.

–converts, with the sacrospinous ligament, the lesser sciatic notch into the lesser sciatic foramen.

B. Sacrospinous ligament

–extends from the ischial spine to the lower sacrum and coccyx.

–converts the greater sciatic notch into the greater sciatic foramen.

C. Sciatic foramina

1. Greater sciatic foramen

–provides a pathway for the piriformis muscle, superior and inferior gluteal vessels and nerves, internal pudendal vessels and pudendal nerve, sciatic nerve, posterior femoral cutaneous nerve, and the nerves to the obturator internus and quadratus femoris muscles.

2. Lesser sciatic foramen

–provides a pathway for the tendon of the obturator internus, the nerve to the obturator internus, and the internal pudendal vessels and pudendal nerve.

3. **Structures that pass through both the greater and lesser sciatic foramina**

–include the pudendal nerve, the internal pudendal vessels, and the nerve to the obturator internus.

D. **Iliotibial tract**

–is a thick lateral portion of the **fascia lata.**
–provides insertion for the gluteus maximus and tensor fasciae latae muscles.
–helps form the **fibrous capsule of the knee joint** and is important in maintaining posture and locomotion.

E. **Fascia lata**

–is a membranous, deep fascia covering muscles of the thigh and forms the **lateral and medial intermuscular septa** by its inward extension to the femur.
–is attached to the pubic symphysis, pubic crest, pubic rami, ischial tuberosity, inguinal and sacrotuberous ligaments, and the sacrum and coccyx.

II. Muscles of the Gluteal Region (Table 3-1; Figure 3-9)

Table 3–1. Muscles of the Gluteal Region

Muscle	Origin	Insertion	Nerve	Action
Gluteus maximus	Ilium; sacrum; coccyx; sacrotuberous ligament	Gluteal tuberosity; iliotibial tract	Inferior gluteal	Extends and rotates thigh laterally
Gluteus medius	Ilium between iliac crest, and anterior and posterior gluteal lines	Greater trochanter	Superior gluteal	Abducts and rotates thigh medially; stabilizes pelvis
Gluteus minimus	Ilium between anterior and inferior gluteal lines	Greater trochanter	Superior gluteal	Abducts and rotates thigh medially
Tensor fasciae latae	Iliac crest; anterior–superior iliac spine	Iliotibial tract	Superior gluteal	Flexes, abducts, and rotates thigh medially
Piriformis	Pelvic surface of sacrum; sacrotuberous ligament	Upper end of greater trochanter	Sacral (S1–S2)	Rotates thigh laterally
Obturator internus	Ischiopubic rami; obturator membrane	Greater trochanter	Nerve to obturator internus	Abducts and rotates thigh laterally
Superior gemellus	Ischial spine	Obturator internus tendon	Nerve to obturator internus	Rotates thigh laterally
Inferior gemellus	Ischial tuberosity	Obturator internus tendon	Nerve to quadratus femoris	Rotates thigh laterally
Quadratus femoris	Ischial tuberosity	Intertrochanteric crest	Nerve to quadratus femoris	Rotates thigh laterally

III. Posterior Muscles of the Thigh (Table 3-2; see Figure 3-9)

Table 3–2. Posterior Muscles of the Thigh*

Muscle	Origin	Insertion	Nerve	Action
Semitendinosus	Ischial tuberosity	Medial surface of upper part of tibia	Tibial portion of sciatic nerve	Extends thigh; flexes and rotates leg medially
Semimembranosus	Ischial tuberosity	Medial condyle of tibia	Tibial portion of sciatic nerve	Extends thigh; flexes and rotates leg medially
Biceps femoris	Long head from ischial tuberosity; short head from linea aspera and upper supracondylar line	Head of fibula	Tibial (long head) and common peroneal (short head) divisions of sciatic nerve	Extends thigh; flexes and rotates leg laterally

*These three muscles collectively are called hamstrings.

IV. Nerves of the Gluteal Region

  A. Superior gluteal nerve (see Nerves and Vasculature: I C)

  B. Inferior gluteal nerve (see Nerves and Vasculature: I D)

  C. Posterior femoral cutaneous nerve (see Nerves and Vasculature: I E)

  D. Sciatic nerve (see Nerves and Vasculature: I F 1–2)

V. Arteries of the Gluteal Region

  A. Superior gluteal artery (see Nerves and Vasculature: II A)

  B. Inferior gluteal artery (see Nerves and Vasculature: II B)

VI. Hip (Coxal) Joint (see Joints and Ligaments: I A–B; see Figures 3-1, 3-2, and 3-3)

Anterior Thigh and Leg

I. Fibrous Structures of the Anterior Thigh

A. Femoral triangle

  –is bounded by the inguinal ligament superiorly, the sartorius muscle laterally, and the adductor longus muscle medially.

  –contains the femoral nerve and vessels. The pulsation of the femoral artery may be felt just inferior to the midpoint of the inguinal ligament.

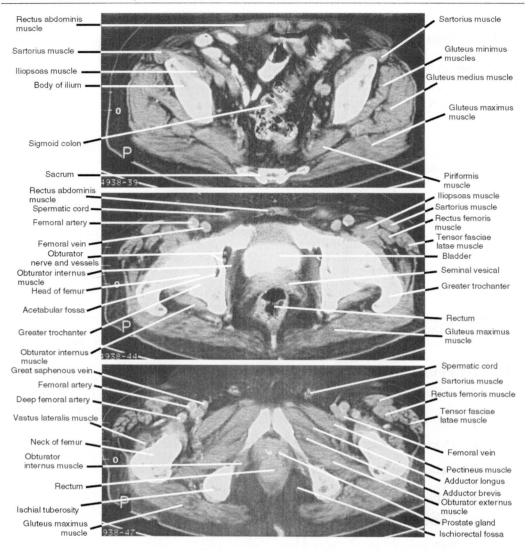

Figure 3–9. Computed tomography (CT) scans of the hip, thigh, and pelvis.

B. Femoral ring

–is the abdominal opening of the femoral canal.

–is bounded by the inguinal ligament anteriorly, the femoral vein laterally, the lacunar ligament medially, and the pectineal ligament posteriorly.

C. Femoral canal

–lies medial to the femoral vein in the femoral sheath.

–contains fat, areolar connective tissue, and lymph nodes.

–transmits **lymphatics** from the lower limb and perineum to the peritoneal cavity.

–is a potential weak area and a site of **femoral herniation,** which occurs most frequently in women because of the greater width of the superior pubic ramus of the female pelvis.

   D. Femoral sheath

   –is formed by a prolongation of the **transversalis** and **iliac fasciae** in the thigh.

   –contains the femoral artery and vein, the femoral branch of the genitofemoral nerve, and the femoral canal. (The femoral nerve lies outside the femoral sheath, lateral to the femoral artery.)

   –reaches the level of the proximal end of the saphenous opening with its distal end.

   E. Adductor canal

   –begins at the apex of the femoral triangle and ends at the **adductor hiatus** (hiatus tendineus).

   –lies between the adductor magnus and longus muscles and the vastus medialis muscle and is covered by the sartorius muscle and fascia.

   –contains the femoral vessels, the saphenous nerve, and the nerve to the vastus medialis.

   F. Adductor hiatus (hiatus tendineus)

   –is the aperture in the tendon of insertion of the adductor magnus.

   –allows the passage of the femoral vessels into the popliteal fossa.

   G. Saphenous opening (saphenous hiatus) **or fossa ovalis**

   –is an oval gap in the fascia lata below the inguinal ligament that is covered by the cribriform fascia.

   –provides a pathway for the greater saphenous vein.

   H. Popliteal fossa

   –is bounded superomedially by the semitendinosus and semimembranosus muscles and superolaterally by the biceps muscle.

   –is bounded inferolaterally by the lateral head of the gastrocnemius muscle and inferomedially by the medial head of the gastrocnemius muscle.

   –has a floor that is composed of the femur, the oblique popliteal ligament, and the popliteus muscle.

   –contains the popliteal vessels, the common peroneal and tibial nerves, and the small saphenous vein.

II. Anterior Muscles of the Thigh (Table 3-3; see Figure 3-9)

III. Medial Muscles of the Thigh (Table 3-4; see Figure 3-9)

IV. Anterior and Lateral Muscles of the Leg (Table 3-5)

V. Posterior Muscles of the Leg (Table 3-6)

VI. Knee Joint (see Figures 3-5 and 3-6)

   A. Anterior cruciate ligament (see Joints and Ligaments: II A 1 a)

   B. Posterior cruciate ligament (see Joints and Ligaments: II A 1 b)

   C. Medial meniscus (see Joints and Ligaments: II A 1 c)

   D. Lateral meniscus (see Joints and Ligaments: II A 1 d)

   E. Medial (tibial) collateral ligament (see Joints and Ligaments: II A 2 a)

   F. Lateral (fibular) collateral ligament (see Joints and Ligaments: II A 2 b)

Table 3–3. Anterior Muscles of the Thigh

Muscle	Origin	Insertion	Nerve	Action
Iliacus	Iliac fossa; ala of sacrum	Lesser trochanter	Femoral	Flexes thigh (with Psoas major)
Sartorius	Anterior–superior iliac spine	Upper medial side of tibia	Femoral	Flexes and rotates thigh laterally; flexes and rotates leg medially
Rectus femoris	Anterior–inferior iliac spine; posterior–superior rim of acetabulum	Base of patella; tibial tuberosity	Femoral	Flexes thigh; extends leg
Vastus medialis	Intertrochanteric line; linea aspera; medial intermuscular septum	Medial side of patella; tibial tuberosity	Femoral	Extends leg
Vastus lateralis	Intertrochanteric line; greater trochanter; linea aspera; gluteal tuberosity; lateral intermuscular septum	Lateral side of patella; tibial tuberosity	Femoral	Extends leg
Vastus intermedius	Upper shaft of femur; lower lateral intermuscular septum	Upper border of patella; tibial tuberosity	Femoral	Extends leg

Table 3–4. Medial Muscles of the Thigh

Muscle	Origin	Insertion	Nerve	Action
Adductor longus	Body of pubis below its crest	Middle third of linea aspera	Obturator	Adducts and flexes thigh
Adductor brevis	Body and inferior pubic ramus	Pectineal line; upper part of linea aspera	Obturator	Adducts and flexes thigh
Adductor magnus	Ischiopubic ramus; ischial tuberosity	Linea aspera; medial supracondylar line; adductor tubercle	Obturator and sciatic (tibial part)	Adducts, flexes, and extends thigh
Pectineus	Pectineal line of pubis	Pectineal line of femur	Obturator and femoral	Adducts and flexes thigh
Gracilis	Body and inferior pubic ramus	Medial surface of upper quarter of tibia	Obturator	Adducts and flexes thigh; flexes and rotates leg medially
Obturator externus	Margin of obturator foramen and obturator membrane	Intertrochanteric fossa of femur	Obturator	Rotates thigh laterally

Table 3–5. Anterior and Lateral Muscles of the Leg

Muscle	Origin	Insertion	Nerve	Action
Anterior				
Tibialis anterior	Lateral tibial condyle; interosseous membrane	First cuneiform; first metatarsal	Deep peroneal	Dorsiflexes and inverts foot
Extensor hallucis longus	Middle half of anterior surface of fibula; interosseous membrane	Base of distal phalanx of big toe	Deep peroneal	Extends big toe; dorsiflexes and inverts foot
Extensor digitorum longus	Lateral tibial condyle; upper two-thirds of fibula; interosseous membrane	Bases of middle and distal phalanges	Deep peroneal	Extends toes; dorsiflexes and everts foot
Peroneus tertius	Distal one-third of fibula; interosseous membrane	Base of fifth metatarsal	Deep peroneal	Dorsiflexes and everts foot
Lateral				
Peroneus longus	Lateral tibial condyle; head and upper lateral side of fibula	Base of first metatarsal; medial cuneiform	Superficial peroneal	Everts and plantar flexes foot
Peroneus brevis	Lower lateral side of fibula; intermuscular septa	Base of fifth metatarsal	Superficial peroneal	Everts and plantar flexes foot

Foot

I. Fascial Structures

A. Superior extensor retinaculum

–is a **broad band of deep fascia** extending between the tibia and fibula, above the ankle.

B. Inferior extensor retinaculum

–is a **Y-shaped band of deep fascia,** which forms a loop for the tendons of the extensor digitorum longus and the peroneus tertius and then divides into an upper band, which attaches to the medial malleolus, and a **lower band,** which attaches to the deep fascia of the foot and the plantar aponeurosis.

C. Flexor retinaculum

–is a deep fascial band that passes between the medial malleolus and the medial surface of the calcaneus.

–holds three tendons in place beneath it: the tibialis posterior, flexor digitorum longus, and flexor hallucis longus.

–provides a pathway for the tibial nerve and posterior tibial artery beneath it.

Table 3–6. Posterior Muscles of the Leg

Muscle	Origin	Insertion	Nerve	Action
Superficial group				
Gastrocnemius	Lateral (lateral head) and medial (medial head) femoral condyles	Posterior aspect of calcaneus via tendo calcaneus	Tibial	Flexes knee; plantar flexes foot
Soleus	Upper fibula head; soleal line on tibia	Posterior aspect of calcaneus via tendo calcaneus	Tibial	Plantar flexes foot
Plantaris	Lower lateral supracondylar line	Posterior surface of calcaneus	Tibial	Flexes and rotates leg medially
Deep group				
Popliteus	Lateral condyle of femur; popliteal ligament	Upper posterior side of tibia	Tibial	Flexes and rotates leg medially
Flexor hallucis longus	Lower two-thirds of fibula; interosseous membrane; intermuscular septa	Base of distal phalanx of big toe	Tibial inv.	Plantar flexes foot; flexes distal phalanx of big toe
Flexor digitorum longus	Middle posterior aspect of tibia	Distal phalanges of lateral four toes	Tibial inv.	Flexes lateral four toes; plantar flexes foot
Tibialis posterior	Interosseous membrane; upper parts of tibia and fibula	Tuberosity of navicular; sustentacula tali; three cuneiforms; cuboid; bases of metatarsals 2–4	Tibial	Plantar flexes and inverts foot

    D. Tendo calcaneus (Achilles tendon)

        –is the tendon of insertion of the **triceps surae** (gastrocnemius and soleus) into the tuberosity of the calcaneus.

    E. Plantar aponeurosis

        –is a thick fascia investing the plantar muscles.

        –radiates from the **calcaneal tuberosity** (tuber calcanei) toward the toes and provides attachment to the short flexor muscles of the toes.

II. Muscles (Table 3-7)

III. Arches (Figure 3-10)

    –consist of medial and lateral longitudinal arches and proximal and distal transverse arches.

    –support the body in the erect position and act as a spring in locomotion.

    A. Medial longitudinal arch

        –is formed and maintained by the interlocking of the talus, calcaneus, navicular, cuneiform bones, and three medial metatarsal bones.

Table 3–7. Muscles of the Foot

Muscle	Origin	Insertion	Nerve	Action
Dorsum of foot				
Extensor digitorum brevis	Dorsal surface of calcaneus	Tendons of extensor digitorum longus	Deep peroneal	Extends toes
Extensor hallucis brevis	Dorsal surface of calcaneus	Base of proximal phalanx of big toe	Deep peroneal	Extends big toe
Sole of foot				
First layer				
Abductor hallucis	Medial tubercle of calcaneus	Base of proximal phalanx of big toe	Medial plantar	Abducts big toe
Flexor digitorum brevis	Medial tubercle of calcaneus	Middle phalanges of lateral four toes	Medial plantar	Flexes middle phalanges of lateral four toes
Abductor digiti minimi	Medial and lateral tubercles of calcaneus	Proximal phalanx of little toe	Lateral plantar	Abducts little toe
Second layer				
Quadratus plantae	Medial and lateral side of calcaneus	Tendons of flexor digitorum longus	Lateral plantar	Aids in flexing toes
Lumbricals (4)	Tendons of flexor digitorum longus	Proximal phalanges; extensor expansion	First by medial plantar; lateral three by lateral plantar	Flex metatarsophalangeal joints and extend interphalangeal joints
Third layer				
Flexor hallucis brevis	Cuboid; third cuneiform	Proximal phalanx of big toe	Medial plantar	Flexes big toe
Adductor hallucis:				
Oblique head	Bases of metatarsals 2–4	Proximal phalanx of big toe	Lateral plantar	Adducts big toe
Transverse head	Capsule of lateral four metatarsophalangeal joints			
Flexor digiti minimi brevis	Base of metatarsal 5	Proximal phalanx of little toe	Lateral plantar	Flexes little toe
Fourth layer				
Plantar interossei (3)	Medial sides of metatarsals 3–5	Medial sides of base of proximal phalanges 3–5	Lateral plantar	Adduct toes; flex proximal and extend distal phalanges
Dorsal interossei (4)	Adjacent shafts of metatarsals	Proximal phalanges of second toes (medial and lateral sides), and third and fourth toes (lateral sides)	Lateral plantar	Abduct toes; flex proximal and extend distal phalanges

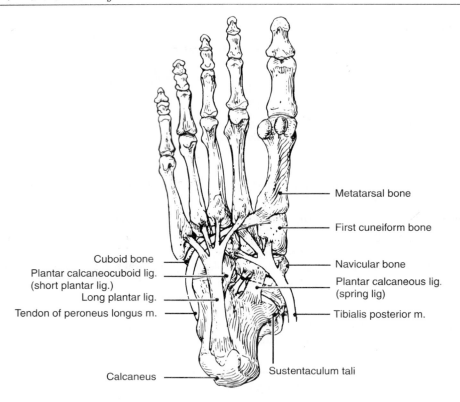

Cuboid bone
Plantar calcaneocuboid lig.
(short plantar lig.)
Long plantar lig.
Tendon of peroneus longus m.

Metatarsal bone
First cuneiform bone
Navicular bone
Plantar calcaneous lig.
(spring lig)
Tibialis posterior m.

Calcaneus
Sustentaculum tali

Figure 3–10. Plantar ligaments.

–has, as its **keystone,** the **head of the talus,** which is located at the summit between the sustentaculum tali and the navicular bone.

–is supported by the spring ligament and the tendon of the flexor hallucis longus.

B. Lateral longitudinal arch

–is formed by the calcaneus, the cuboid bone, and the lateral two metatarsal bones. The **keystone** is the **cuboid bone.**

–is supported by the peroneus longus tendon and the long and short plantar ligaments.

–supports the body in the erect position and acts as a spring in locomotion.

C. Transverse arch

1. Proximal (metatarsal) arch

–is formed by the navicular bone, the three cuneiform bones, the cuboid bone, and the bases of the five metatarsal bones of the foot.

–is supported by the tendon of the **peroneus longus.**

2. Distal arch

–is formed by the heads of five metatarsal bones.

–is maintained by the **transverse head** of the **adductor hallucis.**

IV. Ligaments

A. Long plantar (plantar calcaneocuboid) ligament

–extends from the plantar aspect of the calcaneus in front of its tuberosity to the tuberosity of the cuboid bone and the base of the metatarsals and forms a canal for the tendon of the peroneus longus.

–supports the lateral side of the longitudinal arch of the foot.

B. Short plantar (plantar calcaneocuboid) ligament

–extends from the front of the plantar surface of the calcaneus to the plantar surface of the cuboid bone.

–lies deep to the long plantar ligament and supports the lateral longitudinal arch.

C. Spring (plantar calcaneonavicular) ligament

–passes from the sustentaculum tali of the calcaneus to the navicular bone.

–supports the **head of the talus** and the medial longitudinal arch.

–is called the spring ligament because it contains considerable numbers of elastic fibers to give elasticity to the arch and spring to the foot.

–is supported by the tendon of the tibialis posterior.

V. Ankle Joint

A. Articular capsule (see Joints and Ligaments: IV A)

B. Ligaments (see Joints and Ligaments: IV B)

1. Medial (deltoid) ligament

2. Lateral ligament

Nerves and Vasculature

I. Nerves (Figure 3-11)

A. Obturator nerve

–arises from the **lumbar plexus** (L3–L4) and enters the thigh through the obturator foramen.

–divides into anterior and posterior branches.

1. Anterior branch

–descends between the adductor longus and adductor brevis muscles.

–innervates the adductor longus, adductor brevis, gracilis, and pectineus muscles.

2. Posterior branch

–descends between the adductor brevis and adductor magnus muscles.

–innervates the obturator externus and adductor magnus muscles.

B. Femoral nerve

–arises from the **lumbar plexus** (L2–L4) within the substance of the psoas major, emerges between the iliacus and psoas major muscles, and enters the thigh by passing deep to the inguinal ligament and lateral to the femoral sheath.

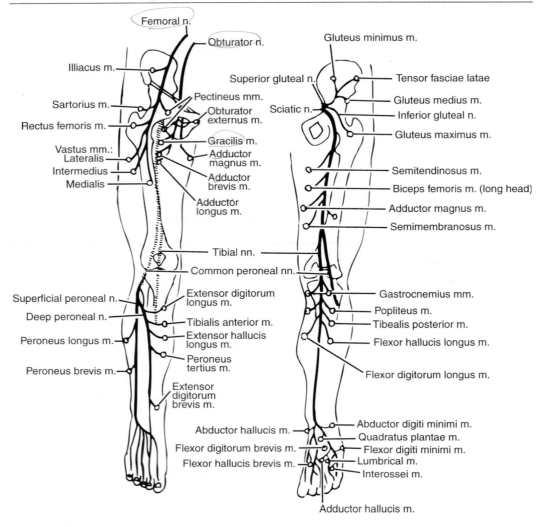

Figure 3–11. Innervation of the lower limb.

–gives rise to **muscular branches; articular branches** to the hip and knee joints; and **cutaneous branches,** including the anterior femoral cutaneous nerve and the saphenous nerve, which descends through the femoral triangle and accompanies the femoral vessels in the adductor canal.

C. Superior gluteal nerve

–arises from the **sacral plexus** (L4–S1) and enters the buttock through the greater sciatic foramen above the piriformis.

–passes between the gluteus medius and minimus muscles and divides into numerous branches.

–innervates the gluteus medius and minimus, the tensor fasciae latae, and the hip joint.

D. Inferior gluteal nerve

  –arises from the **sacral plexus** (L5–S2) and enters the buttock through the
  greater sciatic foramen below the piriformis.
  –divides into numerous branches.
  –innervates the overlying gluteus maximus.

E. Posterior femoral cutaneous nerve

  –arises from the **sacral plexus** (S1–S3) and enters the buttock through the
  greater sciatic foramen below the piriformis.
  –runs deep to the gluteus maximus and emerges from the inferior border of
  this muscle.
  –descends on the posterior thigh.
  –innervates the skin of the buttock, thigh, and calf.

F. Sciatic nerve

  –arises from the **sacral plexus** (L4–S3) and is the **largest nerve in the
  body.**
  –divides at the superior border of the popliteal fossa into the **tibial nerve,**
  which runs through the fossa to disappear deep to the gastrocnemius, and
  the **common peroneal nerve,** which runs along the medial border of the
  biceps femoris and superficial to the lateral head of the gastrocnemius.
  –enters the buttock through the greater sciatic foramen below the piriformis.
  –descends over the obturator internus gemelli and quadratus femoris muscles
  between the ischial tuberosity and the greater trochanter.
  –**innervates the hamstring muscles** by its tibial division, except for the
  short head of the biceps femoris, which is innervated by its common peroneal
  division.
  –provides articular branches to the hip and knee joints.

  1. Common peroneal (fibular) nerve

    –arises as the smaller terminal portion of the sciatic nerve at the apex of
    the popliteal fossa, descends through the fossa, and superficially crosses
    the lateral head of the gastrocnemius muscle.
    –passes behind the head of the fibula, then winds laterally around the neck
    of the fibula, and pierces the peroneus longus, where it divides into the
    deep peroneal and superficial peroneal nerves.
    –is **vulnerable to injury as it winds around the neck of the fibula,**
    where it also can be palpated.
    –gives rise to the **lateral sural cutaneous nerve,** which supplies the
    skin on the lateral part of the back of the leg, and the **recurrent articular
    branch** to the knee joint.

    a. Superficial peroneal nerve (see Cutaneous Nerves, Superficial
    Nerves, and Lymphatics: I H)

      –arises from the common peroneal nerve in the substance of the peroneus
      longus on the lateral side of the neck of the fibula, and thus it is **less
      vulnerable** to injury than the common peroneal nerve.
      –descends in the lateral compartment and innervates the skin of the
      lower leg and foot.
      –innervates the peroneus longus and brevis muscles and then emerges
      between the peroneus longus and brevis muscles by piercing the deep
      fascia at the lower third of the leg to become subcutaneous.

b. Deep peroneal nerve

–arises from the common peroneal nerve between the peroneus longus and the neck of the fibula.

–gives rise to a recurrent branch to the knee joint.

–passes around the neck of the fibula and through the extensor digitorum longus muscle.

–descends on the **interosseous membrane** between the extensor digitorum longus and the tibialis anterior and then between the extensor digitorum longus and the extensor hallucis longus muscles.

–innervates the anterior muscles of the leg and divides into a **lateral branch,** which supplies the extensor digitorum brevis, and a **medial branch,** which accompanies the dorsalis pedis artery to supply adjacent sides of the first and second toes.

2. Tibial nerve

–descends through the popliteal fossa and then lies on the popliteus muscle.

–gives rise to **three articular branches,** which accompany the medial superior genicular, middle genicular, and medial inferior genicular arteries to the knee joint.

–gives rise to **muscular branches** to the posterior muscles of the leg.

–gives rise to the medial sural cutaneous nerve, the medial calcaneal branch to the skin of the heel and sole, and the articular branches to the ankle joint.

–terminates beneath the flexor retinaculum by dividing into the **medial** and **lateral plantar nerves.**

a. Medial plantar nerve

–arises beneath the flexor retinaculum, deep to the posterior portion of the abductor hallucis muscle as the larger terminal branch from the tibial nerve.

–passes distally between the abductor hallucis and flexor digitorum brevis muscles and innervates them.

–gives rise to **common digital branches** that divide into proper digital branches, which supply the flexor hallucis brevis and the first lumbrical and the skin of the medial three and one-half toes.

b. Lateral plantar nerve

–is the smaller terminal branch of the tibial nerve.

–runs distally and laterally between the quadratus plantae and the flexor digitorum brevis, innervating the quadratus plantae and the abductor digiti minimi muscles.

–divides into a **superficial branch,** which innervates the flexor digiti minimi brevis, and a **deep branch,** which innervates the plantar and dorsal interossei, the lateral three lumbricals, and the adductor hallucis.

II. Arteries (Figure 3-12)

A. Superior gluteal artery

–arises from the **internal iliac artery,** passes between the lumbosacral trunk and the first sacral nerve, and enters the buttock through the greater sciatic foramen above the piriformis muscle.

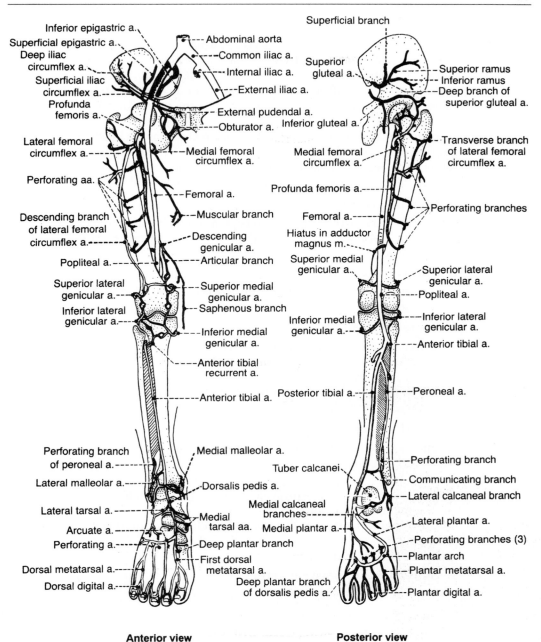

Inferior epigastric a.
Superficial epigastric a.
Deep iliac circumflex a.
Superficial iliac circumflex a.
Profunda femoris a.
Lateral femoral circumflex a.
Perforating aa.
Descending branch of lateral femoral circumflex a.
Popliteal a.
Superior lateral genicular a.
Inferior lateral genicular a.
Perforating branch of peroneal a.
Lateral malleolar a.
Lateral tarsal a.
Arcuate a.
Perforating a.
Dorsal metatarsal a.
Dorsal digital a.

Superficial branch
Abdominal aorta
Common iliac a.
Internal iliac a.
External iliac a.
External pudendal a.
Obturator a.
Medial femoral circumflex a.
Femoral a.
Muscular branch
Descending genicular a.
Articular branch
Superior medial genicular a.
Saphenous branch
Inferior medial genicular a.
Anterior tibial recurrent a.
Anterior tibial a.
Medial malleolar a.
Tuber calcanei
Dorsalis pedis a.
Medial calcaneal branches
Medial tarsal aa.
Medial plantar a.
Deep plantar branch
First dorsal metatarsal a.
Deep plantar branch of dorsalis pedis a.

Superior gluteal a.
Inferior gluteal a.
Medial femoral circumflex a.
Profunda femoris a.
Femoral a.
Hiatus in adductor magnus m.
Superior medial genicular a.
Inferior medial genicular a.
Posterior tibial a.

Superior ramus
Inferior ramus
Deep branch of superior gluteal a.
Transverse branch of lateral femoral circumflex a.
Perforating branches
Superior lateral genicular a.
Popliteal a.
Inferior lateral genicular a.
Anterior tibial a.
Peroneal a.
Perforating branch
Communicating branch
Lateral calcaneal branch
Lateral plantar a.
Perforating branches (3)
Plantar arch
Plantar metatarsal a.
Plantar digital a.

Anterior view   **Posterior view**

Figure 3–12. Blood supply to the lower limb.

–runs deep to the gluteus maximus muscle and divides into a **superficial branch,** which forms numerous branches to supply the gluteus maximus, and a **deep branch,** which runs between the gluteus medius and minimus muscles and supplies these muscles and the tensor fasciae latae.

–anastomoses with the lateral and medial circumflex and inferior gluteal arteries.

B. Inferior gluteal artery

–arises from the **internal iliac artery,** usually passes between the first and second sacral nerves, and enters the buttock through the greater sciatic foramen below the piriformis.

–enters the deep surface of the gluteus maximus and descends on the medial side of the sciatic nerve, in company with the posterior femoral cutaneous nerve.

–supplies the gluteus maximus, the lateral rotators of the hips, the hamstrings (upper part), and the hip joint.

–enters the cruciate anastomosis, and anastomoses with the medial femoral circumflex, inferior gluteal, and internal pudendal and obturator arteries.

C. Obturator artery

–arises from the **internal iliac artery** in the pelvis and passes through the obturator foramen, where it divides into **anterior and posterior branches.**

1. Anterior branch

–descends in front of the adductor brevis muscle and gives rise to muscular branches.

2. Posterior branch

–descends behind the adductor brevis muscle to supply the adductor muscles, and gives rise to the **acetabular branch,** which passes through the acetabular notch.

–provides an **artery to the head of the femur,** which accompanies the ligament of the head of the femur.

D. Femoral artery

–begins as the continuation of the **external iliac artery** distal to the inguinal ligament, descends through the femoral triangle, and enters the adductor canal.

–has a **palpable pulsation,** which may be felt just inferior to the midpoint of the inguinal ligament.

–is **vulnerable to injury** because of its relatively superficial position in the femoral triangle.

–includes several branches:

1. Superficial epigastric artery

–runs subcutaneously upward toward the umbilicus.

2. Superficial circumflex iliac artery

–runs laterally almost parallel with the inguinal ligament.

3. External pudendal artery

–emerges through the saphenous ring, runs medially over the spermatic cord (or the round ligament of the uterus), and sends inguinal branches and anterior scrotal (or labial) branches.

4. Profunda femoris (deep femoral) artery

–arises from the **femoral artery** within the femoral triangle.

–descends in front of the pectineus, adductor brevis, and adductor magnus muscles, but behind the adductor longus muscle.

–gives rise to the medial and lateral femoral circumflex and muscular branches.

–provides, in the adductor canal, **four perforating arteries** that perforate and supply the adductor magnus and hamstring muscles.

–forms the **cruciate anastomosis** of the buttock with its **first perforating branch** (ascending branch), which anastomoses with the **inferior gluteal** artery and the **transverse branches** of the **medial** and **lateral femoral circumflex** arteries.

5. **Medial femoral circumflex artery**

–arises from the **femoral or profunda femoris artery** in the femoral triangle.

–runs between the pectineus and iliopsoas muscles, continues between the obturator externus and adductor brevis muscles, and enters the gluteal region between the adductor magnus and quadratus femoris muscles.

–gives rise to **muscular branches** and an **acetabular branch** to the hip joint and then divides into an **ascending branch,** which anastomoses with branches of the superior and inferior gluteal arteries, and a **transverse branch,** which joins the **cruciate anastomosis**.

–is clinically important because its branches run through the neck to reach the head. It thus supplies most of the **blood to the head and neck** of the femur.

6. **Lateral femoral circumflex artery**

–arises from the **femoral or profunda femoris artery** and passes laterally deep to the sartorius and rectus femoris muscles.

–divides into three branches: an **ascending branch,** which forms a vascular circle with branches of the medial femoral circumflex artery around the femoral neck, and also anastomoses with the superior gluteal artery; a **transverse branch,** which joins the cruciate anastomosis; and a **descending branch,** which anastomoses with the superior lateral genicular branch of the popliteal artery.

7. **Descending genicular artery**

–arises from the **femoral artery** just before it passes through the adductor canal.

–divides into the **articular branch,** which enters the anastomosis around the knee, and the **saphenous branch,** which supplies the superficial tissue and skin on the medial side of the knee.

E. **Popliteal artery**

–is a continuation of the **femoral artery** at the adductor hiatus and runs through the popliteal fossa.

–terminates at the lower border of the popliteus muscle by dividing into the anterior and posterior tibial arteries.

–may be felt by gentle palpation in the depth of the popliteal fossa.

–is vulnerable to injury from fracture of the femur and dislocation of the knee joint.

–gives rise to five genicular arteries:

1. **Superior lateral genicular artery,** which passes deep to the biceps femoris tendon

2. **Superior medial genicular artery,** which passes deep to the semimembranosus and semitendinosus muscles and enters the substance of the vastus medialis

3. **Inferior lateral genicular artery,** which passes laterally above the head of the fibula and then deep to the fibular collateral ligament

4. **Inferior medial genicular artery,** which passes medially along the upper border of the popliteus muscle, deep to the popliteus fascia

5. **Middle genicular artery,** which pierces the oblique popliteal ligament and enters the knee joint

F. Posterior tibial artery

–arises from the popliteal artery at the lower border of the popliteus, between the tibia and the fibula.

–is accompanied by two venae comitantes and the tibial nerve on the posterior surface of the tibialis posterior muscle.

–gives rise to the **peroneal (fibular) artery,** which descends between the tibialis posterior and the flexor hallucis longus muscles and supplies the lateral muscles in the posterior compartment. The peroneal artery passes behind the lateral malleolus, gives rise to the **posterior lateral malleolar branch,** and ends in branches to the ankle and heel.

–also gives rise to the posterior medial malleolar, perforating, and muscular branches and terminates by dividing into the **medial** and **lateral plantar arteries.**

1. Medial plantar artery

–is the smaller terminal branch of the posterior tibial artery.

–runs between the abductor hallucis and the flexor digitorum brevis muscles.

–gives rise to a **superficial branch,** which supplies the big toe, and a **deep branch,** which forms three superficial digital branches.

2. Lateral plantar artery

–is the larger terminal branch of the posterior tibial artery.

–runs forward laterally in company with the lateral plantar nerve between the quadratus plantae and the flexor digitorum brevis muscles and then between the flexor digitorum brevis and the adductor digiti minimi muscles.

–forms the **plantar arch** by joining the deep plantar branch of the dorsalis pedis artery. The plantar arch gives rise to four plantar metatarsal arteries.

G. Anterior tibial artery

–arises from the **popliteal artery** and enters the anterior compartment by passing through the gap between the tibia and fibula at the upper end of the interosseous membrane.

–descends on the interosseous membrane between the tibialis anterior and extensor digitorum longus muscles.

–gives rise to the **anterior tibial recurrent artery,** which ascends to the knee joint, and the **anterior medial** and **lateral malleolar arteries** at the ankle.

–runs distally and ends at the ankle midway between the lateral and medial malleoli, where it becomes the dorsalis pedis artery.

H. Dorsalis pedis artery

–begins anterior to the ankle joint midway between the two malleoli as the continuation of the **anterior tibial artery.**

–descends on the dorsum of the foot between the tendons of the extensor hallucis longus and extensor digitorum longus muscles.

–gives rise to the **medial tarsal, lateral tarsal, arcuate,** and **first dorsal metatarsal arteries.** The **arcuate artery** gives rise to the second, third, and fourth dorsal metatarsal arteries.

–terminates as the **deep plantar artery,** which enters the sole of the foot by passing between the two heads of the first dorsal interosseous muscle and joins the lateral plantar artery to form the **plantar arch.**

–exhibits a pulsation that may be felt on the navicular and cuneiform bones lateral to the tendon of the flexor hallucis longus.

III. Deep Veins

A. Deep veins of the leg

–are the venae comitantes to the anterior and posterior tibial arteries.

B. Popliteal vein

–ascends through the popliteal fossa behind the popliteal artery.

–receives the small saphenous vein and those veins corresponding to the branches of the popliteal artery.

C. Femoral vein

–accompanies the femoral artery as a continuation of the popliteal vein through the upper two-thirds of the thigh.

–has valves, receives tributaries corresponding to branches of the femoral artery, and is joined by the great saphenous vein, which passes through the saphenous opening.

Clinical Considerations

I. Reflexes

A. Knee-jerk (patellar) reflex

–occurs when the patellar ligament is tapped, resulting in a sudden contraction of the quadriceps femoris.

–tests the L2–L4 spinal nerves by activating muscle spindles in the quadriceps; afferent impulses travel in the femoral nerve to the spinal cord, and efferent impulses are transmitted to the quadriceps via motor fibers in the femoral nerve.

B. Ankle-jerk (Achilles) reflex

–is a reflex twitch of the **triceps surae** (i.e., the medial and lateral heads of the gastrocnemius and the soleus muscles).

–is induced by tapping the tendo calcaneus.

–has a reflex center in the fifth lumbar and first sacral segments of the spinal cord.

II. Syndromes and Abnormal Signs

A. Femoral hernia

–is more common in women than in men.

–lies lateral and inferior to the pubic tubercle and deep to the inguinal ligament, and its sac is formed by the parietal peritoneum.

–passes through the femoral ring and canal.

B. Gluteal gait (gluteus medius limp)

–is a **waddling gait,** characterized by the pelvis falling (or drooping) toward the unaffected side at each step.

–results from **paralysis of the gluteus medius muscle,** which normally functions to stabilize the pelvis when the opposite foot is off the ground.

C. Trendelenburg's sign

–is seen in a fracture of the femoral neck, dislocated hip joint, or weakness and paralysis of the gluteus medius muscle.

–is characterized by the following appearance: If the right gluteus medius and minimum muscles are paralyzed, the unsupported left side (sound side) of the pelvis falls (sags) instead of rising; normally, the pelvis rises.

D. Congenital dislocation of the hip joint

–is characterized by movement of the head of the femur out of the acetabulum through the ruptured capsule onto the gluteal surface of the ilium.

–occurs because of **faulty development of the upper lip of the acetabulum.**

–results in **shortening, adduction,** and **medial rotation** of the affected limb.

E. Traumatic dislocation of the hip joint

–is usually produced by trauma (severe enough to fracture the acetabulum), when the thigh is in the flexed position because the hip joint is less stable.

1. Anterior dislocation

–is characterized by tearing of the joint capsule anteriorly with movement of the femoral head out from the acetabulum; the femoral head lies inferior to the pubic bone.

2. Posterior dislocation

–is characterized by posterior tearing of the joint capsule, moving the femoral head out from the acetabulum, and resting the fractured femoral head on the posterior surface of the ischium.

–results in probable rupture of both the posterior acetabular labrum and the ligamentum capitis femoris and, usually, injury of the sciatic nerve.

3. Medial or intrapelvic dislocation

–is characterized by tearing of the joint capsule medially and dislocation of the femoral head; this may be accompanied by acetabular fracture and rupture of the bladder.

F. "Unhappy triad" of the knee joint

–may occur when a football player's cleated shoe is planted firmly in the turf and the knee is struck from the lateral side.

–is indicated by a knee that is markedly swollen, particularly in the suprapatellar region.

–results in tenderness on application of pressure along the extent of the tibial collateral ligament.

–is characterized by:

1. **Rupture of the tibial collateral ligament,** as a result of excessive abduction

2. **Tearing of the anterior cruciate ligament,** as a result of forward displacement of the tibia

3. **Injury to the medial meniscus,** as a result of the tibial collateral ligament attachment

G. Prepatellar bursitis (housemaid's knee)

–is inflammation and swelling of the prepatellar bursa.

H. Popliteal (Baker's) cyst

–is a **swelling behind the knee,** caused by escape of synovial fluid posteriorly through the joint capsule.

–impairs flexion and extension of the knee joint.

I. Knock-knee (genu valgum)

–is a deformity in which the tibia is bent or twisted outward.

–may occur as a result of collapse of the lateral compartment of the knee and rupture of the medial collateral ligament.

J. Bowleg (genu varum)

–is a deformity in which the tibia is bent inward.

–may occur as a result of collapse of the medial compartment of the knee and rupture of the lateral collateral ligament.

K. Anterior tibial compartment syndrome

–is characterized by **ischemic necrosis** of the muscles of the anterior tibial compartment of the leg.

–occurs, presumably, as a result of compression of arteries by swollen muscles, following excessive exertion.

–is accompanied by extreme tenderness and pain on the anterolateral aspect of the leg.

L. Shin splint

–is a painful condition of the anterior compartment of the leg along the shin bone (tibia) caused by swollen muscles (or strain of the flexor digitorum longus) following athletic overexertion.

–may be a mild form of the anterior compartment syndrome.

M. Pott's fracture (Dupuytren's fracture)

–is a fracture of the lower end of the fibula, often accompanied by fracture of the medial malleolus or rupture of the deltoid ligament.

–is caused by forced eversion of the foot.

N. Flat foot (pes planus or talipes planus)

–is characterized by a **waddling gait** with the feet turned out.

–results in disappearance or collapse of the medial portion of the longitudinal arch with eversion and abduction of the forefoot.

–causes greater wear on the inner border of the soles and heels of shoes than on the outer border.

–causes pain as a result of stretching of the plantar muscles and straining of the spring ligament and the long and short plantar ligaments.

O. Clubfoot (talipes equinovarus)

–is a congenital deformity of the foot, which is twisted from its natural position, in which the foot is plantarflexed **(equinus)** or dorsiflexed **(calcaneus).**

–may involve a deformity in which the heel is turned laterally **(valgus)** or medially **(varus),** where the heel is elevated and turned laterally **(equino-valgus)** or medially **(equinovarus),** or where the anterior part of the foot (forefoot) is elevated and the heel is turned laterally **(calcaneovalgus).**

P. Hallux valgus

–is a deviation of the big toe toward the lateral side of the foot.

–is frequently accompanied by swelling (bunion) on the medial aspect of the first metatarsophalangeal joint.

–contrasts with **hallux varus,** which is a medial deviation of the big toe.

III. Lesions of Peripheral Nerves

A. Damage to the femoral nerve

–causes impaired flexion of the hip and impaired extension of the leg due to paralysis of the quadriceps femoris.

B. Damage to the obturator nerve

–causes a weakness of adduction and a **lateral swinging of the limb during walking** because of the unopposed abductors.

C. Damage to the sciatic nerve

–causes impaired extension at the hip and impaired flexion at the knee, loss of dorsiflexion at the ankle and of eversion of the foot, and **peculiar gait** because of increased flexion at the hip to lift the dropped foot off the ground.

D. Damage to the common peroneal nerve

–results in **foot drop** and loss of sensation on the dorsum of the foot and lateral aspect of the leg.

–causes **paralysis** of all of the dorsiflexor and evertor muscles of the foot.

E. Damage to the tibial nerve

–causes loss of plantar flexion of the foot and impaired inversion due to paralysis of the tibialis posterior.

–causes a difficulty in getting the heel off the ground and a **shuffling of the gait.**

–results in a **characteristic clawing of the toes** and secondary loss on the sole of the foot, affecting posture and locomotion.

F. Damage to the deep peroneal nerve

–results in **foot drop** and hence a characteristic **high-stepping gait.**

G. Damage to the superficial peroneal nerve

–causes no foot drop but loss of eversion of the foot.

Summary of Muscle Actions of the Lower Limb

Movements at the Hip Joint (Ball-and-Socket Joint)

Flexion—iliopsoas, tensor fasciae latae, rectus femoris, adductors, sartorius, pectineus, gracilis

Extension—hamstrings, gluteus maximus, adductor magnus

Adduction—adductor magnus, adductor longus, adductor brevis, pectineus, gracilis

Abduction—gluteus medius, gluteus minimus

Medial rotation—tensor fasciae latae, gluteus medius, gluteus minimus

Lateral rotation—obturator internus, obturator externus, gemelli, piriformis, quadratus femoris, gluteus maximus

Movements at the Knee Joint (Hinge Joint)

Flexion—hamstrings, gracilis, sartorius, gastrocnemius, popliteus

Extension—quadriceps femoris

Medial rotation—semitendinosus, semimembranosus, popliteus

Lateral rotation—biceps femoris

Movements at the Ankle Joint (Hinge Joint)

Dorsiflexion—anterior tibialis, extensor digitorum longus, extensor hallucis longus, peroneus tertius

Plantar flexion—triceps surae, plantaris, posterior tibialis, peroneus longus and brevis, flexor digitorum longus, flexor hallucis longus (when the knee is fully flexed)

Movements at the Intertarsal Joint (Talocalcaneal, Transverse Tarsal Joint)

Inversion—tibialis posterior, tibialis anterior, triceps surae, extensor hallucis longus

Eversion—peroneus longus, brevis and tertius, extensor digitorum longus

Movements at the Metatarsophalangeal Joint (Ellipsoid Joint)

Flexion—lumbricals, interossei, flexor hallucis brevis, flexor digiti minimi brevis

Extension—extensor digitorum longus and brevis, extensor hallucis longus

Movements at the Interphalangeal Joint (Hinge Joint)

Flexion—flexor digitorum longus and brevis, flexor hallucis longus

Extension—extensor digitorum longus and brevis, extensor hallucis longus

Summary of Muscle Innervations of the Lower Limb

Muscles of the Thigh

Muscles of the Anterior Compartment: Femoral Nerve

Sartorius

Quadriceps femoris–rectus femoris; vastus medialis; vastus intermedius; and vastus lateralis

Muscles of the Medial Compartment: Obturator Nerve

Adductor longus; adductor brevis; adductor magnus (obturator and tibial nerves)[*]; gracilis; obturator externus; pectineus (femoral and obturator nerves)[*]

---

[*]Indicates exception.

Muscles of the Posterior Compartment: Tibial Part of Sciatic Nerve

Semitendinosus; semimembranosus; biceps femoris, long head; biceps femoris, short head (common peroneal part of sciatic nerve)*; adductor magnus (tibial part of sciatic and obturator nerve)*

Muscles of the Lateral Compartment

Gluteus maximus (inferior gluteal nerve)
Gluteus medius (superior gluteal nerve)
Gluteus minimus (superior gluteal nerve)
Tensor fasciae latae (superior gluteal nerve)
Piriformis (nerve to piriformis)
Obturator internus (nerve to obturator internus)
Superior gemellus (nerve to obturator internus)
Inferior gemellus (nerve to quadratus femoris)
Quadratus femoris (nerve to quadratus femoris)

Muscles of the Leg

Muscles of the Anterior Compartment: Deep Peroneal Nerve

Tibialis anterior; extensor digitorum longus; extensor hallucis longus; peroneus tertius

Muscles of the Lateral Compartment: Superficial Peroneal Nerve

Peroneus longus; peroneus brevis

Muscles of the Posterior Compartment: Tibial Nerve

Superficial layer—gastrocnemius; soleus; plantaris
Deep layer—popliteus; tibialis posterior; flexor digitorum longus; flexor hallucis longus

Review Test

Directions: Each of the numbered items or incomplete statements in this section is followed by answers or by completions of the statement. Select the **one** lettered answer or completion that is **best** in each case.

1. If there is a loss of skin sensation and paralysis of muscles on the plantar aspect of the medial side of the foot, which of the following nerves is damaged?

(A) Common peroneal
(B) Tibial
(C) Superficial peroneal
(D) Deep peroneal
(E) Sural

2. A patient walks with a waddling gait that is characterized by the pelvis falling toward one side at each step. Which of the following nerves is damaged?

(A) Obturator nerve
(B) Nerve to obturator internus
(C) Superior gluteal nerve
(D) Inferior gluteal nerve
(E) Femoral nerve

3. A patient is unable to prevent anterior displacement of the femur on the tibia when the knee is flexed. Which of the following ligaments is most likely damaged?

(A) Anterior cruciate
(B) Fibular collateral
(C) Patellar
(D) Posterior cruciate
(E) Tibial collateral

4. Lesion of the femoral nerve results in which of the following conditions?

(A) Paralysis of the psoas major muscle
(B) Loss of skin sensation on the lateral side of the foot
(C) Loss of skin sensation over the greater trochanter
(D) Paralysis of the vastus lateralis muscle
(E) Paralysis of the tensor fasciae latae

5. A patient is unable to invert the foot, indicating lesions of which of the following nerves?

(A) Superficial and deep peroneal
(B) Deep peroneal and tibial
(C) Superficial peroneal and tibial
(D) Medial and lateral plantar
(E) Obturator and tibial

6. A 22-year-old patient is unable to "unlock" the knee joint to permit flexion of the leg. Which of the following muscles is most likely damaged?

(A) Rectus femoris
(B) Semimembranosus
(C) Popliteus
(D) Gastrocnemius
(E) Biceps femoris

7. A patient presents with sensory loss on adjacent sides of the great and second toes and impaired dorsiflexion of the foot. These signs probably indicate damage to which of the following nerves?

(A) Superficial peroneal
(B) Lateral plantar
(C) Deep peroneal
(D) Sural
(E) Tibial

8. When the superficial peroneal nerve is severed near its origin by a deep gash as a result of a fall from a motorcycle, which of the following muscles is paralyzed?

(A) Peroneus longus
(B) Extensor hallucis longus
(C) Extensor digitorum longus
(D) Peroneus tertius
(E) Extensor digitorum brevis

9. To avoid damaging the sciatic nerve during an intramuscular injection in the right gluteal region, the needle should be inserted in which of the following areas?

(A) Over the sacrospinous ligament
(B) Midway between the ischial tuberosity and the lesser trochanter
(C) Midpoint of the gemelli muscles
(D) Upper right quadrant of the gluteal region
(E) Lower right quadrant of the gluteal region

119

10. Which of the following muscles is damaged if a patient cannot flex and medially rotate the thigh during running and climbing?

(A) Semimembranosus
(B) Sartorius
(C) Rectus femoris
(D) Vastus intermedius
(E) Tensor fasciae latae

11. A motorcycle accident results in destruction of the groove in the lower surface of the cuboid bone. Which of the following muscle tendons is most likely damaged?

(A) Flexor hallucis longus
(B) Peroneus brevis
(C) Peroneus longus
(D) Tibialis anterior
(E) Tibialis posterior

12. A construction worker sustains a fracture of the groove on the undersurface of the sustentaculum tali of the calcaneus bone as a result of falling feet first from a roof. Which of the following muscle tendons is most likely torn?

(A) Flexor digitorum brevis
(B) Flexor digitorum longus
(C) Flexor hallucis brevis
(D) Flexor hallucis longus
(E) Tibialis posterior

13. The great saphenous vein runs

(A) posterior to the medial malleolus
(B) into the popliteal vein
(C) anterior to the medial condyles of the tibia and femur
(D) superficial to the fascia lata of the thigh
(E) along with the femoral vessels

14. The inability to extend the leg at the knee joint indicates paralysis of which of the following muscles?

(A) Semitendinosus
(B) Sartorius
(C) Gracilis
(D) Quadriceps femoris
(E) Biceps femoris

15. Which of the following muscles is damaged if a patient experiences weakness in dorsiflexing and inverting the foot?

(A) Peroneus longus
(B) Peroneus brevis
(C) Tibialis anterior
(D) Extensor digitorum longus
(E) Peroneus tertius

Questions 16–20

A 62-year-old woman slips and falls on the bathroom floor, which results in a posterior dislocation of the hip joint and a fracture of the neck of the femur.

16. Rupture of the ligamentum teres capitis femoris may lead to damage to a branch of which of the following arteries?

(A) Medial circumflex femoral
(B) Lateral circumflex femoral
(C) Obturator
(D) Superior gluteal
(E) Inferior gluteal

17. Fracture of the neck of the femur results in avascular necrosis of the femoral head, probably owing to lack of blood supply from which of the following arteries?

(A) Obturator and inferior gluteal
(B) Superior gluteal and femoral
(C) Inferior gluteal and superior gluteal
(D) Lateral and medial femoral circumflex
(E) Medial femoral circumflex and obturator

18. If the acetabulum is fractured at its posterosuperior margin by dislocation of the hip joint, which of the following bones could be involved?

(A) Ilium and pubis
(B) Ischium and sacrum
(C) Ilium and ischium
(D) Pubis and sacrum
(E) Pubis and head of the femur

19. The woman experiences weakness when abducting and medially rotating the thigh following this accident. Which of the following muscles is most likely damaged?

(A) Piriformis
(B) Obturator internus
(C) Quadratus femoris
(D) Gluteus maximus
(E) Gluteus minimus

20. The woman undergoes hip surgery. If all of the arteries that are part in the cruciate anastomosis of the upper thigh are ligated, which of the following arteries maintains blood flow?

(A) Medial femoral circumflex
(B) Lateral femoral circumflex
(C) Superior gluteal
(D) Inferior gluteal
(E) First perforating

21. Which of the following conditions most likely occurs as the result of occlusion of the dorsalis pedis artery at its origin? *Ø a.tibial a*

(A) Ischemia in the peroneus longus muscle
(B) Aneurysm in the plantar arterial arch
(C) Reduction of blood flow in the medial tarsal artery
(D) Low blood pressure in the anterior tibial artery
(E) High blood pressure in the arcuate artery

22. A patient experiences paralysis of the muscle that originates from the femur and contributes directly to the stability of the knee joint. Which of the following muscles is involved?

(A) Vastus lateralis
(B) Semimembranosus
(C) Sartorius
(D) Biceps femoris (long head)
(E) Rectus femoris

23. Which of the following structures remains intact if the structures that pass deep to the inferior or superior extensor retinaculum of the ankle are damaged?

(A) Anterior tibial nerve
(B) Extensor digitorum longus muscle
(C) Dorsalis pedis artery
(D) Peroneus tertius muscle
(E) Superficial peroneal nerve

24. A knife wound penetrates the superficial vein that terminates in the popliteal vein. Bleeding occurs from which of the following vessels?

(A) Posterior tibial vein
(B) Anterior tibial vein
(C) Peroneal vein
(D) Great saphenous vein
(E) Lesser saphenous vein

25. A 10-year-old boy falls from a tree house, causing heavy compression of the sole of his foot against the ground with fracture of the head of the talus. Which of the following structures is unable to function normally?

(A) Transverse arch
(B) Medial longitudinal arch
(C) Lateral longitudinal arch
(D) Tendon of the peroneus longus
(E) Long plantar ligament

26. A 24-year-old woman complains of weakness associated with extending her thigh and rotating it laterally. Which of the following muscles is paralyzed? *Ø extension Ø lat. rot.*

(A) Obturator externus
(B) Sartorius
(C) Tensor fasciae latae
(D) Gluteus maximus *pos hamstings*
(E) Semitendinosus

27. A radiograph reveals a blood clot in the popliteal artery at its distal end. Blood may reach the foot by way of which of the following arteries?

(A) Anterior tibial
(B) Posterior tibial
(C) Peroneal
(D) Lateral circumflex femoral
(E) Superior medial genicular

28. Pus in the adductor canal damages the enclosed structures. Which of the following structures remains intact?

(A) Femoral artery
(B) Femoral vein
(C) Saphenous nerve
(D) Great saphenous vein
(E) Nerve to the vastus medialis

29. Hypertrophy of the extensor muscles of the leg may cause ischemia due to compression of which of the following arteries?

(A) Popliteal
(B) Deep femoral
(C) Anterior tibial
(D) Posterior tibial
(E) Peroneal

30. Which of the following muscles functions normally even if the greater trochanter of the femur is fractured?

(A) Piriformis
(B) Obturator internus
(C) Gluteus medius
(D) Gluteus maximus
(E) Gluteus minimus

Questions 31–35

A 20-year-old college student receives a severe blow on the inferolateral side of the left knee joint while playing football. Radiographic examination reveals a fracture of the head and neck of the fibula.

31. Which of the following nerves is damaged?

(A) Sciatic
(B) Tibial
(C) Common peroneal
(D) Deep peroneal
(E) Superficial peroneal

32. Following injury to this nerve, which of the following muscles could be paralyzed?

(A) Gastrocnemius
(B) Popliteus
(C) Extensor hallucis longus
(D) Flexor digitorum longus
(E) Tibialis posterior

33. If the lateral (fibular) collateral ligament is torn by this fracture, which of the following conditions may occur?

(A) Abnormal passive abduction of the extended leg
(B) Abnormal passive adduction of the extended leg
(C) Anterior displacement of the femur on the tibia
(D) Posterior displacement of the femur on the tibia
(E) Maximal flexion of the leg

34. Which of the following arteries could also be damaged by this fracture?

(A) Popliteal
(B) Posterior tibial
(C) Anterior tibial
(D) Peroneal
(E) Lateral inferior genicular

35. Which of the following conditions would occur from this fracture?

(A) Ischemia in the gastrocnemius
(B) Loss of plantar flexion
(C) Trendelenburg's sign
(D) Anterior tibial compartment syndrome
(E) Flat foot

36. Which of the following muscles is able to dorsiflex and invert the foot?

(A) Extensor digitorum longus
(B) Tibialis anterior
(C) Tibialis posterior
(D) Peroneus longus
(E) Peroneus brevis

37. The obturator and sciatic (tibial portion) nerves both innervate which of the following muscles?

(A) Semitendinosus
(B) Biceps femoris
(C) Pectineus
(D) Adductor magnus
(E) Adductor longus

38. A lesion of which of the following muscles most likely causes weakness in flexing the hip joint and extending the knee joint?

(A) Sartorius
(B) Gracilis
(C) Rectus femoris
(D) Vastus medialis
(E) Semimembranosus

39. The obturator nerve is the sole source of innervation for which of the following muscles?

(A) Pectineus
(B) Adductor magnus
(C) Adductor longus
(D) Biceps femoris
(E) Semimembranosus

40. Which of the following bones forms the keystone for the lateral longitudinal arch of the foot?

(A) Calcaneus
(B) Cuboid bone
(C) Head of the talus
(D) Sustenaculum tali
(E) Navicular bone

41. While playing football, a 19-year-old college student receives a twisting injury to his knee when being tackled from the lateral side. Which of the following conditions most likely has occurred?

(A) Tear of the medial meniscus
(B) Ruptured fibular collateral ligament
(C) Tenderness on pressure along the fibular collateral ligament
(D) Ruptured posterior cruciate ligament
(E) Swelling on the back of the knee joint

42. Injury to which of the following muscles most likely causes weakness in flexing both the thigh and leg?

(A) Rectus femoris
(B) Semitendinosus
(C) Biceps femoris
(D) Sartorius
(E) Adductor longus

43. A 35-year-old man has difficulty dorsiflexing the foot. Which of the following muscles is most likely damaged?

(A) Tibialis posterior
(B) Flexor digitorum longus
(C) Tibialis anterior
(D) Peroneus longus
(E) Peroneus brevis

44. If inversion of the foot is impaired, which of the following muscles is most likely paralyzed?

(A) Tibialis posterior
(B) Peroneus longus
(C) Peroneus brevis
(D) Peroneus tertius
(E) Extensor digitorum longus

45. If an orthopedic surgeon ligates the posterior tibial artery at its origin, which of the following arteries maintains normal blood flow immediately after ligation?

(A) Peroneal
(B) Dorsalis pedis
(C) Medial plantar
(D) Lateral plantar
(E) Deep plantar arterial arch

46. Before knee surgery, a surgeon ligates arteries participating in the anastomosis around the knee joint. Which of the following arteries is most likely spared?

(A) Lateral superior genicular
(B) Medial inferior genicular
(C) Descending branch of the lateral femoral circumflex
(D) Saphenous branch of the descending genicular
(E) Anterior tibial recurrent

47. A lesion of the obturator nerve most likely causes complete paralysis of which of the following muscles?

(A) Vastus medialis
(B) Gracilis
(C) Adductor magnus
(D) Pectineus
(E) Sartorius

48. A thrombosis in the popliteal vein most likely causes reduction of blood flow in which of the following veins?

(A) Greater saphenous
(B) Lesser saphenous
(C) Femoral
(D) Posterior tibial
(E) Anterior tibial

Directions: Each set of matching questions in this section consists of four to seven lettered options (in the figures) and several numbered items. For each numbered item, select the ONE lettered option that is most closely associated with it. To avoid spending too much time on matching sets with large numbers of options, it is generally advisable to begin each set by reading the list of options. Then, for each item in the set, try to generate the correct answer and locate it in the option list, rather than evaluating each option individually. Each lettered option may be selected once, more than once, or not at all.

Questions 49–51

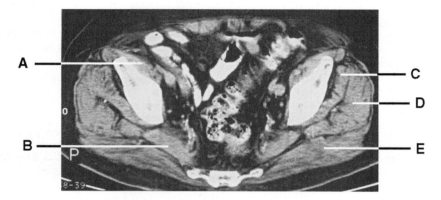

Questions 49–51. CT scan

Match the following scenarios with the appropriate lettered structure in this computed tomography (CT) image of the hip and pelvis.

49. A 62-year-old woman stands on her left limb, and her pelvis (buttock) on the right side falls instead of rising. Which muscle is most likely paralyzed?

50. A 34-year-old man with a fracture of the lesser trochanter has difficulty in flexing his thigh. Which muscle is most likely paralyzed?

51. A 41-year-old woman is diagnosed with a large tumor in the lateral pelvic wall. Which muscle that passes through the greater sciatic foramen is ischemic by tumor-induced arterial compression is most likely paralyzed?

Questions 52–54

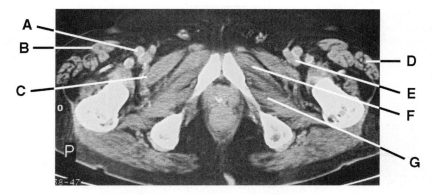

Questions 52–54. CT scan

Match the following descriptions with the appropriate lettered structure in this computed tomography (CT) image of the hip.

52. A muscle that, if paralyzed, impairs <u>flexion</u> of the <u>thigh and leg</u> *Sartorius B*

53. A muscle that, if paralyzed, results from a lesion of the superior gluteal nerve *G s. glutealn. ᵍ lifts thigh mallus*

54. A vessel that receives blood from the popliteal and greater saphenous veins

fem. A.

Questions 55–57

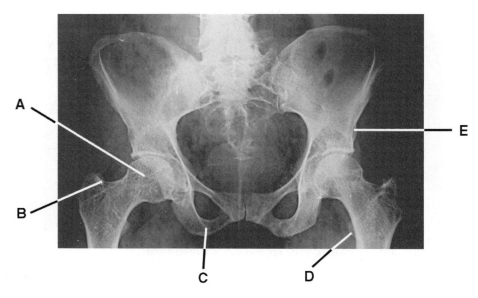

Questions 55–57. Radiograph

Match the following descriptions with the appropriate lettered structure in this radiograph of the hip and pelvis.

55. May be fractured, resulting in loss of the chief flexor of the thigh   *D*

56. Provides site for insertion of the muscle that can rotate the thigh laterally and its tendon passes through the lesser sciatic foramen

obturator internus

B

57. Provides site for attachment of the adductor magnus

C

Questions 58–60

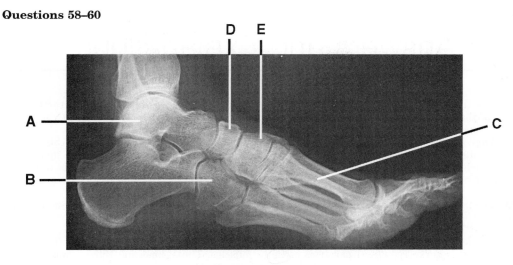

Questions 58–60. Radiograph

Match the following descriptions with the appropriate lettered structure in the radiograph of the ankle and foot.

58. A bone with a groove for the flexor hallucis longus tendon

59. A bone that is most likely fractured if the lateral longitudinal arch of the foot is flattened

60. A bone that is most likely to be fractured if the spring ligament is paralyzed

Answers and Explanations

1–B. The tibial nerve divides into medial and lateral plantar nerves, which innervate the plantar aspect of the foot.

2–C. The superior gluteal nerve innervates the gluteus medius muscle. Paralysis of this muscle causes gluteal gait, a waddling gait characterized by a falling of the pelvis toward the unaffected side at each step. The gluteus medius muscle normally functions to stabilize the pelvis when the opposite foot is off the ground.

3–D. The posterior cruciate ligament is important because it prevents forward displacement of the femur on the tibia when the knee is flexed.

4–D. The femoral nerve innervates the quadratus femoris, sartorius, and vastus muscles. Therefore, damage to this nerve results in paralysis of these muscles. The second and third lumbar nerves innervate the psoas major muscle, the sural nerve innervates the skin on the lateral side of the foot, the iliohypogastric nerve and superior clunial nerves supply the skin over the greater trochanter, and the superior gluteal nerve innervates the tensor fasciae latae.

5–B. The tibialis anterior and extensor hallucis longus muscles, which are innervated by the deep peroneal nerve, and the tibialis posterior and triceps surae, which are innervated by the tibial nerve, produce inversion of the foot.

6–C. The popliteus muscle rotates the femur laterally ("unlocks" the knee) or rotates the tibia medially, depending on which bone is fixed. This action results in unlocking of the knee joint to initiate flexion of the leg at the joint.

7–C. The deep peroneal nerve supplies the anterior muscles of the leg, including the tibialis anterior, extensor hallucis longus, extensor digitorum longus, and peroneus tertius muscles, which dorsiflex the foot. The medial branch of the deep peroneal nerve supplies adjacent sides of the great and second toes.

8–A. The superficial peroneal nerve supplies the peroneous longus and brevis muscles.

9–D. To avoid damaging the sciatic nerve during an intramuscular injection, the clinician should insert the needle in the upper right quadrant of the gluteal region.

10–E. The rectus femoris can flex the thigh and extend the leg. The hamstring muscles (semitendinosus, semimembranosus, and biceps femoris) can extend the thigh and flex the leg. The sartorius can flex the thigh and leg. The vastus medialis can extend the leg. The tensor fasciae latae can flex and medially rotate the thigh.

11–C. The groove in the lower surface of the cuboid bone is occupied by the tendon of the peroneus longus muscle.

12–D. The tendon of the flexor hallucis longus muscle occupies first the groove on the posterior surface of the talus and then the groove on the undersurface of the sustentaculum tali.

13–D. The greater saphenous vein courses anterior to the medial malleolus, medial to the tibia, and posterior to the medial condyles of the tibia and femur; ascends superficial to the fascia lata; and terminates in the femoral vein by passing through the saphenous opening.

14–D. The quadriceps femoris muscle includes the rectus femoris muscle and the vastus medialis, intermedialis, and lateralis muscles. They extend the leg at the knee joint. The semitendinosus, semimembranosus, and biceps femoris muscles (the hamstrings) extend the thigh and flex the leg. The sartorius and gracilis muscles can flex the thigh and the leg.

15–C. The tibialis anterior can dorsiflex and invert the foot. The peroneus longus and brevis muscles can plantar flex and evert the foot, the peroneus tertius can dorsiflex and evert the foot, and the extensor digitorum longus can dorsiflex the foot and extend the toes.

16–C. The obturator artery gives rise to a branch that follows the round ligament of the head of the femur, particularly in young persons.

17–D. In adults, the chief arterial supply to the head of the femur is from the branches of the medial and lateral femoral circumflex arteries. The posterior branch of the obturator artery gives rise to the artery of the head of the femur, which is usually insufficient to supply the head of the femur (in adults).

18–C. The acetabulum is a cup-shaped cavity on the lateral side of the hip bone and is formed superiorly by the ilium, posteroinferiorly by the ischium, and anteromedially by the pubis.

19–E. The gluteus medius or minimus abducts and rotates the thigh medially. The piriformis, obturator internus, quadratus femoris, and gluteus maximus muscles can rotate the thigh laterally.

20–C. The superior gluteal artery does not participate in the cruciate anastomosis of the thigh. The inferior gluteal artery, transverse branches of the medial and lateral femoral circumflex arteries, and an ascending branch of the first perforating artery form the cruciate anastomosis of the thigh.

21–C. The medial and lateral malleolar arteries are branches of the anterior tibial artery. The dorsalis pedis artery, which begins anterior to the ankle joint midway between the two malleoli as the continuation of the anterior tibial artery, gives off the medial tarsal, lateral tarsal, arcuate, and first dorsal metatarsal arteries and terminates as the deep plantar artery.

22–A. The vastus lateralis muscles arise from the femur and all other muscles originate from the hip (coxal) bone. The biceps femoris inserts on the fibula and other muscles insert on the tibia, and thus all of them contribute to the stability of the knee joint.

23–E. The superficial peroneal nerve emerges between the peroneus longus and peroneus brevis muscles and descends superficial to the extensor retinaculum of the ankle, innervating the skin of the lower leg and foot. Other structures pass deep to the extensor retinaculum.

24–E. The lesser (small) saphenous vein ascends on the back of the leg in company with the sural nerve and terminates in the popliteal vein.

25–B. The keystone of the medial longitudinal arch of the foot is the head of the talus, which is located at the summit between the sustentaculum tali and the navicular bone. The medial longitudinal arch is supported by the spring ligament and the tendon of the flexor hallucis longus muscle.

26–D. The gluteus maximus can extend and rotate the thigh laterally. The obturator externus rotates the thigh laterally. The sartorius can flex both the hip and knee joints. The tensor fasciae latae can flex and medially rotate the thigh. The semitendinosus can extend the thigh and medially rotate the leg.

27–D. If the distal popliteal artery is blocked, blood may reach the foot by way of the descending branch of the lateral circumflex femoral artery. Other blood vessels are direct or indirect branches of the popliteal artery.

28–D. The adductor canal contains the femoral vessels, the saphenous nerve, and the nerve to the vastus medialis.

29–C. A muscular spasm or hypertrophy of the extensor muscles of the leg may compress the anterior tibial artery, causing ischemia.

30–D. The gluteus maximus is inserted into the gluteal tuberosity of the femur and the iliotibial tract.

31–C. The common peroneal nerve is vulnerable to injury as it winds around the neck of the fibula and pierces the peroneus longus muscle, where it divides into the deep and superficial peroneal nerves.

32–C. The extensor hallucis longus is innervated by the deep peroneal nerve, whereas other muscles are innervated by the posterior tibial nerve.

33–B. The lateral (fibular) collateral ligament prevents adduction at the knee. Therefore, a torn lateral collateral ligament can be recognized by abnormal passive adduction of the extended leg.

34–C. The anterior tibial artery, which arises from the popliteal artery, enters the anterior compartment by passing through the gap between the fibula and tibia at the upper end of the interosseous membrane.

35–D. Anterior tibial compartment syndrome is characterized by ischemic necrosis of the muscles of the anterior tibial compartment of the leg due to damage to the anterior tibial artery. The gastrocnemius receives blood from sural branches of the popliteal artery.

36–B. The tibialis anterior can dorsiflex and invert the foot. The extensor digitorum longus can dorsiflex and evert the foot, the tibialis posterior can plantar flex and invert the foot, and the peroneus longus and brevis can plantar flex and evert the foot.

37–D. The biceps femoris is innervated by both tibial and common peroneal portions of the sciatic nerve, whereas the pectineus is innervated by both the femoral and obturator nerves. The adductor magnus is innervated by both the obturator and sciatic (tibial portion) nerves.

38–C. The sartorius can flex both the hip and knee joints. The gracilis adducts and flexes the thigh and flexes the leg; the vastus medialis extends the knee joint; and the semimembranosus extends the hip joint and flexes the knee joint.

39–C. The adductor longus is innervated only by the obturator nerve. The pectineus is innervated by both the obturator and femoral nerves. The adductor magnus is innervated by both the obturator nerve and tibial part of the sciatic nerve. The biceps femoris is innervated by tibial portion (long head) and common peroneal portion (short head) of the sciatic nerve. The obturator internus is innervated by the nerve to the obturator internus.

40–B. The keystone for the lateral longitudinal arch is the cuboid bone, whereas the keystone for the medial longitudinal arch is the head of the talus.

41–A. The "unhappy triad" of the knee joint is characterized by tear of the medial meniscus, rupture of the tibial collateral ligament, and rupture of the anterior cruciate ligament. This injury may occur when a football player's cleated shoe is planted firmly in the turf and the knee is struck from the lateral side. Tenderness along the medial collateral ligament and over the medial meniscus and swelling on the front of the joint are due to excessive production of synovial fluid, which fills the joint cavity and the suprapatellar bursa.

42–D. The sartorius can flex the thigh and flex the leg. It originates from the anterior–superior iliac spine and inserts on superior side of the tibia.

43–C. The tibialis anterior muscle can dorsiflex the foot, whereas all other muscles are able to plantar flex the foot.

44–A. The tibialis posterior inverts the foot. The peroneus longus, brevis, and tertius and extensor digitorum longus can evert the foot.

45–B. The dorsalis pedis artery begins anterior to the ankle as the continuation of the anterior tibial artery.

46–D. The descending genicular artery gives off the articular branch, which enters the anastomosis around the knee joint, and the saphenous branch, which supplies the superficial tissue and skin on the medial side of the knee.

47-B. The vastus medialis is innervated by the femoral nerve. The gracilis is innervated by the obturator nerve. The adductor magnus is innervated by the obturator and sciatic (tibial portion) nerves. The pectineus is innervated by the femoral and obturator nerves. The sartorius is innervated by the femoral nerve.

48–C. The popliteal vein drains blood into the femoral vein.

49–D. When a patient with paralysis of the gluteus medius stands on the affected limb, the pelvis falls or sags on the sound side. Normally, the pelvis rises.

50–A. The iliopsoas muscle inserts on the lesser trochanter and is a chief flexor of the thigh.

51–B. The piriformis muscle passes through the greater sciatic foramen and inserts on the greater trochanter.

52–B. The sartorius can flex both the thigh and the knee, whereas the rectus femoris can flex the thigh and extend the knee.

53–D. The tensor fasciae latae is innervated by the superior gluteal nerve.

54–E. The femoral vein receives the greater saphenous vein, which passes through the saphenous ring.

55–D. The iliopsoas muscle is the chief flexor of the thigh and inserts on the lesser trochanter.

56–B. The greater trochanter is the site for insertion of the obturator internus muscle tendon, which leaves the pelvis through the lesser sciatic foramen.

57–C. The ischiopubic ramus and ischial tuberosity provide attachment for the adductor magnus.

58–A. The body of the talus has a groove on its posterior surface for the flexor hallucis longus tendon. This tendon also occupies the groove on the undersurface of the sustentaculum tali.

59–B. The cuboid bone serves as the keystone in the center of the lateral longitudinal arch of the foot.

60–D. The spring (plantar calcaneonavicular) ligament extends from the sustentaculum tali of the calcaneus to the navicular bone.

4

Thorax

Thoracic Wall

I. Skeleton of the Thorax (Figure 4-1)

A. Sternum

1. Manubrium

–has a superior margin, the **jugular notch,** which can be readily palpated at the root of the neck.

–has a **clavicular notch** on each side for articulation with the clavicle.

–also articulates with the cartilage of the first rib, the upper half of the second rib, and the body of the sternum at the **manubriosternal joint,** or sternal angle.

2. Sternal angle (angle of Louis)

–is the junction between the manubrium and the body of the sternum.

–is located at the level where:

a. The second ribs articulate with the sternum.

b. The aortic arch begins and ends.

c. The trachea bifurcates into the right and left bronchi.

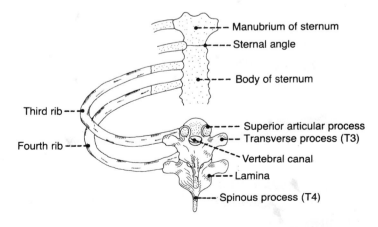

Figure 4-1. Articulations of the ribs with the vertebrae and the sternum.

    d. The inferior border of the superior mediastinum is demarcated.

    e. A transverse plane can pass through the vertebral column between T4 and T5.

3. Body of the sternum

    –articulates with the second to seventh costal cartilages.

    –also articulates with the xiphoid process at the **xiphosternal joint,** which is level with the ninth thoracic vertebra.

4. Xiphoid process

    –is a flat, cartilaginous process at birth that ossifies slowly from the central core and unites with the body of the sternum after middle age.

    –can be palpated in the epigastrium.

    –is attached via its pointed caudal end to the **linea alba.**

B. Ribs

–consist of 12 pairs of bones that form the main part of the **thoracic cage,** extending from the vertebrae to or toward the sternum.

–**increase the anteroposterior and transverse diameters of the thorax** by their movements.

1. Structure

    –Each rib is divided into head, neck, tubercle, and body (shaft).

    –The **head** articulates with the corresponding vertebral bodies and intervertebral disks and suprajacent vertebral bodies.

    –The **tubercle** articulates with the transverse processes of the corresponding vertebrae, with the exception of ribs 11 and 12.

2. Classification

    a. True ribs

        –are the first seven ribs (**ribs 1 to 7**), which are attached to the sternum by their costal cartilages.

    b. False ribs

        –are the lower five ribs (**ribs 8 to 12**); ribs 8 to 10 are connected to the costal cartilages immediately above them to form the **anterior costal margin.**

    c. Floating ribs

        –are the last two ribs (**ribs 11 and 12**), which are connected only to the vertebrae.

3. First rib

    –is the broadest and shortest of the true ribs.

    –has a single articular facet on its head, which articulates with the first thoracic vertebra.

    –has a **scalene tubercle** for the insertion of the anterior scalene muscle and two **grooves** for the subclavian artery and vein.

4. Second rib

    –has two articular facets on its head, which articulate with the bodies of the first and second thoracic vertebrae.

–is about twice as long as the first rib.

5. Tenth rib

–has a single articular facet on its head, which articulates with the tenth thoracic vertebra.

6. Eleventh and twelfth ribs

–have a single articular facet on their heads.
–have no neck or tubercle.

II. Articulations of the Thorax (see Figure 4-1)

A. Sternoclavicular joint

–provides the only bony attachment between the appendicular and axial skeletons.
–is a saddle-type synovial joint but has the movements of a ball-and-socket joint.
–has a fibrocartilaginous articular surface and contains two separate synovial cavities.

B. Sternocostal (sternochondral) joints

–are synchondroses in which the sternum articulates with the first seven costal cartilages.

C. Costochondral joints

–are synchondroses in which the ribs articulate with their respective costal cartilages.

III. Muscles of the Thoracic Wall (Table 4-1)

Table 4–1. Muscles of the Thoracic Wall

Muscle	Origin	Insertion	Nerve	Action
External intercostals	Lower border of ribs	Upper border of rib below	Intercostal	Elevate ribs in inspiration
Internal intercostals	Lower border of ribs	Upper border of rib below	Intercostal	Elevate ribs (interchondral part); depress ribs (costal part)
Innermost intercostals	Lower border of ribs	Upper border of rib below	Intercostal	Elevate ribs
Transverse thoracis	Posterior surface of lower sternum and xiphoid	Inner surface of costal cartilages 2–6	Intercostal	Depresses ribs
Subcostalis	Inner surface of lower ribs near their angles	Upper borders of ribs 2 or 3 below	Intercostal	Elevates ribs
Levator costarum	Transverse processes of T7–T11	Subjacent ribs between tubercle and angle	Dorsal primary rami of C8–T11	Elevates ribs

VAN in b/w

IV. Nerves and Blood Vessels of the Thoracic Wall

A. Intercostal nerves

–are the **anterior primary rami** of the first 11 thoracic spinal nerves. The anterior primary ramus of the 12th thoracic spinal nerve is the **subcostal nerve,** which runs beneath the 12th rib.

–run between the internal and innermost layers of muscles, with the intercostal veins and arteries above [**Veins, Arteries, Nerves (VAN)**].

–are lodged in the **costal grooves** on the inferior surface of the ribs.

–give rise to lateral and anterior cutaneous branches and muscular branches.

B. Internal thoracic artery

–usually arises from the **first part of the subclavian artery** and descends directly behind the first six costal cartilages, just lateral to the sternum.

–gives rise to two anterior intercostal arteries in each of the upper six intercostal spaces and terminates at the sixth intercostal space by dividing into the superior epigastric and musculophrenic arteries.

1. Pericardiophrenic artery

–accompanies the phrenic nerve between the pleura and the pericardium to the diaphragm.

–supplies the pleura, pericardium, and diaphragm (upper surface).

2. Anterior intercostal arteries

–are **twelve small arteries,** two in each of the upper six intercostal spaces that run laterally, one each at the upper and lower borders of each space. The upper one in each intercostal space anastomoses with the **posterior intercostal artery,** and the lower one joins the **collateral branch** of the posterior intercostal artery.

–supply the upper six intercostal spaces.

–provide muscular branches to the intercostal, serratus anterior, and pectoral muscles.

3. Anterior perforating branches

–perforate the internal intercostal muscles in the upper six intercostal spaces, course with the anterior cutaneous branches of the intercostal nerves, and supply the pectoralis major muscle and the skin and subcutaneous tissue over it.

–provide the **medial mammary branches** (second, third, and fourth branches).

4. Musculophrenic artery

–follows the **costal arch** on the inner surface of the costal cartilages.

–gives rise to two anterior arteries in the seventh, eighth, and ninth spaces; perforates the diaphragm; and ends in the tenth intercostal space, where it anastomoses with the **deep circumflex iliac artery.**

–supplies the pericardium, diaphragm, and muscles of the abdominal wall.

5. Superior epigastric artery

–descends on the deep surface of the rectus abdominis muscle within the rectus sheath; supplies this muscle and anastomoses with the **inferior epigastric artery.**

–supplies the diaphragm, peritoneum, and anterior abdominal wall.

C. Thoracoepigastric vein

–is a venous connection between the lateral thoracic vein and the superficial epigastric vein.

V. Lymphatic Drainage of the Thorax

A. Sternal or parasternal (internal thoracic) nodes

–are placed along the **internal thoracic artery.**
–receive lymph from the medial portion of the breast, intercostal spaces, diaphragm, and supraumbilical region of the abdominal wall.
–drain into the junction of the internal jugular and subclavian veins.

B. Intercostal nodes

–lie near the heads of the ribs.
–receive lymph from the intercostal spaces and the pleura.
–drain into the **cisterna chyli** or the **thoracic duct.**

C. Phrenic nodes

–lie on the thoracic surface of the diaphragm.
–receive lymph from the pericardium, diaphragm, and liver.
–drain into the sternal and posterior mediastinal nodes.

Mediastinum, Pleura, and Organs of Respiration

I. Mediastinum (Figure 4-2)

–is an **interpleural space** (area between the pleural cavities) in the thorax and is bounded laterally by the pleural cavities, anteriorly by the sternum and the transverse thoracis muscles, and posteriorly by the vertebral column (does not contain the lungs).
–consists of the superior mediastinum above the pericardium and the three lower divisions: anterior, middle, and posterior.

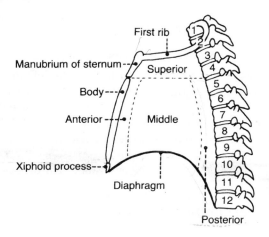

Figure 4-2. Mediastinum.

A. Superior mediastinum

–is bounded superiorly by the oblique plane of the first rib and inferiorly by the imaginary line running from the sternal angle to the intervertebral disk between the fourth and fifth thoracic vertebrae.

–contains the superior vena cava, brachiocephalic veins, arch of the aorta, thoracic duct, trachea, esophagus, thymus, vagus nerve, left recurrent laryngeal nerve, and phrenic nerve.

B. Anterior mediastinum

–lies anterior to the pericardium and posterior to the sternum and the transverse thoracic muscles.

–contains the remnants of the thymus gland, lymph nodes, fat, and connective tissue.

C. Middle mediastinum

–lies between the right and left pleural cavities

–contains the heart, pericardium, phrenic nerves, roots of the great vessels (aorta, pulmonary arteries and veins, and vena cavae), arch of the azygos vein, and main bronchi.

D. Posterior mediastinum (see Structures in the Posterior Mediastinum)

–lies posterior to the pericardium between the mediastinal pleurae

–contains the esophagus, thoracic aorta, azygos and hemiazygos veins, thoracic duct, vagus nerves, sympathetic trunk, and splanchnic nerves.

II. Trachea and Bronchi (Figure 4-3)

A. Trachea

–begins at the inferior border of the **cricoid cartilage** (C6).

–has **16 to 20 incomplete hyaline cartilaginous rings** that prevent the trachea from collapsing and that open posteriorly.

–is about 9–15 cm in length and bifurcates into the right and left main stem bronchi at the level of the **sternal angle** (junction of T4 and T5).

–has a structure called the **carina,** a downward and backward projection of the last tracheal cartilage, which forms a keel-like ridge separating the openings of the right and left main bronchi.

B. Right main (primary) bronchus

–is shorter, wider, and more vertical than the left main bronchus; therefore, more foreign bodies that enter through the trachea are lodged in this bronchus.

–runs under the arch of the azygos vein and divides into the **superior, middle, and inferior lobar (secondary) bronchi.** The right superior lobar (secondary) bronchus is known as the **eparterial bronchus** because it passes above the level of the pulmonary artery. All others are the **hyparterial bronchi.**

C. Left main (primary) bronchus

–crosses anterior to the esophagus and divides into **two lobar (secondary) bronchi,** the upper and lower.

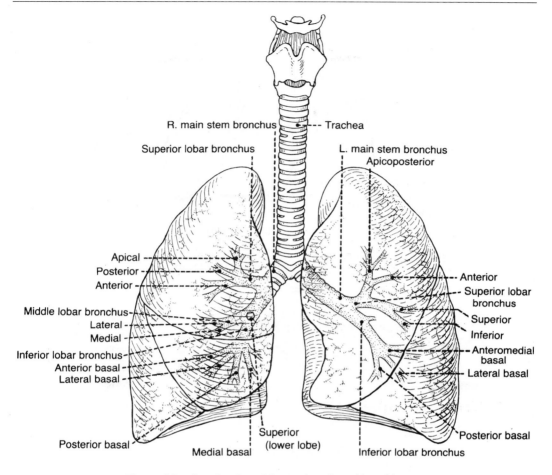

Figure 4-3. Anterior view of the trachea, bronchi, and lungs.

III. Pleurae and Pleural Cavities (Figures 4-4 and 4-5)

A. Pleura

–is a thin serous membrane that consists of a parietal pleura and a visceral pleura.

1. Parietal pleura

–lines the inner surface of the thoracic wall and the mediastinum, and has costal, diaphragmatic, mediastinal, and cervical parts. The cervical pleura **(cupula)** is the dome of the pleura, projecting into the neck above the neck of the first rib. It is reinforced by **Sibson's fascia,** which is a thickened portion of the endothoracic fascia, and is attached to the first rib and the transverse process of the seventh cervical fascia.

–is separated from the thoracic wall by the **endothoracic fascia,** which is an extrapleural fascial sheet lining the thoracic wall.

–are innervated by the **intercostal nerves** (costal pleura and the peripheral portion of the diaphragmatic pleura) and the **phrenic nerves** (central portion of the diaphragmatic pleura and the mediastinal pleura). The pleura is **very sensitive to pain.**

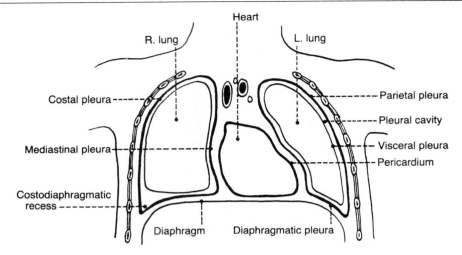

Figure 4-4. Frontal section of the thorax.

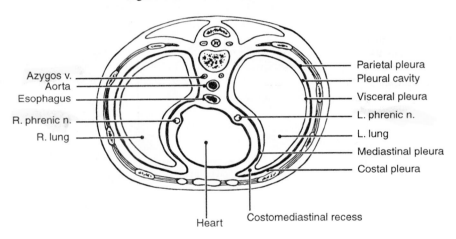

Figure 4-5. Horizontal section through the thorax.

–is supplied by branches of the internal thoracic, superior phrenic, posterior intercostal, and superior intercostal arteries. However, the visceral pleura is supplied by the bronchial arteries.

–forms the **pulmonary ligament,** a two-layered vertical fold of mediastinal pleura, which extends along the mediastinal surface of each lung from the **hilus** to the **base** (diaphragmatic surface) and ends in a free falciform border. It supports the lungs in the **pleural sac** by retaining the lower parts of the lungs in position.

2. Visceral pleura (pulmonary pleura)

–intimately invests the lungs and dips into all of the fissures.

–is supplied by bronchial arteries, but its venous blood is drained by pulmonary veins.

–is insensitive to pain but is sensitive to stretch and contains vasomotor fibers and sensory endings of vagal origin, which may be involved in respiratory reflexes.

B. Pleural cavity

–is a **potential space** between the parietal and visceral pleurae.

–represents a closed sac with no communication between right and left parts.

–contains a film of fluid that lubricates the surface of the pleurae and facilitates the movement of the lungs.

1. Costodiaphragmatic recesses

–are the **pleural recesses** formed by the reflection of the costal and diaphragmatic pleurae.

–can accumulate fluid when in the erect position.

–allow the lungs to be pulled in and expanded during inspiration.

2. Costomediastinal recesses

–are part of the pleural cavity where the costal and mediastinal pleurae meet.

IV. Lungs (see Figure 4-3)

–are the **essential organs of respiration** and are attached to the heart and trachea by their roots and the pulmonary ligaments.

–contain nonrespiratory tissues, which are nourished by the **bronchial arteries** and drained by the **bronchial veins** for the larger subdivisions of the bronchi and by the **pulmonary veins** for the smaller subdivisions of the bronchial tree.

–have **bases** that rest on the convex surface of the diaphragm, descend during inspiration, and ascend during expiration.

–receive parasympathetic fibers that innervate the smooth muscle and glands of the bronchial tree and probably are excitatory to these structures (bronchoconstrictor and secretomotor).

–receive sympathetic fibers that innervate blood vessels, smooth muscle, and glands of the bronchial tree and probably are inhibitory to these structures (bronchodilator and vasoconstrictor).

–have some sensory endings of vagal origin, which are stimulated by the stretching of the lung during inspiration and are concerned in the reflex control of respiration.

A. Right lung

–has an **apex** that projects into the root of the neck and is smaller than that of the left lung.

–is heavier and shorter than the left lung (because of the higher right dome of the diaphragm) and is wider because the heart bulges more to the left.

–is divided into upper, middle, and lower lobes by the **oblique** and **horizontal fissures** but usually receives a single bronchial artery. The **oblique fissure** usually begins at the head of the fifth rib and follows roughly the line of the **sixth rib**.

–has three lobar (secondary) bronchi and ten segmental (tertiary) bronchi.

–has grooves for various structures (e.g., superior vena cava, arch of azygos vein, esophagus).

B. Left lung

–is divided into upper and lower lobes by an **oblique fissure** that follows the line of the sixth rib, is usually more vertical in the left lung than in the right lung, and usually receives two bronchial arteries.

–contains the **lingula,** a tongue-shaped portion of the upper lobe that corresponds to the middle lobe of the right lung.

–contains a **cardiac impression**, a **cardiac notch** (a deep indentation of the anterior border of the **superior lobe** of the left lung), and **grooves** for various structures (e.g., arch of aorta, descending aorta, left subclavian artery).

–has two lobar (secondary) bronchi and eight or ten segmental bronchi.

C. Bronchopulmonary segment

–is the anatomical, functional, and surgical unit (subdivision) of the lungs.

–consists of a segmental (tertiary or lobular) bronchus, a segmental branch of the pulmonary artery, and a segment of the lung tissue, surrounded by a delicate connective-tissue septum (intersegmental septum).

–refers to the **portion of the lung supplied by each segmental bronchus and segmental artery.** The pulmonary veins are intersegmental.

–is clinically important because a surgeon can remove a segment of the lung without seriously disrupting the surrounding lung tissue.

V. Lymphatic Vessels of the Lung (Figure 4-6)

–drain the bronchial tree, pulmonary vessels, and connective-tissue septa.

–run along the bronchiole and bronchi toward the hilus, where they drain to the **pulmonary** (intrapulmonary) and then **bronchopulmonary** nodes, which in turn drain to the inferior (carinal) and superior **tracheobronchial** nodes, the **tracheal** (paratracheal) nodes, **bronchomediastinal** nodes and trunks, and

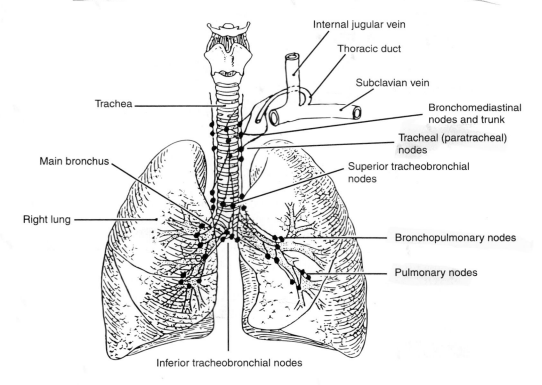

Figure 4-6. The trachea, bronchi, and lungs, plus associated lymph nodes.

eventually to the **thoracic duct** on the left and right lymphatic duct on the right.

–are not present in the walls of the pulmonary alveoli.

VI. Blood Vessels of the Lung (Figure 4-7)

A. Pulmonary trunk

–extends upward from the **conus arteriosus** of the right ventricle of the heart.

–passes superiorly and posteriorly from the front of the ascending aorta to its left side for about 5 cm and bifurcates into the right and left pulmonary arteries.

–has much lower blood pressure than that in the aorta and is partially invested with fibrous pericardium.

1. Left pulmonary artery

–carries unoxygenated blood to the left lung.

–is shorter and narrower than the right pulmonary artery.

–is connected to the arch of the aorta by the **ligamentum arteriosum,** the fibrous remains of the ductus arteriosus.

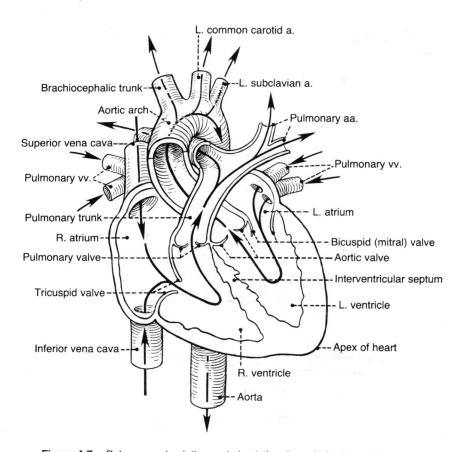

Figure 4-7. Pulmonary circulation and circulation through the heart chambers.

2. Right pulmonary artery

–runs horizontally toward the hilus of the right lung under the arch of the aorta behind the ascending aorta and superior vena cava and anterior to the right bronchus.

B. Pulmonary veins

–are **intersegmental** in drainage (do not accompany the bronchi or the segmental artery within the parenchyma of the lungs).

–leave the lung as five pulmonary veins, one from each lobe of the lungs. However, the right upper and middle veins usually join so that only four veins enter the **left atrium.**

–collect oxygenated blood from the respiratory part of the lung and deoxygenated blood from the visceral pleura and from a part of the bronchi.

C. Bronchial arteries

–arise from the **thoracic aorta;** usually there is one artery for the right lung and two for the left lung.

–supply oxygenated blood to the **nonrespiratory conducting tissues of the lungs** and the visceral pleura. Anastomoses occur between the capillary beds of the bronchial and pulmonary systems.

D. Bronchial veins

–receive blood from the larger subdivisions of the bronchi and empty into the **azygos vein** on the right and into the **accessory hemiazygos vein** on the left.

–may receive twigs (small vessels) from the tracheobronchial lymph nodes.

VII. Respiration

–is the vital exchange of oxygen and carbon dioxide that occurs in the lungs.

A. Inspiration

–includes the following **muscles:** the **diaphragm**, external, internal (interchondral part) and innermost intercostal muscles, sternocleidomastoid, levator scapulae, serratus anterior, scalenus, pectoralis major and minor, levator costarum, and serratus posterior superior muscles.

–involves the following processes:

1. Contraction of the diaphragm

–pulls the dome inferiorly into the abdomen, thereby **increasing the vertical diameter** of the thorax.

2. Enlargement of the **pleural cavities** and **lungs**

–**reduces** the **intrapulmonary pressure** (creates a **negative pressure),** thus allowing air to rush into the lungs passively as a result of atmospheric pressure.

3. Forced inspiration

–involves **contraction of the intercostal muscles** and **elevation of the ribs** (superolateral movement), with the sternum moving anteriorly like a **bucket-handle.** (When the handle is raised, the convexity moves laterally.)

–results in **increased transverse and anteroposterior diameters** of the thoracic cavity. The abdominal volume is decreased with an **increased abdominal pressure.**

B. Expiration

–involves the following muscles: the **muscles of the anterior abdominal wall**, **internal intercostal** (costal part) muscles, and serratus posterior inferior muscles.

–involves the following processes:

1. Overall process

–involves relaxation of the diaphragm, the internal intercostal muscles (costal part), and other muscles; decrease in thoracic volume; and increases in the intrathoracic pressure. The **abdominal pressure is decreased** and the **ribs are depressed.**

2. Elastic recoil of the lungs

–produces a **subatmospheric pressure** in the pleural cavities. Thus, much of the air is expelled. (**Quiet expiration** is a passive process caused by the **elastic recoil** of the lungs, whereas **quiet inspiration** results from contraction of the **diaphragm.**)

3. Forced expiration

–requires contraction of the anterior abdominal muscles and the internal intercostals (costal part).

VIII. Nerve Supply to the Lung

A. Pulmonary plexus

–receives afferent and efferent (parasympathetic preganglionic) fibers from the vagus nerve, joined by branches (sympathetic postganglionic fibers) from the sympathetic trunk and cardiac plexus.

–is divided into the **anterior pulmonary plexus,** which lies in front of the root of the lung, and the **posterior pulmonary plexus,** which lies behind the root of the lung.

–has branches that accompany the blood vessels and bronchi into the lung.

–has sympathetic nerve fibers that dilate the lumina of the bronchi, and parasympathetic fibers constrict the lumina and increase glandular secretion.

B. Phrenic nerve

–arises from the third through fifth cervical nerves (C3–C5) and lies in front of the anterior scalene muscle.

–enters the thorax by passing deep to the subclavian vein and superficial to the subclavian arteries.

–runs anterior to the root of the lung, whereas the vagus nerve runs posterior to the root of the lung.

–is accompanied by the pericardiophrenic vessels of the internal thoracic vessels and descends between the mediastinal pleura and the pericardium.

–innervates the pericardium, the mediastinal and diaphragmatic pleurae, and the diaphragm.

IX. Clinical Considerations

A. Disorders of the lungs and pleurae

1. Pneumothorax

–is the presence of **air in the pleural cavity;** thus, a negative pressure cannot be generated.

–results from an injury to the thoracic wall or to the lung.

   2. Emphysema
   –is an accumulation of **air in the terminal bronchioles and alveolar sacs**.
   –reduces the surface area available for gas exchange and thereby reduces oxygen absorption.

   3. Pneumonia (pneumonitis)
   –is an **inflammation of the lungs**.

   4. Pleurisy (pleuritis)
   –is an **inflammation of the pleura** with exudation (escape of fluid from blood vessels) into the pleural cavity.

B. Pulmonary embolism
   –is an obstruction of the pulmonary artery or one of its branches by an embolus (such as air, blood clot, fat, tumor cells, or other foreign material), which frequently occurs following an operation.

C. Asthma
   –is a condition of dyspnea (difficulty in breathing), with wheezing due to spasmotic contraction of smooth muscles in the bronchi and bronchioles, narrowing the airways.
   –may be caused by vagal stimulation, and thus epinephrine (bronchodilator) relieves the bronchial spasm by blocking the vagal stimuli.

D. Pleural tap (thoracentesis or pleuracentesis)
   –is a surgical puncture of the thoracic wall into the pleural cavity for aspiration of fluid. An accumulation of fluid in the pleural cavity has a clinical name such as a hydrothorax (water), a hemothorax (blood), a chylothorax (lymph), and a pyothorax (pus).
   –is performed posterior to the midaxillary line one or two intercostal spaces below the fluid level but not below the ninth intercostal space.

E. Lesion of the phrenic nerve
   –may not produce complete paralysis of the corresponding half of the diaphragm because the **accessory phrenic nerve,** derived from the fifth cervical nerve as a branch of the nerve to the subclavius, usually joins the phrenic nerve in the root of the neck or in the upper part of the thorax.

F. Hiccup
   –is an **involuntary spasmodic sharp contraction of the diaphragm,** accompanied by the approximation of the vocal folds and closure of the glottis of the larynx.
   –may occur as a result of the stimulation of nerve endings in the digestive tract or the diaphragm.
   –when chronic, can be stopped by **sectioning or crushing the phrenic nerve.**

Pericardium and Heart

I. Pericardium
   –is a fibroserous sac that encloses the heart and the roots of the great vessels and occupies the **middle mediastinum.**

–is composed of the fibrous pericardium and serous pericardium.

–receives blood from the pericardiophrenic, bronchial, and esophageal arteries.

–is innervated by vasomotor and sensory fibers from the phrenic and vagus nerves and the sympathetic trunks.

A. Fibrous pericardium

–is a strong, dense, fibrous layer that blends with the adventitia of the roots of the great vessels and the central tendon of the diaphragm.

B. Serous pericardium

–consists of the **parietal layer,** which lines the inner surface of the fibrous pericardium, and the **visceral layer,** which forms the outer layer (epicardium) of the heart wall and the roots of the great vessels.

C. Pericardial cavity

–is a **potential space** between the visceral layer of the serous pericardium (epicardium) and the parietal layer of the serous pericardium lining the inner surfaces of the fibrous pericardium.

D. Pericardial sinuses

1. Transverse sinus

–is a subdivision of the **pericardial sac,** lying posterior to the ascending aorta and pulmonary trunk and anterosuperior to the left atrium and the pulmonary veins.

–is of great importance to the cardiac surgeon, because while performing surgery on the aorta or pulmonary artery, a surgeon can pass a finger and make a ligature through the sinus between the arteries and veins, thus stopping the blood circulation with the ligature.

2. Oblique sinus

–is a subdivision of the **pericardial sac** behind the heart, surrounded by the reflection of the serous pericardium around the right and left pulmonary veins and the inferior vena cava.

II. Heart (Figures 4-8, 4-9, and 4-10)

A. General characteristics

–The **apex of the heart** lies in the left fifth intercostal space slightly medial to the midclavicular (or nipple) line, about 9 cm from the midline. This location is useful clinically for determining the left border of the heart and for **ausculating the mitral valve.**

–Its posterior aspect, called the **base,** is formed primarily by the left atrium and only partly by the posterior right atrium.

–Its **right (acute) border** is formed by the superior vena cava, right atrium, and inferior vena cava, and its **left (obtuse) border** is formed by the left ventricle.

–The heart wall consists of three layers: inner **endocardium,** middle **myocardium,** and outer **epicardium.**

–The **sulcus terminalis,** a groove on the external surface of the right atrium, marks the junction of the primitive sinus venosus with the atrium in the embryo and corresponds to a ridge on the internal heart surface, the **crista terminalis.**

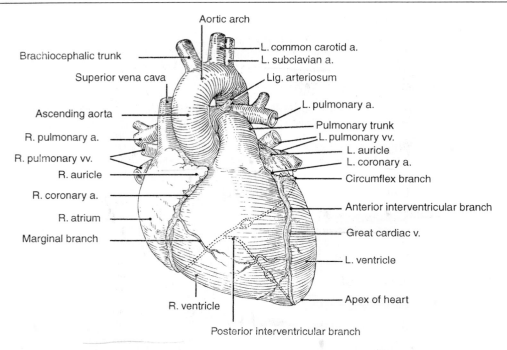

Figure 4-8. Anterior view of the heart with coronary arteries.

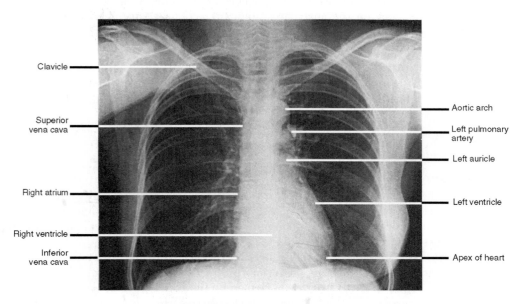

Figure 4-9. Posterior–anterior radiograph of the thorax showing the heart and great vessels.

–The **coronary sulcus,** a groove on the external surface of the heart, marks the division between the atria and the ventricles. The **crux** is the point at which the interventricular and interatrial sulci cross the coronary sulcus.

–The **cardiovascular silhouette,** or cardiac shadow, is the contour of the heart and great vessels seen on **posterior–inferior chest radiographs.**

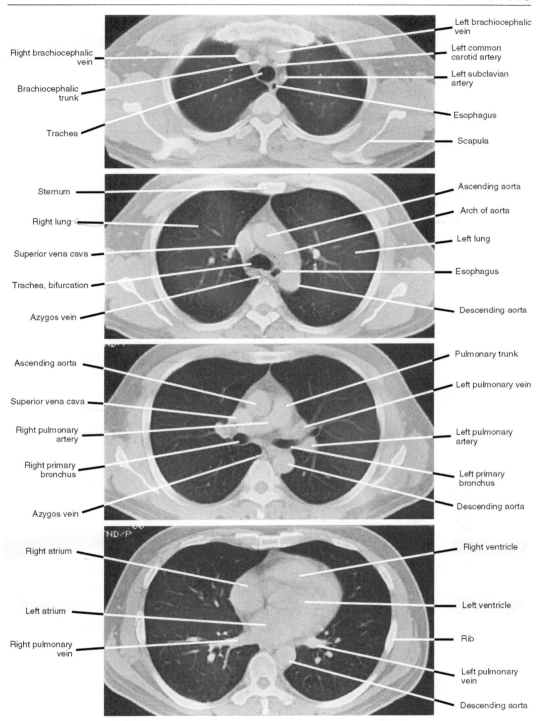

Figure 4-10. Contrast-enhanced computed tomography (CT) scan of the thorax at a setting that demonstrates soft tissues.

Its **right border** is formed by the superior vena cava, the right atrium, and the inferior vena cava. Its **left border** is formed by the aortic arch (which produces the **aortic knob**), the pulmonary trunk, the left auricle, and the left ventricle. Its **inferior border** is formed by the right ventricle and the **left atrium** shows **no border**.

B. **Internal anatomy of the heart** (Figure 4-11; see Figures 4-9 and 4-10)

1. **Right atrium**

   –has relatively smooth-walled muscles, except for the presence of the pectinate muscles.
   –is larger than the left atrium, but has a thinner wall.
   –has a **right atrial pressure** that is normally slightly lower than left atrial pressure.

   a. **Right auricle**

      –is the conical muscular pouch of the upper anterior portion of the right atrium, which covers the first part of the right coronary artery.

   b. **Sinus venarum (sinus venarum cavarum)**

      –is a posteriorly situated, smooth-walled area that is separated from the more muscular atrium proper by the **crista terminalis.**
      –develops from the embryonic **sinus venosus** and receives the superior vena cava, inferior vena cava, coronary sinus, and anterior cardiac veins.

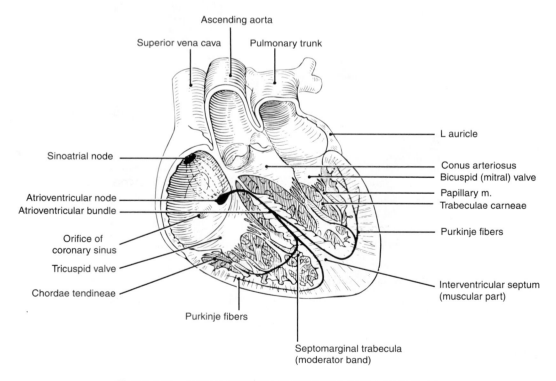

Figure 4-11. Internal anatomy and conducting system of the heart.

c. **Pectinate muscles**

–are **prominent ridges of atrial myocardium** located in the interior of both auricles and the right atrium.

d. **Crista terminalis**

–is a **vertical muscular ridge** running anteriorly along the right atrial wall from the opening of the superior vena cava to the opening of the inferior vena cava, providing the **origin of the pectinate muscles.**

–represents the junction between the primitive sinus venarum (a smooth-walled region) and the right atrium proper and is indicated externally by the **sulcus terminalis.**

e. **Venae cordis minimae**

–are the smallest cardiac veins, which begin in the substance of the heart (endocardium and innermost layer of the myocardium) and end chiefly in the atria at the **foramina venarum minimarum cordis.**

f. **Fossa ovalis**

–represents the position of the **foramen ovale,** through which blood runs from the right to the left atrium before birth.

2. **Left atrium**

–is **smaller** and has **thicker walls** than the right atrium, but its walls are smooth, except for a few pectinate muscles in the auricle.

–is the **most posterior** of the four chambers lying anterior to the esophagus and shows no structural borders on a posteroanterior radiograph.

–receives oxygenated blood through four pulmonary veins.

3. **Right ventricle**

–makes up the major portion of the anterior surface of the heart.

–contains the following structures:

a. **Trabeculae carneae cordis**

–are anastomosing muscular ridges of myocardium in the ventricles.

b. **Papillary muscles**

–are cone-shaped muscles enveloped by endocardium.

–extend from the anterior and posterior ventricular walls and the septum, and their apices are attached to the **chordae tendineae.**

–contract to tighten the chordae tendineae, preventing the cusps of the **tricuspid valve** [right atrioventricular (AV) valve] from being everted into the atrium by the pressure developed by the pumping action of the heart. This prevents regurgitation of ventricular blood into the right atrium.

c. **Chordae tendineae**

–extend from one papillary muscle to more than one cusp of the tricuspid valve.

–prevent eversion of the valve cusps into the atrium during ventricular contractions.

d. **Conus arteriosus (infundibulum)**

–is the upper end of the right ventricle.

–has smooth walls and leads into the pulmonary orifice.

   e. Septomarginal trabecula (moderator band)
   –is an isolated band of trabeculae carneae that forms a bridge between the **interventricular septum** and the base of the anterior papillary muscle of the right ventricle.
   –is called the **moderator band** for its ability to **prevent overdistention** of the ventricle.
   –carries the right limb of the **AV bundle** from the septum to the sternocostal wall of the ventricle.

   f. Interventricular septum
   –is the place of origin of the septal papillary muscle.
   –is mostly muscular but has a small membranous upper part, which is a common site of ventricular septal defects.

4. Left ventricle
   –is divided into the left ventricle proper and the **aortic vestibule,** which is the upper anterior part of the left ventricle and leads into the aorta.
   –contains two **papillary muscles** (anterior and posterior) with their **chordae tendineae** and a meshwork of muscular ridges, the **trabeculae carneae cordis.**
   –performs more work than the right ventricle; its wall is usually twice as thick.
   –is longer, narrower, and more conical-shaped than the right ventricle.

C. Heart valves (Figure 4-12)

1. Pulmonary valve
   –lies behind the medial end of the left third costal cartilage and adjoining part of the sternum.
   –is most audible over the **left second intercostal space** just lateral to the sternum.

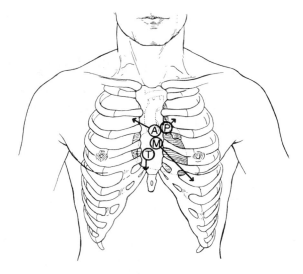

Figure 4-12.   Positions of the valves of the heart and heart sounds. *P* = pulmonary valve; *A* = aortic valve; *M* = mitral valve; *T* = tricuspid valve. *Arrows* indicate positions of the heart sounds.

–is opened by the ventricular systole and shut slightly after closure of the aortic valve.

2. Aortic valve

–lies behind the left half of the sternum opposite the third intercostal space.

–is closed during the ventricular diastole; **its closure** at the beginning of ventricular diastole causes the **second ("dub") heart sound.**

–is most audible over the **right second intercostal space** just lateral to the sternum.

3. Tricuspid (right AV) valve

–lies between the right atrium and ventricle, behind the right half of the sternum opposite the fourth intercostal space and is covered by endocardium.

–is most audible over the **right lower part of the body of the sternum.**

–has **anterior, posterior, and septal cusps,** which are attached by the chordae tendineae to three papillary muscles that keep the valves against the pressure developed by the pumping action of the heart.

–is closed during the ventricular systole (contraction); **its closure** contributes to the **first ("lub") heart sound.**

4. Bicuspid (left AV) valve

–is called the **"mitral valve"** because it is shaped like a bishop's miter.

–lies between the left atrium and ventricle, behind the left half of the sternum at the fourth costal cartilage, and has two cusps: a larger anterior and a smaller posterior.

–is closed slightly before the tricuspid valve by the ventricular contraction (systole); **its closure** at the onset of ventricular systole causes the **first ("lub") heart sound**.

–is most audible over the apical region of the heart in the **left fifth intercostal space at the midclavicular line.**

D. Heart sounds

1. First ("lub") sound

–is caused by the closure of the **tricuspid** and **mitral valves** at the onset of ventricular systole.

2. Second ("dub") sound   *filling occurs b/w*

–is caused by the closure of the **aortic** and **pulmonary valves** (and vibration of walls of the heart and major vessels) at the onset of ventricular diastole.

E. Conducting system of the heart (see Figure 4-11)

1. Sinoatrial (SA) node

–is a small mass of specialized cardiac muscle fibers that lies in the myocardium at the upper end of the crista terminalis near the opening of the superior vena cava in the right atrium.

–is known as the **"pacemaker"** of the heart and initiates the heartbeat, which can be altered by autonomic nervous stimulation (sympathetic stimulation speeds it up and vagal stimulation slows it down).

–is supplied by the **sinus node artery,** which is usually a branch of the **right coronary artery.**

2. AV node

–lies in the interatrial septum, superior and medial to the opening of the coronary sinus in the right atrium.

–is supplied by the AV nodal artery, which usually arises from the **right coronary artery** opposite the origin of the posterior interventricular artery.

–is innervated by autonomic nerve fibers, although the cardiac muscle fibers lack motor endings.

3. AV bundle (bundle of His)

–begins at the **AV node** and runs along the membranous part of the interventricular septum.

–splits into right and left branches, which descend into the muscular part of the interventricular septum, and breaks up into terminal conducting fibers **(Purkinje fibers)** to spread out into the ventricular walls.

F. Coronary arteries (see Figure 4-8)

–arises from the ascending aorta and is **filled with blood during the ventricular diastole.**

–has **maximal blood flow during diastole** and minimal during systole, owing to compression of the arterial branches in the myocardium during systole.

1. Right coronary artery

–arises from the anterior (right) aortic sinus of the ascending aorta, runs between the root of the pulmonary trunk and the right auricle, and generally supplies the right atrium and ventricle.

–gives rise to the following:

a. Sinus node artery

–passes between the right atrium and the opening of the superior vena cava and supplies the SA node and the right atrium.

b. Marginal artery

–runs along the inferior border toward the apex and supplies the right ventricle.

c. Posterior interventricular (posterior descending) artery

–is a larger terminal branch and supplies a part of the interventricular septum and the AV node.

d. AV nodal artery

–arises opposite the origin of its posterior interventricular artery and supplies the AV node.

2. Left coronary artery

–arises from the left aortic sinus of the ascending aorta, just above the **aortic semilunar valve.**

–is shorter than the right coronary artery and usually is distributed to more of the myocardium.

–gives rise to the following:

a. Anterior interventricular (left anterior descending) artery

–generally supplies anterior aspects of the right and left ventricles and is the chief source of blood to the interventricular septum.

b. Circumflex artery

–runs in the coronary sulcus, gives off the left marginal artery, supplies the left atrium and left ventricle, and anastomoses with the terminal branch of the right coronary artery.

G. Cardiac veins and coronary sinus (Figure 4-13)

1. Coronary sinus

–is the **largest vein draining the heart** and lies in the **coronary sulcus,** which separates the atria from the ventricles.
–opens into the right atrium between the opening of the inferior vena cava and the AV opening.
–has a one-cusp valve at the right margin of its aperture.
–receives the great, middle, and small cardiac veins; the oblique vein of the left atrium; and the posterior vein of the left ventricle.

2. Great cardiac vein

–begins at the apex of the heart and ascends in the anterior interventricular groove.
–drains upward alongside the anterior interventricular branch of the left coronary artery.
–turns to the left to lie in the coronary sinus and continues as the **coronary sinus.**

3. Middle cardiac vein

–begins at the apex of the heart and ascends in the **posterior interventricular groove,** accompanying the posterior interventricular branch of the right coronary artery.
–drains into the right end of the coronary sinus.

4. Small cardiac vein

–runs along the right margin of the heart in company with the marginal artery and then posteriorly in the coronary sulcus to end in the right end of the coronary sinus.

AV suclus →Coronary sinus

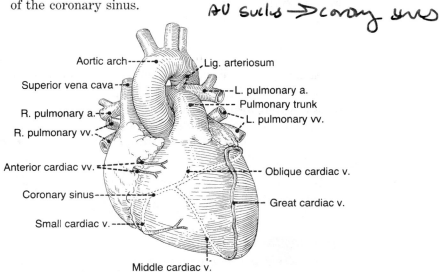

Aortic arch - - - - •
Superior vena cava - -
R. pulmonary a. -
R. pulmonary vv. -
Anterior cardiac vv. -
Coronary sinus - - -
Small cardiac v. - - -

Lig. arteriosum
- - L. pulmonary a.
- - - Pulmonary trunk
- - - L. pulmonary vv.

- - Oblique cardiac v.
- Great cardiac v.

Middle cardiac v.

Figure 4-13. Anterior view of the heart.

5. Oblique vein of the left atrium

–descends to empty into the coronary sinus, near its left end.

6. Anterior cardiac vein

–drains the anterior right ventricle, crosses the coronary groove, and ends directly in the right atrium.

7. Smallest cardiac veins (venae cordis minimae)

–begin in the wall of the heart and empty directly into its chambers.

H. Lymphatic vessels of the heart

–receive lymph from the myocardium and epicardium.
–follow the right coronary artery to empty into the **anterior mediastinal nodes** and follow the left coronary artery to empty into a tracheobronchial node.

I. Cardiac plexus

–receives the superior, middle, and inferior cervical and thoracic cardiac nerves from the sympathetic trunks and vagus nerves.
–is divisible into the **superficial cardiac plexus,** which lies beneath the arch of the aorta, in front of the pulmonary artery, and the **deep cardiac plexus,** which lies posterior to the arch of the aorta, in front of the bifurcation of the trachea.
–richly innervates the conducting system of the heart: the right sympathetic and parasympathetic branches terminate chiefly in the region of the **SA node,** and the left branches end chiefly in the region of the **AV node.** The cardiac muscle fibers are devoid of motor endings and are activated by the conducting system.
–supplies the heart with **sympathetic fibers,** which increase the heart rate and the force of the heartbeat, causing dilation of the coronary arteries; and **parasympathetic fibers,** which decrease the heart rate.

J. Clinical considerations

1. Disorders of the heart and pericardium

a. Angina pectoris

–is characterized by attacks of **chest pain originating** in the heart and felt beneath the sternum, in many cases radiating to the left shoulder and down the arm.
–is caused by an **insufficient supply of oxygen to the heart muscle** owing to coronary artery disease.
–generates pain impulses that travel in visceral afferent fibers through the middle and inferior cervical and thoracic cardiac branches of the sympathetic nervous system before entering the thoracic segment of the spinal cord.

b. Myocardial infarction

–is a **necrosis** of the myocardium due to local **ischemia** resulting from obstruction of the blood supply, most commonly by a thrombus or embolus in the coronary arteries.

c. Coronary atherosclerosis

–is characterized by the presence of **sclerotic plaques** containing cholesterol and lipoid material that impairs myocardial blood flow, leading to ischemia and **myocardial infarction**.

d. Coronary angioplasty

–is an angiographic reconstruction (radiographic view of vessels after the injection of a radiopaque material) of a blood vessel made by enlarging a narrowed coronary arterial lumen.

–is performed by peripheral introduction of a balloon-tip catheter and **dilating the lumen on withdrawal of the inflated catheter tip.**

e. Coronary bypass

–involves the grafting of a section of vein or other conduit between the aorta and a coronary artery distal to an obstruction in the coronary artery, shunting blood from the aorta to the coronary arteries.

f. Cardiac murmur

–is a characteristic sound generated by turbulence of blood flow through an orifice of the heart.

2. Pericardiac tamponade

–is an **acute compression of the heart** caused by a rapid **accumulation of fluid** or blood in the pericardial sac from **wounds** to the heart or **pericardial effusion** (passage of fluid from the pericardial capillaries into the pericardial sac).

–causes **compression of venous return** to the heart, resulting in **decreased diastolic capacity,** reduced cardiac output with an increased heart rate, increased venous pressure with jugular vein distention, hepatic enlargement, and peripheral edema.

3. Pericarditis

–is an **inflammation of the parietal serous pericardium,** which may result in cardiac tamponade and precordial and epigastric pain.

–causes the surfaces of the pericardium to become rough; the resulting friction sounds like the rustle of silk (**pericardial murmur**), which can be heard on auscultation.

4. Pericardiocentesis

–is a **surgical puncture of the pericardial cavity** for the aspiration of fluid, which is necessary to relieve the pressure of accumulated fluid on the heart. A needle is inserted into the pericardial sac through the fifth or sixth intercostal spaces adjacent to the sternum.

5. Cardiopulmonary resuscitation (CPR)

–is a restoration of cardiac output and pulmonary ventilation following cardiac arrest and apnea (cessation of breathing) by external cardiac massage.

–is performed by applying firm pressure to the chest vertically downward over the inferior part of the sternum to move it posteriorly, forcing blood out of the heart into the great vessels. After taking a deep breath, the resuscitator should place his or her mouth tightly over that of the patient's and blow forcefully into the lungs.

Structures in the Posterior Mediastinum

I. Esophagus

–is a muscular tube that is continuous with the pharynx in the neck and enters the thorax behind the trachea.

–has **three constrictions:** one at the level of the sixth cervical vertebra, where it begins; one at the crossing of the left main stem bronchus; and one at the tenth thoracic vertebra, where it pierces the diaphragm. The left atrium also presses against the anterior surface of the esophagus.

–receives blood from three branches of the aorta (the **inferior thyroid, bronchial, and esophageal arteries**) and from the left gastric and inferior phrenic arteries.

II. Blood Vessels and Lymphatic Vessels (see Figures 4-9 and 4-10)

A. Thoracic aorta

–begins at the level of the fourth thoracic vertebra.

–descends on the left side of the vertebral column and then approaches the median plane to end in front of the vertebral column by passing through the **aortic hiatus** of the diaphragm.

–gives rise to nine pairs of **posterior intercostal arteries** and one pair of **subcostal arteries.** The first two intercostal arteries arise from the highest intercostal arteries of the costocervical trunk. The posterior intercostal artery gives rise to a collateral branch, which runs along the upper border of the rib below the space.

–also gives rise to pericardial, bronchial (one right and two left), esophageal, mediastinal, and superior phrenic branches.

B. Azygos venous system (Figure 4-14)

1. Azygos vein

–is formed by the union of the **right ascending lumbar and right subcostal veins.** Its lower end is **connected to the inferior vena cava.**

–enters the thorax through the aortic opening of the diaphragm.

–receives the right intercostal veins, the **right superior intercostal vein,** the hemiazygos, and accessory hemiazygos veins.

–**arches over the root of the right lung** and **empties into the superior vena cava,** of which it is the first tributary.

2. Hemiazygos vein

–is formed by the union of the **left subcostal and ascending lumbar veins.** Its lower end is **connected to the left renal vein.**

–ascends on the left side of the vertebral bodies behind the thoracic aorta, receiving the lower four posterior intercostal veins.

3. Accessory hemiazygos vein

–begins at the fourth intercostal space, usually receives the fifth to eighth intercostal veins, descends in front of the posterior intercostal arteries, and terminates in the azygos vein.

4. Posterior intercostal veins

–The first intercostal vein on each side drains into the corresponding brachiocephalic vein.

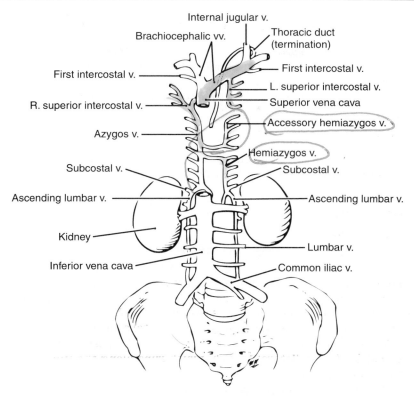

Figure 4-14. Azygos venous system.

–The second, third, and often the fourth intercostal veins join to form the **superior intercostal vein,** which drains into the **azygos vein on the right** and into the **brachiocephalic vein on the left**.

–The rest of the veins drain into the azygos vein on the right and into the hemiazygos or accessory hemiazygos veins on the left.

C. Lymphatics

1. Thoracic duct (Figure 4-15; see Figures 4-10 and 4-14)

–begins in the abdomen at the **cisterna chyli,** which is the dilated junction of the intestinal, lumbar, and descending intercostal trunks.

–is usually beaded because of its numerous valves and may often be double or even triple.

–drains the lower limbs, pelvis, abdomen, left thorax, left upper limb, and left side of the head and neck.

–passes through the aortic opening of the diaphragm and ascends through the posterior mediastinum between the aorta and the azygos vein.

–arches laterally over the apex of the left pleura and between the left carotid sheath in front and the vertebral artery behind, runs behind the left internal jugular vein, and then usually empties into the junction of the left internal jugular and subclavian veins.

2. Right lymphatic duct

–drains the right sides of the thorax, upper limb, head and neck, and empties into the junction of the right internal jugular and subclavian veins.

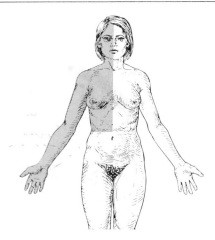

Figure 4-15. All areas except the *shaded area* (upper right quadrant) are drained by the thoracic duct.

III. Autonomic Nervous System in the Thorax (Figure 4-16)

–is composed of motor, or efferent, nerves through which **cardiac muscle, smooth muscle, and glands** are innervated.

–involves two neurons: **preganglionic** and **postganglionic.**

–also includes **general visceral afferent (GVA) fibers** that run along with **general visceral efferent (GVE) fibers.**

–consists of sympathetic (or thoracolumbar outflow) and parasympathetic (or craniosacral outflow) systems.

–consists of **cholinergic** fibers (sympathetic preganglionic, parasympathetic preganglionic and postganglionic) that use acetylcholine as the neurotransmitter, and **adrenergic** fibers (sympathetic postganglionic) that use norepinephrine as the neurotransmitter [except those to sweat glands (cholinergic)].

A. Sympathetic nervous system

–enables the body to cope with crises or emergencies and thus often is referred to as the **fight-or-flight division.**

–contains preganglionic cell bodies that are located in the lateral horn or intermediolateral cell column of the spinal cord segments between T1 and L2.

–has preganglionic fibers that pass through the white rami communicantes and enter the sympathetic chain ganglion, where they synapse.

–has postganglionic fibers that join each spinal nerve by way of the gray rami communicantes and supply the blood vessels, hair follicles (arrector pili muscles), and sweat glands.

1. Sympathetic trunk

–is composed primarily of ascending and descending preganglionic sympathetic fibers and visceral afferent fibers, and contains the cell bodies of the postganglionic sympathetic (GVE) fibers.

–descends in front of the neck of the ribs and the posterior intercostal vessels.

–contains the **cervicothoracic (or stellate) ganglion,** which is formed by fusion of the inferior cervical ganglion with the first thoracic ganglion.

–enters the abdomen through the crus of the diaphragm or behind the medial lumbocostal arch.

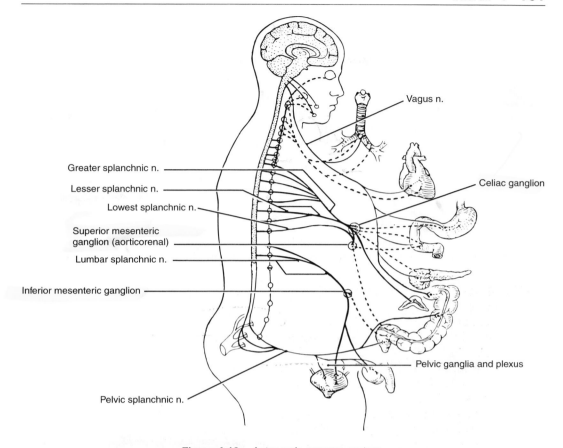

Greater splanchnic n.

Lesser splanchnic n.

Lowest splanchnic n.

Superior mesenteric
ganglion (aorticorenal)

Lumbar splanchnic n.

Inferior mesenteric ganglion

Pelvic splanchnic n.

Vagus n.

Celiac ganglion

Pelvic ganglia and plexus

Figure 4-16. Autonomic nervous system.

–gives rise to cardiac, pulmonary, mediastinal, and splanchnic branches.
–is connected to the thoracic spinal nerves by gray and white rami communicantes.

2. Rami communicantes

a. White rami communicantes

–contain preganglionic sympathetic (GVE; myelinated) fibers with cell bodies located in the lateral horn (intermediolateral cell column) of the spinal cord, and GVA fibers with cell bodies located in the dorsal root ganglia.
–are connected to the spinal nerves, limited to the spinal cord segments between T1 and L2.

b. Gray rami communicantes

–contain postganglionic sympathetic (GVE; unmyelinated) fibers that supply the blood vessels, sweat glands, and arrector pili muscles of hair follicles.
–are connected to every spinal nerve and contain fibers with cell bodies located in the sympathetic trunk.

3. Thoracic splanchnic nerves

–contain sympathetic preganglionic fibers with cell bodies located in the lateral horn (intermediolateral cell column) of the spinal cord and visceral afferent fibers with cell bodies located in the dorsal root ganglia.

a. Greater splanchnic nerve

–arises usually from the fifth through ninth thoracic sympathetic ganglia, perforates the crus of the diaphragm or occasionally passes through the aortic hiatus, and ends in the **celiac ganglion.**

b. Lesser splanchnic nerve

–is derived usually from the tenth and eleventh thoracic ganglia, pierces the crus of the diaphragm, and ends in the **aorticorenal ganglion.**

c. Least splanchnic nerve

–is derived usually from the twelfth thoracic ganglion, pierces the crus of the diaphragm, and ends in the ganglia of the **renal plexus.**

B. Parasympathetic nervous system

–promotes quiet and orderly processes of the body, thereby conserving energy.

–is not as widely distributed over the entire body as sympathetic fibers; the body wall and extremities have no parasympathetic nerve supply.

–has preganglionic fibers running in cranial nerves (CNs) III, VII, and IX that pass to cranial autonomic ganglia (i.e., the ciliary, submandibular, pterygopalatine, and otic ganglia), where they synapse with postganglionic neurons.

–has preganglionic fibers in CN X and in pelvic splanchnic nerves (originating from S2–S4)that pass to terminal ganglia, where they synapse.

–has parasympathetic fibers in the **vagus nerve** that supply all of the thoracic and abdominal viscerae, except the descending and sigmoid colons and other pelvic viscerae. These structures are innervated by the pelvic splanchnic nerves (S2–S4). The vagus nerve contains the parasympathetic preganglionic fibers with cell bodies located in the medulla oblongata, and the GVA fibers with cell bodies located in the inferior (nodose) ganglion.

–decreases the heart rate, constricts bronchial lumen, and stimulates gastrointestinal (GI) motility and secretion.

1. Right vagus nerve

–gives rise to the **right recurrent laryngeal nerve,** which hooks around the right subclavian artery and ascends into the neck between the trachea and the esophagus.

–crosses anterior to the right subclavian artery, runs posterior to the superior vena cava, and descends at the right surface of the trachea and then posterior to the right main bronchus.

–contributes to the cardiac, pulmonary, and esophageal plexuses.

–forms the vagal trunks (or gastric nerves) at the lower part of the esophagus and enters the abdomen through the esophageal hiatus.

2. Left vagus nerve

–enters the thorax between the left common carotid and subclavian arteries and behind the left brachiocephalic vein and descends on the arch of the aorta.

–gives rise to the left recurrent laryngeal nerve, which hooks around the arch of the aorta to the left of the ligamentum arteriosum. It ascends through the superior mediastinum in the groove between the trachea and the esophagus.

–gives rise to the thoracic cardiac branches, breaks up into the pulmonary plexuses, and then continues into the esophageal plexus.

IV. Clinical Considerations

A. Disorders

1. Aneurysm of the aortic arch

–is a sac formed by dilation of the aortic arch that compresses the left recurrent laryngeal nerve, leading to coughing, hoarseness, and paralysis of the ipsilateral vocal cord.

–may cause **dysphagia** (difficulty in swallowing) due to pressure on the esophagus, and **dyspnea** (difficulty in breathing) due to pressure on the trachea, root of the lung, or phrenic nerve.

2. Coarctation of the aorta (Figure 4-17)

–usually occurs distal to the point of entrance of the ductus arteriosus into the aorta, in which case an adequate collateral circulation develops before birth. If this condition occurs proximal to the origin of the left subclavian artery of the ductus arteriosus, adequate collateral circulation does not develop.

postductal

–results in tortuous and enlarged blood vessels, especially the internal thoracic, intercostal, epigastric, and scapular arteries.

–results in elevated blood pressure in the radial artery and decreased pressure in the femoral artery.

↑ *u. body*
p

–causes the femoral pulse to occur after the radial pulse. (Normally, the femoral pulse occurs slightly before the radial pulse and is under about the same pressure.)

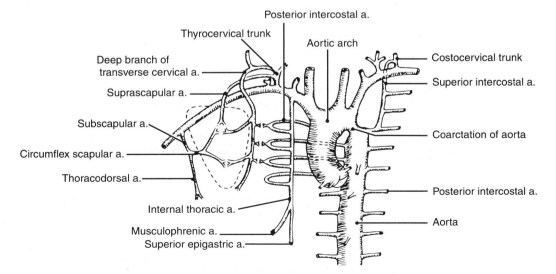

Figure 4-17. Coarctation of the aorta.

–leads to the development of the important **collateral circulation** over the thorax. It occurs between the:

a. **Anterior intercostal** branches of the internal thoracic artery and the **posterior intercostal** arteries

b. **Superior epigastric** branch of the internal thoracic artery and the **inferior epigastric** artery

c. **Posterosuperior intercostal** branch of the costocervical trunk and the **third posterior intercostal** artery

d. **Posterior intercostal** arteries and the **descending scapular** (or dorsal scapular) artery, which anastomoses with the suprascapular and circumflex scapular arteries around the scapula

3. **Rupture of the thoracic duct**

–can be caused by fracture of the thoracic vertebrae, leading to **chylothorax,** an accumulation of chyle in the pleural sac.

4. **Achalasia (of esophagus)**

–is a condition characterized by **impaired esophageal contractions** due to failure of relaxation of the inferior esophageal sphincter, resulting from degeneration of myenteric (Auerbach's) plexus in the esophagus.

B. **Vagotomy**

–is transection of the vagus nerves at the lower portion of the esophagus in an attempt to reduce gastric secretion in the treatment of peptic ulcer.

C. **Stellate block**

–is an injection of local anesthetic in the vicinity of the stellate ganglion by placing the tip of the needle near the neck of the first rib.

–produces a temporary interruption of sympathetic function such as in a patient with excess vasoconstriction in the upper limb.

Review Test

Directions: Each of the numbered items or incomplete statements in this section is followed by answers or by completions of the statement. Select the **one** lettered answer or completion that is **best** in each case.

1. On the surface of the chest, a physician is able to locate the apex of the heart

(A) at the level of the sternal angle
(B) in the left fourth intercostal space
(C) in the left fifth intercostal space
(D) in the right fifth intercostal space
(E) at the level of the xiphoid process of the sternum

2. Normal, quiet expiration is achieved by contraction of the

(A) elastic tissue in the thoracic wall and lungs
(B) serratus posterior superior muscles
(C) pectoralis minor muscles
(D) serratus anterior muscles
(E) diaphragm

3. Which of the following nerve fibers would be injured if the greater splanchnic nerves were severed?

(A) General somatic afferent (GSA) and preganglionic sympathetic fibers
(B) General visceral afferent (GVA) and postganglionic sympathetic fibers
(C) GVA and preganglionic sympathetic fibers
(D) General somatic efferent (GSE) and postganglionic sympathetic fibers
(E) GVA and GSE fibers

4. A stab wound that severed the white rami communicantes at the level of the sixth thoracic vertebra would result in degeneration of nerve cell bodies in which of the following structures?

(A) Dorsal root ganglion and anterior horn of the spinal cord
(B) Sympathetic chain ganglion and dorsal root ganglion
(C) Sympathetic chain ganglion and posterior horn of the spinal cord
(D) Dorsal root ganglion and lateral horn of the spinal cord
(E) Anterior and lateral horns of the spinal cord

5. Where should a physician place the stethoscope to listen to the sound of the mitral valve?

(A) Over the medial end of the second left intercostal space
(B) Over the medial end of the second right intercostal space
(C) In the left fourth intercostal space at the midclavicular line
(D) In the left fifth intercostal space at the midclavicular line
(E) Over the right half of the lower end of the body of the sternum

6. Bleeding comes from the vein that is accompanied by the posterior interventricular artery. Which of the following veins is most likely to be ruptured?

(A) Great cardiac vein
(B) Middle cardiac vein
(C) Anterior cardiac vein
(D) Small cardiac vein
(E) Oblique veins of the left atrium

7. The largest portion of the sternocostal surface of the heart seen on a posterior–anterior chest radiograph is composed of the

(A) left atrium
(B) right atrium
(C) left ventricle
(D) right ventricle
(E) base of the heart

8. If the interventricular septum is damaged, which of the following valves is most likely defective?

(A) Pulmonary valve
(B) Mitral valve
(C) Valve of coronary sinus
(D) Tricuspid valve
(E) Aortic valve

9. An artificial cardiac pacemaker is implanted in a 54-year-old patient. Which of the following conductive tissues of the heart has a defective function?

(A) Atrioventricular (AV) bundle
(B) AV node
(C) Sinoatrial (SA) node
(D) Purkinje fiber
(E) Moderator band

10. Which of the following bronchopulmonary segments must contain cancerous tissues if a thoracic surgeon has to remove the right middle lobar (secondary) bronchus along with lung tissue?

(A) Medial and lateral
(B) Anterior and posterior
(C) Anterior basal and medial basal
(D) Anterior basal and posterior basal
(E) Lateral basal and posterior basal

11. A pulmonary physician finds a small mass of tumor in the eparterial bronchus. Which of the following airways is most likely blocked?

(A) Left superior bronchus
(B) Left inferior bronchus
(C) Right superior bronchus
(D) Right middle bronchus
(E) Right inferior bronchus

12. If a blood clot blocks the circumflex branch of the left coronary artery in a patient with a typical coronary circulation, which area of the heart musculature is most likely to be ischemic?

(A) Anterior part of the left ventricle
(B) Anterior interventricular region
(C) Posterior interventricular region
(D) Posterior part of the left ventricle
(E) Anterior part of the right ventricle

13. Which of the following would most likely occur if the phrenic nerve is severed?

(A) Injury to only general somatic efferent (GSE) fibers
(B) Difficulty in expiration
(C) Loss of sensation in the pericardium and mediastinal pleura
(D) Normal function of the diaphragm
(E) Loss of sensation in the costal part of the diaphragm

14. Which of the following conditions could injure the left recurrent laryngeal nerve?

(A) A pericardial incision medial to the ligamentum arteriosum
(B) Scar tissue in front of the subclavian artery
(C) A tumor in the posterior mediastinum
(D) An aneurysm in the aortic arch
(E) A knife wound on the arch of the azygos vein

15. Which of the following conditions could result from a myocardial infarction limited to the interventricular septum?

(A) Tricuspid valve insufficiency
(B) Pulmonary valve insufficiency
(C) Inferior vena caval valve insufficiency
(D) Mitral valve insufficiency
(E) Aortic valve insufficiency

16. Lung cancer is located in the vicinity of the cardiac notch, a deep indentation on the lung. Which of the following lobes is most likely to be excised?

(A) Superior lobe of the right lung
(B) Middle lobe of the right lung
(C) Inferior lobe of the right lung
(D) Superior lobe of the left lung
(E) Inferior lobe of the left lung

17. Which of the following conditions represents the normal changes that occur in the circulation at or soon after birth?

(A) Decreased blood flow through the lungs
(B) Anatomical closure of the ductus arteriosus
(C) Increased left atrial pressure
(D) Anatomical closure of the foramen ovale
(E) Functional closure of the right umbilical vein

18. Destructive changes in the right atrium could damage which of the following structures?

(A) Papillary muscles
(B) Chordae tendineae
(C) Septomarginal trabecula
(D) Pectinate muscles
(E) Trabeculae carneae cordis

19. A sudden occlusion at the origin of the descending (thoracic) aorta would most likely decrease blood flow in which of the following intercostal arteries?

(A) Upper six anterior
(B) All of the posterior
(C) Upper two posterior
(D) Lower anterior
(E) Lower nine posterior

20. The right coronary artery

(A) is shorter in length than the left one
(B) supplies blood to the sinoatrial (SA) node
(C) causes myocardial infarction in the apex of the heart if it is occluded
(D) provides maximal blood flow during systole and minimal during diastole
(E) arises from the aortic arch

21. Which of the following describes a characteristic of the left lung?

(A) Horizontal fissure
(B) A groove for the superior vena cava
(C) Three lobar (secondary) bronchi
(D) Lingula of lung
(E) A larger capacity than the right lung

22. A victim of an automobile accident experiences difficulty in expiration. Which of the following muscles is most likely injured?

(A) Levator costarum
(B) Innermost intercostal muscle
(C) External intercostal muscle
(D) Diaphragm
(E) Muscles of the abdominal wall

23. In a 78-year-old patient with an advanced cancer in the superior mediastinum, which of the following structures may be spared?

(A) Brachiocephalic veins
(B) Trachea
(C) Lower portion of the left common carotid artery
(D) Arch of the aorta
(E) Hemiazygos vein

24. A tumor located just superior to the root of the right lung may block blood flow in which of the following veins?

(A) Hemiazygos vein
(B) Azygos vein
(C) Right subclavian vein
(D) Right brachiocephalic vein
(E) Accessory hemiazygos vein

25. A lesion of the right vagus nerve near the trachea in the superior mediastinum could cause which of the following conditions?

(A) Loss of sensation carried by the recurrent laryngeal nerve
(B) Lack of parasympathetic fibers in the anterior esophageal plexus
(C) Functional injury to the anterior vagal trunk at the lower part of the esophagus
(D) Reduction in cardiac rate
(E) Injury to parasympathetic preganglionic fibers

26. The ductus arteriosus has which of the following properties?

(A) Anatomical closure right after birth
(B) Carrying highly oxygenated blood during prenatal life
(C) Functional closure several weeks after birth
(D) Connection of the right pulmonary vein to the aorta
(E) Shunt of blood from the pulmonary trunk to the aorta before birth, bypassing the pulmonary circulation

27. Left ventricular hypertrophy could result from which of the following conditions?

(A) A constricted pulmonary trunk
(B) An abnormally small left atrioventricular (AV) opening
(C) Improper closing of the pulmonary valves
(D) An abnormally large right AV opening
(E) Stenosis of the aorta

28. The left primary bronchus

(A) has a larger diameter than the right primary bronchus
(B) often receives more foreign bodies via the trachea than the right primary bronchus
(C) gives rise to the eparterial bronchus
(D) is longer than the right primary bronchus
(E) runs under the arch of the azygos vein

29. The hemiazygos vein

(A) receives the left superior intercostal vein
(B) receives the lower left posterior intercostal veins
(C) empties into the superior vena cava
(D) is connected to the inferior vena cava
(E) enters the thorax through the esophageal opening

30. On posterior–anterior chest radiographs, which of the following structures forms the right border of the cardiovascular silhouette?

(A) Arch of the aorta
(B) Pulmonary trunk
(C) Superior vena cava
(D) Ascending aorta
(E) Left ventricle

31. Which of the following veins typically drains into the right or left brachiocephalic vein?

(A) Azygos
(B) Hemiazygos
(C) Right superior intercostal
(D) Left superior intercostal
(E) Internal thoracic

32. During the cardiac cycle, which of the following events occurs?
(A) Atrioventricular (AV) valves close during diastole
(B) Aortic valve closes during systole
(C) Pulmonary valve opens during diastole
(D) Blood flow in coronary arteries is maximal during diastole
(E) Aortic valve closes at the same time as AV valve

33. Which of the following conditions may occur at or soon after birth?
(A) Anatomical closure of the ductus venosus
(B) Anatomical closure of the foramen ovale
(C) Anatomical closure of the ductus arteriosus
(D) Obliteration of the left umbilical vein
(E) Obliteration of the right umbilical vein

34. Which of the following anatomic features would most likely be found at the level of the sternal angle?
(A) Bifurcation of the trachea
(B) Beginning of the ascending aorta
(C) Middle of the aortic arch
(D) Articulation of the third rib with the sternum
(E) Superior border of the superior mediastinum

35. Which of the following structures would most likely articulate with the third rib?
(A) Manubrium of the sternum
(B) Body of the second thoracic vertebra
(C) Spinous process of the third thoracic vertebra
(D) Body of the fourth thoracic vertebra
(E) Transverse process of the second thoracic vertebra

36. A large tumor confined in the posterior mediastinum may compress which of the following structures?
(A) Ascending aorta
(B) Trachea
(C) Descending aorta
(D) Arch of the aorta
(E) Arch of the azygos vein

37. Which of the following structures is correctly paired with its nerve supply?
(A) Mediastinal pleura–intercostal nerves
(B) Peripheral part of the diaphragmatic pleura–phrenic nerves
(C) Visceral pleura–general visceral afferent (GVA) pain fibers
(D) Glands in the bronchial tree–parasympathetic fibers
(E) Smooth muscle in the pulmonary artery–parasympathetic fibers

38. The near-simultaneous closure of which of the following valves produces the first heart sound?
(A) Aortic and tricuspid
(B) Aortic and pulmonary
(C) Tricuspid and mitral
(D) Mitral and pulmonary
(E) Tricuspid and pulmonary

39. Which of the following structures loops around the arch of the aorta near the ligamentum arteriosum?
(A) Left vagus nerve
(B) Left phrenic nerve
(C) Left sympathetic trunk
(D) Left recurrent laryngeal nerve
(E) Left greater splanchnic nerve

40. The right atrium
(A) receives blood from the oblique cardiac veins
(B) associated with the apex of the heart
(C) contains the sinoatrial (SA) node
(D) enlarges briefly in response to coarctation of the aorta
(E) is hypertrophied by pulmonary stenosis

41. Which of the following structures maintains constant tension on the cusps of the atrioventricular (AV) valves?
(A) Crista terminalis
(B) Septomarginal trabecula
(C) Chordae tendineae
(D) Pectinate muscle
(E) Anulus fibrosus

42. If the right coronary artery is blocked by a fat globule after giving off the right marginal artery, which of the following structures may have oxygen deficiency?
(A) Right atrium
(B) Sinoatrial (SA) node
(C) Atrioventricular (AV) node
(D) Apex of the heart
(E) Root of the pulmonary trunk

43. A surgical resident ligates the phrenic nerve instead of the accompanying artery descending between the mediastinal pleura and the pericardium. Which of the following arteries did he intend to ligate?
(A) Internal thoracic
(B) Musculophrenic
(C) Pericardiacophrenic
(D) Right coronary artery
(E) Superior (supreme) thoracic

44. When the diaphragm contracts, which of the following conditions most likely occurs?
(A) Decreased thoracic volume
(B) Increased abdominal volume
(C) Increased lung volume
(D) Air flow out of the bronchi
(E) Increased thoracic pressure

45. During a pleural tap, a needle may injure the intercostal neurovascular bundle because it is located
(A) above the upper border of the ribs
(B) deep to the upper border of the ribs
(C) beneath the lower border of the ribs
(D) between the external and internal intercostals
(E) between the transverse thoracis and subcostalis

Directions: Each set of matching questions in this section consists of a list of four to twenty-six lettered options (some of which may be in figures) followed by several numbered items. For each numbered item, select the ONE lettered option that is most closely associated with it. To avoid spending too much time on matching sets with large numbers of options, it is generally advisable to begin each set by reading the list of options. Then, for each item in the set, try to generate the correct answer and locate it in the option list, rather than evaluating each option individually. Each lettered option may be selected once, more than once, or not at all.

Questions 46–50

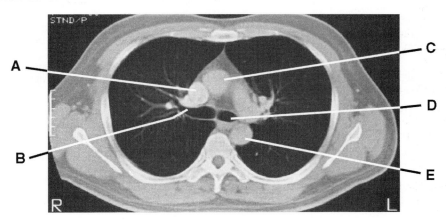

Figure 4-46Q [CT scan of the thorax]

Match each of the following descriptions with the appropriate lettered structure in this computed tomography (CT) scan of the heart from a 42-year-old man who complains of chest pain and breathing problems. His electrocardiogram (ECG) shows left ventricular hypertrophy.

46. Stenosis of this structure may produce left ventricular hypertrophy

47. Structure that is most likely to be removed by a pulmonary surgeon in a surgical resection of a lobe (lobectomy) to remove lung cancer in the apex of the right lung

48. Structure that branches into the bronchial arteries

49. Structure into which the azygos vein drains venous blood

50. Structure from which the left coronary artery arises

Questions 51–55

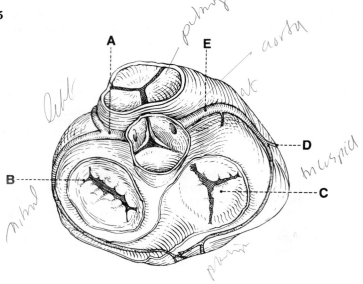

Figure 4-51Q [superior view of the heart]

Match each of the following descriptions with the appropriate lettered structure in the superior cross-sectional view of the heart.

51. Runs toward the apex of the heart and supplies atrial blood to the anterior right ventricle

52. Supplies arterial blood to the sinoatrial (SA) node

53. Arises from the left aortic sinus

54. Gives rise to the anterior interventricular artery

55. Has a sound that is best heard through a stethoscope at the left fifth intercostal space at the midclavicular line

Answers and Explanations

1-C. On the surface of the chest, the apex of the heart can be located in the left fifth intercostal space slightly medial to the midclavicular (or nipple) line.

2-A. Normal, quiet expiration is achieved by contraction of extensible tissue in the lungs and the thoracic wall. The serratus posterior superior muscles, diaphragm, pectoralis major, and serratus anterior are muscles of inspiration.

3-C. The greater splanchnic nerves contain general visceral afferent (GVA) and preganglionic sympathetic general visceral efferent (GVE) fibers.

4-D. The white rami communicantes contain preganglionic sympathetic general visceral efferent (GVE) fibers and general visceral afferent (GVA) fibers whose cell bodies are located in the lateral horn of the spinal cord and the dorsal root ganglia.

5-D. The mitral valve [left atrioventricular (AV) valve] produces the apical beat (thrust) of the heart, which is most audible over the left fifth intercostal space at the midclavicular line.

6-B. The middle cardiac vein ascends in the posterior interventricular groove, accompanied by the posterior interventricular branch of the right coronary artery.

7-D. The right ventricle forms a large part of the sternocostal surface of the heart.

8-D. The septal cusp of the tricuspid valve is attached by a cordae tendineae to the septal papillary muscle, which arises from the interventricular septum.

9-C. The sinoatrial (SA) node initiates the impulse of contraction and is known as the "pacemaker" of the heart.

10-A. The right middle lobar (secondary) bronchus leads to the medial and lateral bronchopulmonary segments.

11-C. The eparterial bronchus is the right superior lobar (secondary) bronchus; all of the other bronchi are hyparterial bronchi.

12-D. The circumflex branch of the left coronary artery supplies the posterior portion of the left ventricle. The anterior interventricular artery supplies the anterior aspects of the right and left ventricles and the anterior interventricular septum.

13-C. The phrenic nerve supplies the pericardium and mediastinal and diaphragmatic (central part) pleurae as well as the diaphragm, an important muscle of inspiration. It contains general somatic efferent (GSE), general somatic afferent (GSA), and general visceral efferent (GVE) [postganglionic sympathetic] fibers. The costal part of the diaphragm receives GSA fibers from the intercostal nerves.

14-D. The left recurrent laryngeal nerve arises from the left vagus nerve in the superior mediastinum and hooks around the aortic arch lateral to the ligamentum arteriosum; therefore, it can be damaged by an aneurysm of the aortic arch, causing paralysis of the laryngeal muscles.

15-A. The three cusps of the tricuspid valve are the anterior, posterior, and septal cusps. The septal cusp lies on the margin of the orifice adjacent to the interventricular septum. There is defective conduction of cardiac impulses because the bundle descends into the interventricular septum. The pulmonary, aortic, and mitral valves are not closely associated with the interventricular septum.

16-D. The cardiac notch is a deep indentation of the anterior border of the superior lobe of the left lung.

17-C. The right umbilical vein is obliterated during the embryonic period. The changes in circulation that occur at, or soon after, birth include obliteration of the umbilical arteries, left umbilical vein, and ductus venosus; functional closure of the ductus arteriosus and the foramen ovale (anatomic closure requires weeks or months); increased blood flow through the lungs; and increased left atrial pressure.

18-D. The pectinate muscles are prominent ridges of atrial myocardium located in the interior of the right atrium and both auricles. Other structures are found in the right and left ventricles, except for the septomarginal trabecula, which is found only in the right ventricle.

19-E. The first two posterior intercostal arteries are branches of the highest (superior) intercostal artery of the costocervical trunk; the remaining nine branches are from the thoracic aorta. The internal thoracic artery gives off the upper six anterior intercostal arteries and is divided into the superior epigastric and musculophrenic arteries, which gives off anterior intercostal arteries in the seventh, eighth, and ninth intercostal spaces, and ends in the tenth intercostal space where it anastomoses with the deep circumflex iliac artery.

20-B. The apex of the heart receives blood typically from the anterior interventricular branch of the left coronary artery. The coronary arteries arise from the ascending aorta immediately above the aortic valve. Blood flow in the coronary arteries is maximal during diastole and minimal during systole, owing to the compression of the arterial branches in the myocardium during systole (ventricular contraction). The diastole is the dilation of the heart chambers, during which they fill with blood.

21-D. The lingula is the tongue-shaped portion of the upper lobe of the left lung. The left lung has grooves for the arch of aorta, descending aorta, and left subclavian artery. The right lung has grooves for the superior vena cava, arch of azygos vein, and esophagus.

22-E. The abdominal muscles are the major muscles of expiration, whereas the other distractors are muscles of inspiration.

23-E. The brachiocephalic veins, trachea, part of the left common carotid artery, and the arch of the aorta are located in the superior mediastinum. The hemiazygos vein is located in the inferior mediastinum.

24-B. The azygos vein arches over the root of the right lung and empties into the superior vena cava.

25-E. The vagus nerve carries parasympathetic preganglionic fibers to the thoracic and abdominal viscerae. The right vagus nerve forms primarily the right pulmonary plexus, it continues to form the posterior esophageal plexus, where it loses its identity. At the lower end of the esophagus, branches of the plexus reunite to form the posterior vagal trunk, which contains parasympathetic preganglionic fibers. The parasympathetic nerve decreases heart rate, constricts bronchial lumen, and stimulates gastrointestinal (GI) motility and secretion.

26-E. Before birth, the ductus arteriosus connects the bifurcation of the pulmonary trunk with the aortic arch and carries poorly oxygenated blood. It is functionally closed shortly after birth; however, anatomic closure requires several weeks or months. After birth, the ductus arteriosus becomes the ligamentum arteriosum, which connects the arch of the aorta to the left pulmonary artery. It shunts blood from the pulmonary trunk to the aorta before birth, bypassing the pulmonary circulation.

27-E. Stenosis of the aorta can cause left ventricular hypertrophy. Right ventricular hypertrophy may occur as a result of pulmonary stenosis, pulmonary and tricuspid valve defects, or mitral valve stenosis.

28-D. The right primary bronchus is shorter than the left one and has a larger diameter. More foreign bodies enter it via the trachea because it is more vertical than the left primary bronchus. The right primary bronchus runs under the arch of the azygos vein and gives rise to the eparterial bronchus.

29-B. The right superior intercostal vein drains into the azygos vein; the left superior intercostal vein drains into the left brachiocephalic vein. The azygos vein may enter the thorax through the aortic opening, arch over the root of the right lung, and empty into the superior vena cava. The azygos vein is connected to the inferior vena cava, whereas the hemiazygos vein is connected to the left renal vein.

30-C. A cardiovascular silhouette or cardiac shadow is the contour of the heart and great vessels seen on posterior–anterior chest radiographs. Its right border is formed by the superior vena cava, right atrium and inferior vena cava, whereas its left border is formed by the aortic arch (aortic knob), pulmonary trunk, left auricle, and left ventricle.

31-D. The left superior intercostal vein is formed by the second, third, and fourth posterior intercostal vein and drains into the left brachiocephalic vein, whereas the right superior intercostal vein drains into the azygos vein, which in turn drains into the superior vena cava.

32-D. During diastole the atrioventricular (AV) valves open and the aortic and pulmonary valves close, whereas during systole the AV valves close and the aortic and pulmonary valves open.

33-D. The right umbilical vein is obliterated during the embryonic period; the left umbilical vein is obliterated after birth to form the ligamentum teres hepatis. Functional closure of the ductus arteriosus, ductus venosus, and foramen ovale occurs at or soon after birth, but their anatomical closure requires several weeks.

34-A. The sternal angle is the junction of the manubrium and the body of the sternum. It is located at the level where the second rib articulates with the sternum, the trachea bifurcates into the right and left bronchi, and the aortic arch begins and ends. It marks the end of the ascending aorta and the beginning of the descending aorta, and it forms the inferior border of the superior mediastinum.

35-B. The third rib articulates with the body of the sternum, bodies of the second and third thoracic vertebrae, and transverse process of the third thoracic vertebra.

36-C. The descending aorta is found in both the superior and posterior mediastina. The superior mediastinum contains the trachea and arch of the aorta, and the middle mediastinum contains the ascending aorta, arch of the azygos vein, and main bronchi.

37-D. Glands and smooth muscles in the bronchial tree are supplied by sympathetic and parasympathetic fibers. The visceral pleura is insensitive to pain. The mediastinal pleura and the central part of the diaphragmatic pleura are innervated by the phrenic nerve, whereas the peripheral part of the diaphragmatic pleura is innervated by the intercostal nerves. The blood vessels are controlled by sympathetic fibers.

38-C. The first heart sound is produced by the closure of the tricuspid and mitral valves, whereas the second heart sound is produced by the closure of the aortic and pulmonary valves.

39-D. The left recurrent laryngeal nerve loops around the arch of the aorta near the ligamentum arteriosum, whereas the right recurrent laryngeal nerve hooks around the right subclavian artery.

40-C. The sinoatrial (SA) and atrioventricular (AV) nodes are in the wall of the right atrium.

41-C. The chordae tendineae are tendinous strands that extend from the papillary muscles to the cusps of the valve. The papillary muscles and chordae tendineae prevent the cusps from being everted into the atrium during ventricular contraction.

42-C. The atrioventricular (AV) node is supplied by the AV nodal artery, which usually arises from the right coronary artery opposite the origin of the posterior interventricular branch.

43-C. The phrenic nerve is accompanied by the pericardiacophrenic vessels of the internal thoracic vessels and descends between the mediastinal pleura and the pericardium to supply the pericardium, the mediastinal and diaphragmatic pleurae, and the diaphragm.

44-C. During inspiration the diaphragm contracts, increasing the vertical diameter of the thorax and decreasing intrathoracic and intrapulmonary pressures.

45-C. The intercostal veins, arteries, and nerves run in the costal groove beneath the inferior border of the ribs between the internal and innermost layers of muscles.

46-C. Ascending aortic stenosis results in left ventricular hypertrophy.

47-B. During surgical treatment for cancer in the apex of the right lung by a lobectomy, the right superior secondary (eparterial) bronchus should be removed.

48-E. The right and left bronchial arteries arise from the descending (thoracic) aorta.

49-A. The azygos vein drains venous blood into the superior vena cava.

50-C. The right and left coronary arteries arise from the ascending aorta.

51-D. The marginal branch of the right coronary artery supplies the anterior wall of the right ventricle.

52-E. The right coronary artery gives rise to the sinus node artery, which supplies the sinoatrial (SA) node. The posterior interventricular artery, a branch of the right coronary artery, gives rise to a branch that supplies the node.

53-A. The left coronary artery arises from the left aortic sinus.

54-A. The left coronary artery branches to form the anterior interventricular artery.

55-B. The mitral valve is best heard through a stethoscope at the left fifth intercostal space at the midclavicular line.

5

Abdomen

Anterior Abdominal Wall

I. Abdomen (Figure 5-1)

–is divided topographically by two transverse and two longitudinal planes into nine regions: **right and left hypochondriac; epigastric; right and left lumbar; umbilical; right and left inguinal (iliac);** and **hypogastric (pubic).**

–is also divided by vertical and horizontal planes through the umbilicus into four quadrants: right and left upper quadrants and right and left lower quadrants. The umbilicus lies at the level of the intervertebral disk between the third and fourth lumbar vertebrae. Its region is innervated by the tenth thoracic nerve.

II. Muscles of the Anterior Abdominal Wall (Table 5-1)

III. Fasciae and Ligaments of the Anterior Abdominal Wall

–are organized into superficial (**tela subcutanea**) and deep layers; the superficial has a thin fatty layer **(Camper's fascia),** and the deep has a membranous layer **(Scarpa's fascia).**

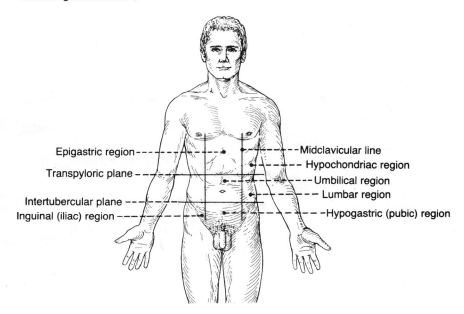

Epigastric region --------- Midclavicular line
Transpyloric plane --------- Hypochondriac region
--------- Umbilical region
Intertubercular plane --------- Lumbar region
Inguinal (iliac) region --------- Hypogastric (pubic) region

Figure 5-1. Planes of subdivision of the abdomen.

Table 5–1. Muscles of the Anterior Abdominal Wall

Muscle	Origin	Insertion	Nerve	Action
External oblique	External surface of lower eight ribs (5–12)	Anterior half of iliac crest; anterior–superior iliac spine; pubic tubercle; linea alba	Intercostal n. (T7–T11); subcostal n. (T12)	Compresses abdomen; flexes trunk; active in forced expiration
Internal oblique	Lateral two-thirds of inguinal ligament; iliac crest; thoracolumbar fascia	Lower four costal cartilages; linea alba; pubic crest; pectineal line	Intercostal n. (T7–T11); subcostal n. (T12); iliohypogastric and ilioinguinal nn. (L1)	Compresses abdomen; flexes trunk; active in forced expiration
Transverse	Lateral one-third of inguinal ligament; iliac crest; thoracolumbar fascia; lower six costal cartilages	Linea alba; pubic crest; pectineal line	Intercostal n. (T7–T12); subcostal n. (T12); iliohypogastric and ilioinguinal nn. (L1)	Compresses abdomen; depresses ribs
Rectus abdominis	Pubic crest and pubic symphysis	Xiphoid process and costal cartilages 5–7	Intercostal n. (T7–T11); subcostal n. (T12)	Depresses ribs; flexes trunk
Pyramidal	Pubic body	Linea alba	Subcostal n. (T12)	Tenses linea alba
Cremaster	Middle of inguinal ligament; lower margin of internal oblique muscle	Pubic tubercle and crest	Genitofemoral n.	Retracts testis

A. Superficial fascia

  1. Superficial layer of the superficial fascia (Camper's fascia)

  –continues over the inguinal ligament to merge with the superficial fascia of the thigh.

  –continues over the pubis and perineum as the superficial layer of the superficial perineal fascia.

  2. Deep layer of the superficial fascia (Scarpa's fascia)

  –is attached to the **fascia lata** just below the inguinal ligament.

  –continues over the pubis and perineum as the membranous layer (**Colles' fascia**) of the superficial perineal fascia.

  –continues over the penis as the **superficial fascia of the penis** and over the scrotum as the **tunica dartos,** which contains smooth muscle.

  –may contain extravasated urine between this fascia and the deep fascia of the abdomen, resulting from rupture of the spongy urethra (see Chapter 6, Perineal Region: VII A).

B. Deep fascia

  –covers the muscles and continues over the spermatic cord at the superficial inguinal ring as the **external spermatic fascia.**

–continues over the penis as the deep fascia of the penis (**Buck's fascia**) and over the pubis and perineum as the **deep perineal fascia.**

C. Linea alba

–is a **tendinous median raphe** between the two rectus abdominis muscles, extending from the xiphoid process to the pubic symphysis.

–is formed by the fusion of the aponeuroses of the external oblique, internal oblique, and transverse muscles of the abdomen.

D. Linea semilunaris

–is a **curved line** along the lateral border of the rectus abdominis.

E. Linea semicircularis (arcuate line)

–is a **crescent-shaped line** marking the termination of the posterior sheath of the rectus abdominis just below the level of the iliac crest.

F. Lacunar ligament (Gimbernat's ligament)

–represents the medial triangular expansion of the inguinal ligament to the pectineal line of the pubis.

–forms the medial border of the femoral ring and the floor of the inguinal canal.

G. Pectineal (Cooper's) ligament

–is a strong fibrous band that extends laterally from the lacunar ligament along the pectineal line of the pubis.

H. Inguinal ligament (Poupart's ligament)

–is the folded lower border of the aponeurosis of the external oblique muscle, extending between the anterior–superior iliac spine and the pubic tubercle.

–forms the floor (inferior wall) of the inguinal canal.

I. Iliopectineal arcus or ligament

–is a **fascial partition** that separates the muscular (lateral) and vascular (medial) lacunae deep to the inguinal ligament.

1. The **muscular lacuna** transmits the iliopsoas muscle.

2. The **vascular lacuna** transmits the femoral sheath and its contents, including the femoral vessels, a femoral branch of the genitofemoral nerve, and the femoral canal.

J. Reflected inguinal ligament

–is formed by certain fibers of the inguinal ligament reflected from the pubic tubercle upward toward the **linea alba.**

–also has some reflection from the lacunar ligament.

K. Falx inguinalis (conjoint tendon)

–is formed by the aponeuroses of the internal oblique and transverse muscles of the abdomen and is inserted into the pubic tubercle.

–strengthens the posterior wall of the medial half of the **inguinal canal.**

L. Rectus sheath (Figure 5-2)

–is formed by fusion of the aponeuroses of the external oblique, internal oblique, and transverse muscles of the abdomen.

–encloses the rectus abdominis and sometimes the pyramidal muscle.

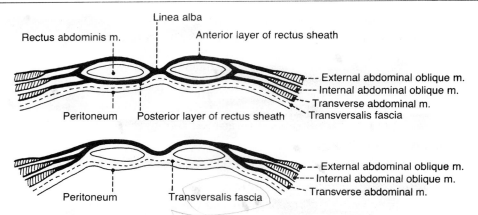

Figure 5-2. Arrangement of the rectus sheath above the umbilicus *(upper)* and below the arcuate line *(lower)*.

–also contains the superior and inferior epigastric vessels and the ventral primary rami of thoracic nerves 7 to 12.

1. Anterior layer of the rectus sheath

a. Above the arcuate line: aponeuroses of the external and internal oblique muscles

b. Below the arcuate line: aponeuroses of the external oblique, internal oblique, and transverse muscles

2. Posterior layer of the rectus sheath

a. Above the arcuate line: aponeuroses of the internal oblique and transverse muscles

b. Below the arcuate line: rectus abdominis is in contact with the transversalis fascia

IV. Inguinal Region

A. Inguinal (Hesselbach's) triangle

–is bounded medially by the linea semilunaris (lateral edge of the rectus abdominis), laterally by the inferior epigastric vessels, and inferiorly by the inguinal ligament.

–is an area of potential weakness and hence is a common site of a **direct inguinal hernia.**

B. Inguinal rings

1. Superficial inguinal ring

–is a **triangular opening** in the aponeurosis of the external oblique muscle that lies just lateral to the pubic tubercle.

2. Deep inguinal ring

–lies in the transversalis fascia, just lateral to the inferior epigastric vessels.

C. Inguinal canal

–begins at the deep inguinal ring and terminates at the superficial ring.

–transmits the spermatic cord or the round ligament of the uterus and the genital branch of the genitofemoral nerve, both of which also run through the **deep inguinal ring** and the **inguinal canal.** An indirect inguinal hernia (if present) also passes through this canal. Although the ilioinguinal nerve runs through the part of the inguinal canal and the superficial inguinal ring, it does not pass through the deep inguinal ring.

1. **Anterior wall:** aponeuroses of the external oblique and internal oblique muscles

2. **Posterior wall:** aponeurosis of the transverse abdominal muscle and transversalis fascia

3. **Superior wall (roof):** arching fibers of the internal oblique and transverse muscles

4. **Inferior wall (floor):** inguinal and lacunar ligaments

V. Spermatic Cord, Scrotum, and Testis

A. Spermatic cord

–is composed of the **ductus deferens; testicular,** cremasteric, and deferential arteries; pampiniform plexus of **testicular veins; genital branch of the genitofemoral** and cremasteric nerves and the testicular sympathetic plexus; and lymph vessels. These are all conjoined by loose connective tissue.
–has several fasciae:

1. **External spermatic fascia,** derived from the aponeurosis of the external oblique muscle

2. **Cremasteric fascia** (cremaster muscle and fascia), originating in the internal oblique muscle

3. **Internal spermatic fascia,** derived from the transversalis fascia

B. Fetal structures

1. **Processus vaginalis testis**
   –is a **peritoneal diverticulum** in the fetus that evaginates into a developing scrotum and forms the visceral and parietal layers of the **tunica vaginalis testis.**
   –normally closes before birth or shortly thereafter and loses its connection with the peritoneal cavity.
   –may result in a **congenital indirect inguinal hernia** if it persists.
   –may cause **fluid accumulation** (hydrocele processus vaginalis) if it is occluded.

2. **Tunica vaginalis**
   –is a **double serous membrane,** a peritoneal sac that covers the front and sides of the **testis** and **epididymis.**
   –is derived from the abdominal peritoneum and forms the **innermost layer of the scrotum.**

3. **Gubernaculum testis**
   –is the **fetal ligament** that connects the bottom of the fetal testis to the developing scrotum.
   –appears to be important in **testicular descent** (pulls the testis down as it migrates).

–is homologous to the ovarian ligament and the round ligament of the uterus.

VI. Inner Surface of the Anterior Abdominal Wall (Figure 5-3)

A. Supravesical fossa

–is a depression on the anterior abdominal wall between the median and medial umbilical folds of the peritoneum.

B. Medial inguinal fossa

–is a depression on the anterior abdominal wall between the medial and lateral umbilical folds of the peritoneum. It lies lateral to the supravesical fossa.

–is the fossa where most **direct inguinal hernias occur.**

C. Lateral inguinal fossa

–is a depression on the anterior abdominal wall, lateral to the lateral umbilical fold of the peritoneum.

D. Umbilical folds or ligaments

1. Median umbilical ligament or fold

–is a fibrous cord, the remnant of the obliterated **urachus,** which forms a **median umbilical fold** of peritoneum.

–lies between the transversalis fascia and the peritoneum and extends from the apex of the bladder to the umbilicus.

2. Medial umbilical ligament or fold

–is a fibrous cord, the remnant of the **obliterated umbilical artery,** which forms a medial umbilical fold and extends from the side of the bladder to the umbilicus.

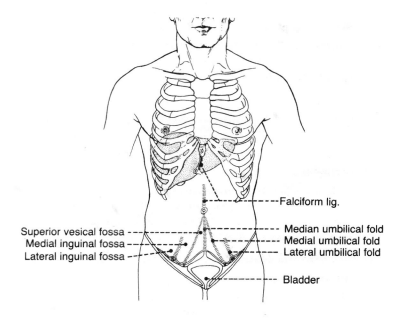

Figure 5-3. Peritoneal folds over the anterior abdominal wall.

3. Lateral umbilical fold

   –is a fold of peritoneum that covers inferior epigastric vessels and extends from the medial side of the deep inguinal ring to the arcuate line.

E. Transversalis fascia

   –is the lining fascia of the entire abdominopelvic cavity between the parietal peritoneum and the inner surface of the abdominal muscles.

   –continues with the diaphragmatic, psoas, iliac, pelvic, and quadratus lumborum fasciae.

   –forms the **deep inguinal ring** and gives rise to the femoral sheath and the internal spermatic fascia.

   –is directly in contact with the rectus abdominis below the arcuate line.

VII. Nerves of the Anterior Abdominal Wall

A. Subcostal nerve

   –is the ventral ramus of the twelfth thoracic nerve and innervates the muscles of the anterior abdominal wall.

   –has a **lateral cutaneous branch** that innervates the skin of the side of the hip.

B. Iliohypogastric nerve

   –arises from the **first lumbar nerve** and innervates the internal oblique and transverse muscles of the abdomen.

   –divides into a **lateral cutaneous branch** to supply the skin of the lateral side of the buttocks and an **anterior cutaneous branch** to supply the skin above the pubis.

C. Ilioinguinal nerve

   –arises from the **first lumbar nerve,** pierces the internal oblique muscle near the deep inguinal ring, and runs medially through the inguinal canal and then through the superficial inguinal ring.

   –innervates the internal oblique and transverse muscles.

   –gives rise to a **femoral branch,** which innervates the upper and medial parts of the thigh, and the **anterior scrotal nerve,** which innervates the skin of the root of the penis (or the skin of the mons pubis) and the anterior part of the scrotum (or the labium majus).

VIII. Lymphatic Drainage of the Anterior Abdominal Wall

A. Lymphatics in the region above the umbilicus drain into the axillary lymph nodes.

B. Lymphatics in the region below the umbilicus drain into the superficial inguinal nodes.

C. Superficial inguinal lymph nodes receive lymph from the lower abdominal wall, buttocks, penis, scrotum, labium majus, and the lower parts of the vagina and anal canal. Their efferent vessels primarily enter the external iliac nodes and, ultimately, the lumbar (aortic) nodes.

IX. Blood Vessels of the Anterior Abdominal Wall

A. Superior epigastric artery

   –arises from the **internal thoracic artery,** enters the rectus sheath, and descends on the posterior surface of the rectus abdominis.

   –anastomoses with the inferior epigastric artery within the rectus abdominis.

B. Inferior epigastric artery

–arises from the **external iliac artery** above the inguinal ligament, enters the rectus sheath, and ascends between the rectus abdominis and the posterior layer of the rectus sheath.

–anastomoses with the superior epigastric artery, providing collateral circulation between the subclavian and external iliac arteries.

–gives rise to the **cremasteric artery,** which accompanies the spermatic cord.

C. Deep circumflex iliac artery

–arises from the **external iliac artery** and runs laterally along the inguinal ligament and the iliac crest between the transverse and internal oblique muscles.

–forms an ascending branch that anastomoses with the **musculophrenic artery.**

D. Superficial epigastric arteries

–arise from the **femoral artery** and run superiorly toward the umbilicus over the inguinal ligament.

–anastomose with branches of the inferior epigastric artery.

E. Superficial circumflex iliac artery

–arises from the **femoral artery** and runs laterally upward, parallel to the inguinal ligament.

–anastomoses with the deep circumflex iliac and lateral femoral circumflex arteries.

F. Superficial (external) pudendal arteries

–arise from the **femoral artery,** pierce the cribriform fascia, and run medially to supply the skin above the pubis.

G. Thoracoepigastric veins

–are longitudinal venous connections between the lateral thoracic vein and the superficial epigastric vein.

–provide a collateral route for venous return if a caval or portal obstruction occurs.

X. Clinical Considerations

A. Inguinal hernia

–occurs superior to the inguinal ligament and medial to the pubic tubercle, whereas a **femoral hernia** occurs inferior to the ligament and lateral to the tubercle.

1. Indirect inguinal hernia

–passes through the deep inguinal ring, inguinal canal, and superficial inguinal ring and descends into the scrotum.

–lies lateral to the inferior epigastric vessels.

–is found more commonly on the right side in men and is more common than a direct inguinal hernia.

–is **congenital** and is associated with the persistence of the processus vaginalis.

–is covered by the peritoneum and the coverings of the spermatic cord.

2. Direct inguinal hernia

–occurs through the **posterior wall of the inguinal canal** (in the region of the inguinal triangle) but does not descend into the scrotum.

–lies medial to the inferior epigastric vessels and protrudes forward to (rarely through) the superficial inguinal ring.

–is **acquired** (develops after birth) and is associated with weakness in the posterior wall of the inguinal canal lateral to the falx inguinalis.

–has a sac that is formed by the peritoneum.

B. Umbilical hernia

–may occur due to failure of the midgut to return to the abdomen early in fetal life **(exomphalos or omphalocele).**

–may also occur as a **protrusion of the bowel or omentum** through the abdominal wall at the umbilicus as a result of incomplete closure of the anterior abdominal wall after ligation of the umbilical cord at birth.

C. Epigastric hernia

–is a **protrusion of extraperitoneal fat or a small piece of greater omentum** through a defect in the linea alba above the umbilicus.

D. Cremasteric reflex

–is a **drawing up of the testis** by contraction of the cremaster muscle when the skin on the upper anteromedial side of the thigh is stroked. The efferent limb (of the reflex arc) is the **genital branch of the genitofemoral nerve;** the afferent limb is **femoral branch of the genitofemoral nerve** and also the ilioinguinal nerve.

Peritoneum and Peritoneal Cavity

I. Peritoneum

–is a **serous membrane** lined by mesothelial cells.

–consists of the **parietal peritoneum** and the **visceral layer.**

A. Parietal peritoneum

–lines the abdominal and pelvic walls and the inferior surface of the diaphragm.

–is innervated by the phrenic, lower intercostal, subcostal, iliohypogastric, and ilioinguinal nerves.

B. Visceral peritoneum

–covers the viscera.

–is innervated by visceral nerves, which travel along autonomic pathways, and is relatively insensitive to pain.

II. Peritoneal Reflections (Figures 5-4 and 5-5)

–support the viscera and provide pathways for associated neurovascular structures.

A. Omentum

1. Lesser omentum

–is a **double layer of peritoneum** extending from the porta hepatis of the liver to the lesser curvature of the stomach and the beginning of the duodenum.

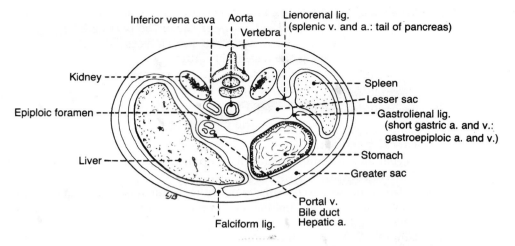

Figure 5-4. Horizontal section of the upper abdomen.

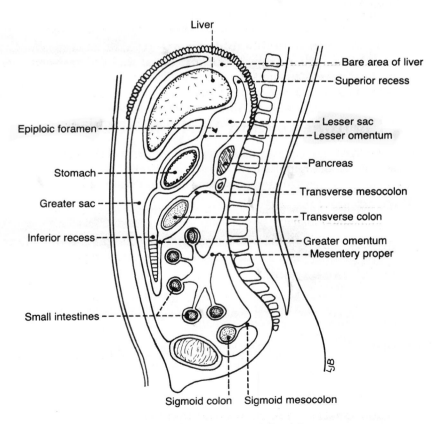

Figure 5-5. Sagittal section of the abdomen.

–consists of the **hepatogastric and hepatoduodenal ligaments** and forms the anterior wall of the lesser sac of the peritoneal cavity.

–acts as a route for the left and right gastric vessels, which run between its two layers along the lesser curvature.

–has a right free margin that contains the **proper hepatic artery, bile duct,** and **portal vein.**

2. Greater omentum

–hangs down like an apron from the greater curvature of the stomach, covering the transverse colon and other abdominal viscera.

–transmits the right and left gastroepiploic vessels along the greater curvature.

–is often referred to by surgeons as the "abdominal policeman" because it plugs the neck of a hernial sac, preventing the entrance of coils of the small intestine.

–adheres to areas of inflammation and wraps itself around the inflamed organs, thus preventing serious diffuse **peritonitis.** Peritonitis is an inflammation of the peritoneum, characterized by an accumulation of peritoneal fluid that contains fibrin and leukocytes (pus).

B. Mesenteries

1. Mesentery of the small intestine (mesentery proper)

–is a fan-shaped **double fold of peritoneum** that suspends the jejunum and ileum from the posterior abdominal wall and transmits nerves and blood vessels to and from the small intestine.

–forms a root that extends from the duodenojejunal flexure to the right iliac fossa and is about 15 cm (6 inches) long.

–has a free border that encloses the **small intestine,** which is about 6 m (20 feet) long.

–contains the superior mesenteric and intestinal (jejunal and ileal) vessels, nerves, and lymphatics.

2. Transverse mesocolon

–connects the posterior surface of the **transverse colon** to the posterior abdominal wall.

–fuses with the greater omentum to form the **gastrocolic ligament.**

–contains the middle colic vessels, nerves, and lymphatics.

3. Sigmoid mesocolon

–is an inverted V-shaped peritoneal fold that connects the **sigmoid colon** to the pelvic wall and contains the sigmoid vessels.

4. Mesoappendix

–connects the **appendix** to the mesentery of the ileum and contains the appendicular vessels.

C. Peritoneal ligaments

1. Lienogastric (gastrosplenic) ligament

–extends from the left portion of the greater curvature of the stomach to the hilus of the spleen.

–contains the short gastric vessels and the left gastroepiploic vessels.

2. Lienorenal (splenorenal) ligament

–runs from the hilus of the spleen to the left kidney.

–contains the splenic vessels and the tail of the pancreas.

3. Gastrophrenic ligament

–runs from the upper part of the greater curvature of the stomach to the diaphragm.

4. Gastrocolic ligament

–runs from the greater curvature of the stomach to the transverse colon.

5. Phrenicocolic ligament

–runs from the colic flexure to the diaphragm.

6. Falciform ligament

–is a **sickle-shaped peritoneal fold** connecting the **liver** to the diaphragm and the anterior abdominal wall.

–appears to demarcate the right lobe from the left lobe of the liver on the diaphragmatic surface.

–contains the **ligamentum teres hepatis** and the **paraumbilical vein,** which connects the left branch of the portal vein with the subcutaneous veins in the region of the umbilicus.

7. Ligamentum teres hepatis (round ligament of the liver)

–lies in the free margin of the falciform ligament and ascends from the umbilicus to the inferior (visceral) surface of the liver, lying in the fissure that forms the left boundary of the quadrate lobe of the liver.

–is formed after birth from the remnant of the **left umbilical vein,** which carries oxygenated blood from the placenta to the left branch of the portal vein in the fetus. (The right umbilical vein is obliterated during the embryonic period.)

8. Coronary ligament

–is a peritoneal reflection from the diaphragmatic surface of the liver onto the diaphragm and encloses a triangular area of the right lobe, the **bare area of the liver.**

–has right and left extensions that form the **right and left triangular ligaments,** respectively.

9. Ligamentum venosum

–is the fibrous remnant of the **ductus venosus.**

–lies in the fissure on the inferior surface of the liver, forming the left boundary of the **caudate lobe of the liver.**

D. Peritoneal folds

–are peritoneal reflections with free edges.

1. Umbilical folds

–are five folds of peritoneum below the umbilicus, including the median, medial, and lateral umbilical folds.

2. Rectouterine fold

–extends from the cervix of the uterus, along the side of the rectum, to the posterior pelvic wall, forming the rectouterine pouch (of Douglas).

3. Ileocecal fold

–extends from the terminal ileum to the cecum.

III. Peritoneal Cavity (see Figures 5-4 and 5-5)

–is a **potential space** between the parietal and visceral peritoneum.

–contains a film of fluid that lubricates the surface of the peritoneum and facilitates free movements of the viscera.

–is a completely closed sac in the male, but it communicates with the exterior through the openings of the uterine tubes in the female.

–is divided into the lesser and greater sacs.

A. Lesser sac (omental bursa)

–is an irregular space that lies behind the liver, lesser omentum, stomach, and upper anterior part of the greater omentum.

–is a closed sac, except for its communication with the greater sac through the **epiploic foramen.**

–presents three recesses:

1. Superior recess

–lies behind the stomach, lesser omentum, and liver.

2. Inferior recess

–lies behind the stomach, extending into the layers of the greater omentum.

3. Splenic recess

–extends to the left at the hilus of the spleen.

B. Greater sac

–extends across the entire breadth of the abdomen and from the diaphragm to the pelvic floor.

–presents numerous recesses into which pus from an abscess may be drained:

1. Subphrenic (suprahepatic) recess

–is a peritoneal pocket between the diaphragm and the anterior and superior part of the liver.

–is separated into right and left recesses by the **falciform ligament.**

2. Subhepatic recess

–is a peritoneal pocket between the liver and the transverse colon.

3. Hepatorenal recess

–is a deep peritoneal pocket between the liver anteriorly and the kidney and suprarenal gland posteriorly.

4. Morison's pouch

–is formed by the right subhepatic recess and the hepatorenal recess.

–communicates with the subphrenic recess, the lesser sac via the epiploic foramen, and the right paracolic gutter, thus the pelvic cavity.

5. Paracolic recesses (gutters)

–lie lateral to the ascending colon (right paracolic gutter) and lateral to the descending colon (left paracolic gutter).

C. Epiploic (Winslow's) foramen

–is a natural opening between the lesser and greater sacs.

–is bounded superiorly by peritoneum on the caudate lobe of the liver, inferiorly by peritoneum on the first part of the duodenum, anteriorly by the free edge of the lesser omentum, and posteriorly by peritoneum covering the inferior vena cava.

Gastrointestinal (GI) Viscera

I. Stomach (Figures 5-6, 5-7, and 5-8; see Figure 5-20)

–rests, in the supine position, on the **stomach bed,** which is formed by the pancreas, spleen, left kidney, left suprarenal gland, transverse colon and its mesocolon, and diaphragm.

–is covered entirely by peritoneum and is located in the left hypochondriac and epigastric regions of the abdomen.

–has **greater and lesser curvatures,** anterior and posterior walls, cardiac and pyloric openings, and cardiac and angular notches.

–is divided into four regions: **cardia, fundus, body,** and **pylorus.** The fundus lies inferior to the apex of the heart at the level of the fifth rib. The pylorus is divided into the **pyloric antrum** and **pyloric canal.** The pyloric orifice is surrounded by the **pyloric sphincter,** which is a group of thickened circular smooth muscles and controls the rate of discharge of stomach contents into the duodenum.

–receives blood from the right and left gastric, right and left gastroepiploic, and short gastric arteries.

–undergoes contraction, which is characterized by the appearance of longitudinal folds of mucous membrane, the **rugae.** The **gastric canal,** a grooved channel along the lesser curvature formed by the rugae, directs fluids toward the pylorus.

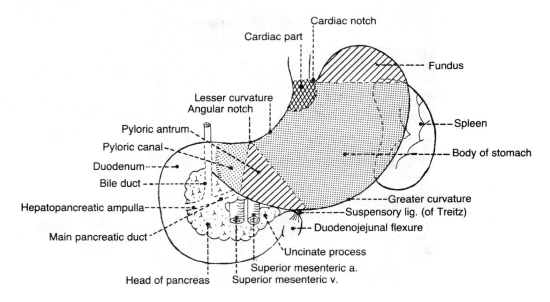

Figure 5-6. Stomach and duodenum.

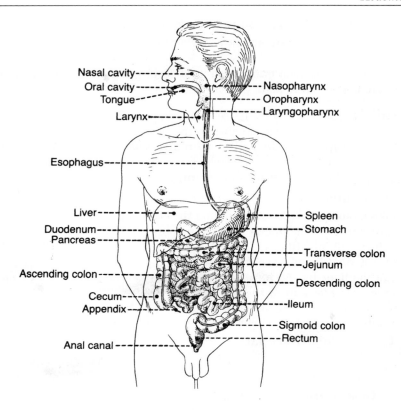

Figure 5-7. Diagram of the digestive system.

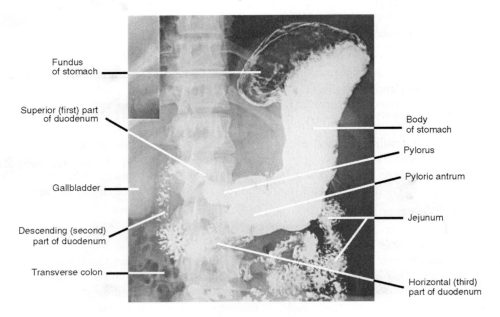

Figure 5-8. Radiograph of the stomach and small intestines.

–produces **hydrochloric acid** (which destroys many organisms present in food and drink) and **pepsin** (which converts proteins to polypeptides) in its fundus and body.

–produces the hormone **gastrin** in its pyloric antrum. Parasympathetic fibers in the vagus nerve stimulate gastric secretion.

II. Small Intestine (see Figures 5-7, 5-8, and 5-20)

–extends from the pyloric opening to the ileocecal junction.

–is the location of **complete digestion and absorption** of most of the products of digestion, as well as water, electrolytes, and minerals such as calcium and iron.

–consists of the **duodenum, jejunum,** and **ileum.**

A. Duodenum

–is a **C-shaped tube** surrounding the head of the pancreas and is the shortest [25 cm (10 inches) long or 12 finger-breadths in length] but widest part of the small intestine.

–is retroperitoneal except for the beginning of the first part, which is connected to the liver by the **hepatoduodenal ligament** of the lesser omentum.

–receives blood from the celiac (foregut) and superior mesenteric (midgut) artery.

–is divided into four parts:

1. Superior (first) part

–has a mobile or free section, termed the **duodenal cap** (because of its appearance on radiographs), into which the pylorus invaginates.

2. Descending (second) part

–contains the **junction of the foregut and midgut,** where the **common bile and main pancreatic ducts** open.

–contains the **greater papilla,** on which terminal openings of the bile and main pancreatic ducts are located, and the **lesser papilla,** which lies 2 cm above the greater papilla and marks the site of entry of the **accessory pancreatic duct.**

3. Transverse (third) part

–is the longest part and crosses the inferior vena cava, aorta, and vertebral column to the left.

–is crossed anteriorly by the superior mesenteric vessels.

4. Ascending (fourth) part

–ascends to the left of the aorta to the level of the second lumbar vertebra and terminates at the duodenojejunal junction, which is fixed in position by the **suspensory ligament (of Treitz),** a surgical landmark. This fibromuscular band is attached to the right crus of the diaphragm.

B. Jejunum

–makes up the proximal two-fifths of the small intestine (the ileum makes up the distal three-fifths).

–is emptier, larger in diameter, and thicker-walled than the ileum.

–has the **plicae circulares** (circular folds), which are tall and closely packed.

–contains no Peyer's patches (aggregations of lymphoid tissue).

–has translucent areas called **windows** between the blood vessels of its mesentery.

–has less prominent **arterial arcades** (anastomotic loops) in its mesentery compared with the ileum.

–has longer **vasa recta** (straight arteries, or arteriae rectae) compared with the ileum.

C. Ileum

–is longer than the jejunum and occupies the **false pelvis** in the right lower quadrant of the abdomen.

–is characterized by the presence of **Peyer's patches** (lower portion), shorter plicae circulares and vasa recta, and more mesenteric fat and arterial arcades when compared with the jejunum.

III. Large Intestine (see Figures 5-7 and 5-20)

–extends from the ileocecal junction to the anus and is approximately 1.5 m (5 feet) long.

–consists of the **cecum, appendix, colon, rectum,** and **anal canal.**

–functions to convert the liquid contents of the ileum into semisolid feces by **absorbing water as well as salts and electrolytes.** It also **lubricates feces** with mucus.

A. Colon

–has **ascending** and **descending** colons that are retroperitoneal, and **transverse** and **sigmoid** colons that are surrounded by peritoneum (they have their own mesenteries, the **transverse mesocolon** and the **sigmoid mesocolon,** respectively). The ascending and transverse colons are supplied by the superior mesenteric artery and the vagus nerve; the descending and sigmoid colons are supplied by the inferior mesenteric artery and the pelvic splanchnic nerves.

–is characterized by the following:

1. **Teniae coli:** three narrow bands of the outer longitudinal muscular coat

2. **Sacculations or haustra:** produced by the teniae, which are slightly shorter than the gut

3. **Epiploic appendages:** peritoneum-covered sacs of fat, attached in rows along the teniae

B. Cecum

–is the **blind pouch of the large intestine.** It lies in the right iliac fossa and is usually surrounded by peritoneum.

C. Appendix

–is a **narrow, hollow, muscular tube** with large aggregations of lymphoid tissue in its wall.

–is suspended from the terminal ileum by a small mesentery, the **mesoappendix,** which contains the appendicular vessels.

–causes spasm and distention when inflamed, resulting in **pain** that is referred to the epigastrium.

–has a base that lies deep to **McBurney's point,** which occurs at the junction of the lateral one-third of a line between the right anterior–superior iliac spine and the umbilicus. This is the site of maximum tenderness in **acute appendicitis.**

D. Rectum and anal canal

–extend from the sigmoid colon to the anus.

–are described as **pelvic organs** (see Chapter 6, Pelvis: VIII).

IV. Accessory Organs of the Digestive System

A. Liver (Figures 5-9 and 5-10; see Figure 5-20)

–is the **largest visceral organ** and the **largest gland** in the body.

–plays an important role in **bile production and secretion; detoxification** (by filtering the blood to remove bacteria and foreign particles that have gained entrance from the intestine); **storage** of carbohydrate as **glycogen; protein synthesis** from amino acids; **production of heparin** (anticoagulant) and **bile pigments** (bilirubin and biliverdin) from the breakdown of hemoglobin; and storage of vitamin, iron, and copper. In the fetus, the liver is important in the manufacture of red blood cells.

–is surrounded by the peritoneum and is attached to the diaphragm by the **coronary and falciform ligaments** and the right and left **triangular ligaments.**

–has a **bare area** on the diaphragmatic surface, which is limited by layers of the coronary ligament but is devoid of peritoneum.

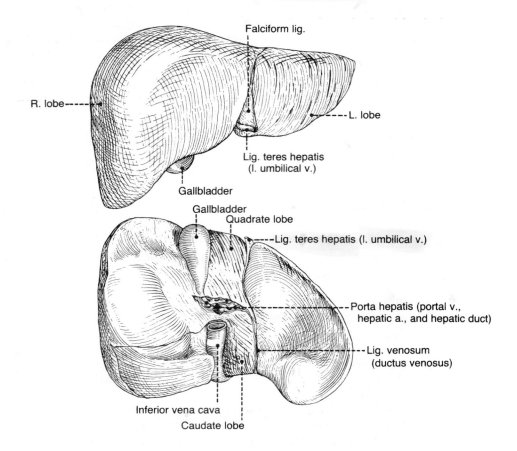

Figure 5-9. Anterior and visceral surfaces of the liver.

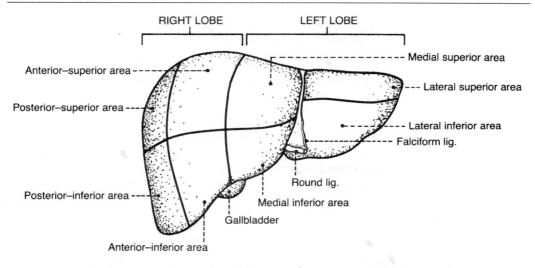

RIGHT LOBE   LEFT LOBE

Anterior–superior area - - - -

Posterior–superior area - - -

Posterior–inferior area - - -

Anterior–inferior area

Medial superior area

Lateral superior area

Lateral inferior area

Falciform lig.

Round lig.

Medial inferior area

Gallbladder

Figure 5-10. Divisions of the liver, based on hepatic drainage and blood supply.

—receives oxygenated blood from the hepatic artery and deoxygenated, nutrient-rich, sometimes toxic blood from the portal vein; its venous blood is drained by the hepatic veins into the inferior vena cava.

—appears to be divided into the right and left lobes on the diaphragmatic surface by the coronary ligament. (These lobes serve as landmarks but do not correspond to the functional units or hepatic segments.)

—is divided, on the basis of hepatic drainage and blood supply, into the **right and left lobes** by the fossae for the gallbladder and the inferior vena cava.

1. **Lobes of the liver**

   a. **Right lobe**

      —is divided into **anterior** and **posterior segments,** each of which is subdivided into superior and inferior areas or segments.

   b. **Left lobe**

      —is divided into **medial** and **lateral segments,** each of which is subdivided into superior and inferior areas (segments).

      —includes the **medial superior (caudate lobe), medial inferior (quadrate lobe), lateral superior,** and **lateral inferior segments.** The **quadrate lobe** receives blood from the left hepatic artery and drains bile into the left hepatic duct, whereas the **caudate lobe** receives blood from the right and left hepatic arteries and drains bile into both right and left hepatic ducts.

2. **Fissures and ligaments of the liver**

   —include an H-shaped group of fissures:

   a. Fissure for the round ligament (**ligamentum teres hepatis**), located between the left lobe and the quadrate lobe

   b. Fissure for the **ligamentum venosum,** located between the left lobe and the caudate lobe

   c. Fossa for the **gallbladder,** located between the quadrate lobe and the major part of the right lobe

d. Fissure for the **inferior vena cava,** located between the caudate lobe and the major part of the right lobe

e. Porta hepatis. This **transverse fissure on the visceral surface** of the liver between the quadrate and caudate lobes lodges the **hepatic ducts, hepatic arteries**, branches of the **portal vein**, hepatic nerves, and lymphatic vessels.

B. Gallbladder (Figure 5-11; see Figures 5-8 and 5-20)

–is located at the junction of the right ninth costal cartilage and lateral border of the rectus abdominis, which is the site of maximum tenderness in acute inflammation of the gallbladder.

–is a **pear-shaped sac** lying on the inferior surface of the liver in a fossa between the right and quadrate lobes with a capacity of about 30–50 ml. It is in contact with the duodenum and transverse colon.

–consists of the **fundus** (the rounded blind end); the **body** (the major part); and the **neck** (the narrow part), which gives rise to the **cystic duct** with **spiral valves** (Heister's valves).

–receives bile, concentrates it by absorbing water and salts, and serves as a reservoir for it.

–**contracts to expel bile** as a result of stimulation by the hormone **cholecystokinin,** which is produced by the duodenal mucosa when food arrives in the duodenum.

–receives blood from the cystic artery, which arises from the right hepatic artery within the **cystohepatic triangle (of Calot),** which is formed by the visceral surface of the liver superiorly, the cystic duct inferiorly, and the common hepatic duct medially.

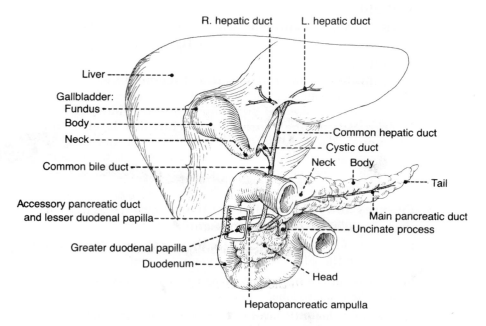

Figure 5-11. Extrahepatic bile passages and pancreatic ducts.

C. Pancreas (see Figures 5-11 and 5-20)

–lies largely in the floor of the lesser sac in the epigastric and left hypochondriac regions, where it forms a major portion of the stomach bed.

–is a retroperitoneal organ except for a small portion of its **tail,** which lies in the **lienorenal ligament.**

–has a **head** that lies within the C-shaped concavity of the duodenum. If tumors are present in the head, bile flow is obstructed, resulting in **jaundice.** Bile pigments accumulate in the blood, giving the skin and eyes a characteristic yellow coloration.

–has an **uncinate process,** which is a projection of the lower part of the head to the left side behind the superior mesenteric vessels.

–receives blood from branches of the splenic artery and from the superior and inferior pancreaticoduodenal arteries.

–is both an **exocrine gland,** which produces digestive enzymes, and an **endocrine gland,** which secretes two hormones, insulin and glucagon.

–has two ducts, the **main pancreatic duct** and the **accessory pancreatic duct.**

1. Main pancreatic duct (duct of Wirsung)

–begins in the tail and runs to the right along the entire pancreas.

–joins the bile duct to form the **hepatopancreatic ampulla (ampulla of Vater)** before entering the second part of the duodenum at the greater papilla.

2. Accessory pancreatic duct (Santorini's duct)

–begins in the lower portion of the head and drains a small portion of the head and body.

–empties at the lesser duodenal papilla about 2 cm above the greater papilla.

D. Duct system for bile passage (see Figure 5-11)

1. Right and left hepatic ducts

–are formed by union of the **intrahepatic ductules** from each lobe of the liver.

–**drain bile** from the corresponding halves of the liver.

2. Common hepatic duct

–is formed by union of the right and left hepatic ducts.

–is accompanied by the proper hepatic artery and the portal vein.

3. Cystic duct

–has spiral folds (valves) to keep it constantly open, and thus bile can pass upward into the **gallbladder** when the common bile duct is closed.

–runs alongside the hepatic duct before joining the common hepatic duct.

–is a common site of impaction of **gallstones.**

4. Common bile duct (ductus choledochus)

–is formed by union of the common hepatic duct and the cystic duct.

–is located lateral to the proper hepatic artery and anterior to the portal vein in the right free margin of the lesser omentum.

–descends behind the first part of the duodenum and runs through the head of the pancreas.

–joins the main pancreatic duct to form the **hepatopancreatic duct (hepatopancreatic ampulla),** which enters the second part of the duodenum at the greater papilla.

–contains the **sphincter of Boyden,** which is a circular muscle layer around the lower end of the duct.

5. Hepatopancreatic duct or ampulla (ampulla of Vater)

–is formed by the union of the common bile duct and the main pancreatic duct and enters the second part of the duodenum at the greater papilla. This represents the junction of the embryonic foregut and midgut.

–contains the **sphincter of Oddi,** which is a circular muscle layer around it in the greater duodenal papilla.

V. Spleen (see Figure 5-20)

–is a **large lymphatic organ** lying against the diaphragm and ribs 9 to 11 in the left hypochondriac region.

–is developed in the dorsal mesogastrium and supported by the **lienogastric and lienorenal ligaments.**

–is composed of **white pulp,** which consists of lymphatic nodules and diffuse lymphatic tissue, and **red pulp,** which consists of venous sinusoids connected by splenic cords.

–is **hematopoietic** in early life and later **destroys aged (i.e., worn-out) red blood cells.**

–**filters blood** (removes particulate matter and cellular residue from the blood), **stores red blood cells,** and **produces lymphocytes and antibodies.**

–is supplied by the splenic artery and is drained by the splenic vein.

–is frequently ruptured by fractured ribs or severe blows to the left hypochondrium. Repair of a ruptured spleen is difficult.

–may be removed surgically with minimal effect on body function because its functions are assumed by other reticuloendothelial organs.

VI. Celiac and Mesenteric Arteries

A. Celiac trunk (Figure 5-12)

–arises from the front of the abdominal aorta immediately below the aortic hiatus of the diaphragm, between the right and left crura.

–divides into the left gastric, splenic, and common hepatic arteries.

1. Left gastric artery

–is the **smallest branch** of the celiac trunk.

–runs upward and to the left toward the cardia, giving rise to **esophageal and hepatic branches,** and then turns to the right and runs along the lesser curvature within the lesser omentum to anastomose with the right gastric artery.

2. Splenic artery

–is the **largest branch** of the celiac trunk.

–runs a highly tortuous course along the superior border of the pancreas and enters the lienorenal ligament.

–gives rise to the following:

a. A number of pancreatic branches, including the **dorsal pancreatic artery**

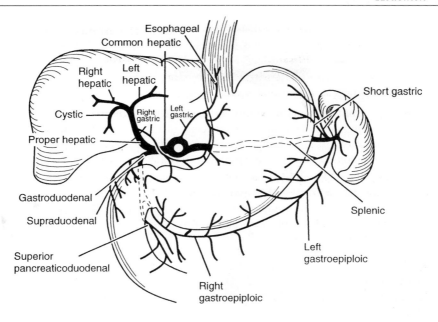

Figure 5-12. Branches of the celiac trunk.

b. A few **short gastric arteries,** which pass through the lienogastric ligament to reach the fundus of the stomach

c. The **left gastroepiploic artery,** which reaches the greater omentum through the lienogastric ligament and runs along the greater curvature of the stomach to distribute to the stomach and greater omentum

3. Common hepatic artery

–runs to the right along the upper border of the pancreas and divides into the proper hepatic artery, the gastroduodenal artery, and possibly the right gastric artery.

a. Proper hepatic artery

–ascends in the free edge of the lesser omentum and divides, near the porta hepatis, into the **left and right hepatic arteries;** the right hepatic artery gives rise to the **cystic artery,** which supplies the gallbladder.

–gives rise, near its beginning, to the right gastric artery.

b. Right gastric artery

–runs to the pylorus and then along the lesser curvature of the stomach and anastomoses with the left gastric artery.

c. Gastroduodenal artery

–descends behind the first part of the duodenum, giving off the supraduodenal artery to its superior aspect and a few retroduodenal arteries to its inferior aspect.

–divides into two major branches:

(1) The **right gastroepiploic artery** runs to the left along the greater curvature of the stomach, supplying the stomach and the greater omentum.

(2) The **superior pancreaticoduodenal artery** passes between the duodenum and the head of the pancreas and further divides into the anterior–superior pancreaticoduodenal artery and the posterior–superior pancreaticoduodenal artery.

B. Superior mesenteric artery (Figure 5-13)

–arises from the aorta behind the neck of the pancreas.

–descends across the uncinate process of the pancreas and the third part of the duodenum and then enters the root of the mesentery behind the transverse colon to run to the right iliac fossa.

–gives rise to the following branches:

1. Inferior pancreaticoduodenal artery

–passes to the right and divides into the anterior–inferior pancreaticoduodenal artery and the posterior–inferior pancreaticoduodenal artery, which

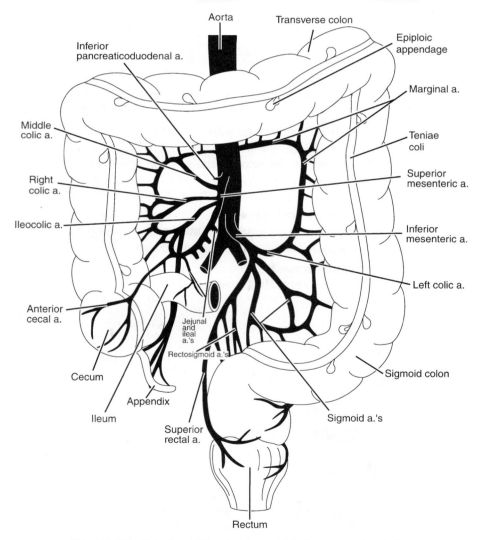

Figure 5-13. Branches of the superior and inferior mesenteric arteries.

anastomose with the corresponding branches of the superior pancreatico-duodenal artery.

2. Middle colic artery

–enters the transverse mesocolon and divides into the **right branch,** which anastomoses with the right colic artery, and the **left branch,** which anastomoses with the ascending branch of the left colic artery. The branches of the mesenteric arteries form an anastomotic channel, the **marginal artery,** along the large intestine.

3. Ileocolic artery

–descends behind the peritoneum toward the right iliac fossa and ends by dividing into the **ascending colic artery,** which anastomoses with the right colic artery, **anterior and posterior cecal arteries, the appendicular artery,** and **ileal branches.**

4. Right colic artery

–arises from the superior mesenteric artery or the ileocolic artery.
–runs to the right behind the peritoneum and divides into **ascending and descending branches,** distributing to the ascending colon.

5. Intestinal arteries

–are 12 to 15 in number and supply the jejunum and ileum.
–branch and anastomose to form a series of arcades in the mesentery.

C. Inferior mesenteric artery (see Figure 5-13)

–passes to the left behind the peritoneum and distributes to the descending and sigmoid colons and the upper portion of the rectum.
–gives rise to:

1. Left colic artery

–runs to the left behind the peritoneum toward the descending colon and divides into **ascending and descending branches.**

2. Sigmoid arteries

–are two to three in number, run toward the sigmoid colon in its mesentery, and divide into **ascending and descending branches.**

3. Superior rectal artery

–is the **termination of the inferior mesenteric artery,** descends into the pelvis, divides into two branches that follow the sides of the rectum, and anastomoses with the middle and inferior rectal arteries. (The middle and inferior rectal arteries arise from the internal iliac and internal pudendal arteries, respectively.)

VII. Hepatic Portal Venous System

–is a system of vessels in which blood collected from the intestinal capillaries passes through the portal vein and then through the liver capillary sinusoids before reaching to the inferior vena cava (systemic circulation).

A. Portal vein (Figure 5-14; see Figure 5-20)

–drains the abdominal part of the gut, spleen, pancreas, and gallbladder and is 8 cm (3.2 inches) long.
–is formed by the union of the **splenic vein** and the **superior mesenteric vein** posterior to the neck of the pancreas. The **inferior mesenteric vein**

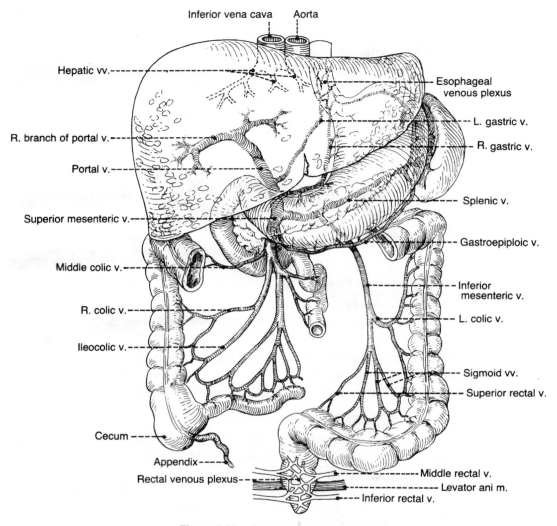

Figure 5-14. Portal venous system.

joins either the splenic or the superior mesenteric vein or the junction of these two veins.

–receives the **left gastric (or coronary) vein.**

–carries deoxygenated blood containing nutrients.

–carries twice as much blood as the hepatic artery and maintains a higher blood pressure than in the inferior vena cava.

–ascends behind the bile duct and hepatic artery within the free margin of the lesser omentum.

1. Superior mesenteric vein

–accompanies the superior mesenteric artery on its right side in the root of the mesentery.

–crosses the third part of the duodenum and the uncinate process of the pancreas and terminates posterior to the neck of the pancreas by joining the splenic vein, thereby forming the portal vein.

–has tributaries that are some of the veins that accompany the branches of the superior mesenteric artery.

2. Splenic vein

–is formed by the union of tributaries from the spleen.

–receives the short gastric, left gastroepiploic, and pancreatic veins.

3. Inferior mesenteric vein

–is formed by the union of the superior rectal and sigmoid veins.

–receives the left colic vein.

4. Left gastric (coronary) vein

–drains normally into the portal vein.

–has **esophageal tributaries** that anastomose with the esophageal veins of the azygos system at the lower part of the esophagus and thereby enter the systemic venous system.

5. Paraumbilical veins

–are found in the **falciform ligament** and are virtually closed; however, they dilate in **portal hypertension.**

–connect the left branch of the portal vein with the small subcutaneous veins in the region of the umbilicus, which are radicles of the superior epigastric, inferior epigastric, thoracoepigastric, and superficial epigastric veins.

B. Important portal-caval (systemic) anastomoses

–occur between:

1. The left gastric vein and the esophageal vein of the azygos system

2. The superior rectal vein and the middle and inferior rectal veins

3. The paraumbilical veins and radicles of the epigastric (superficial and inferior) veins

4. The retroperitoneal veins draining the colon and twigs of the renal, suprarenal, and gonadal veins

VIII. Clinical Considerations

A. Gastric ulcer

–erodes the mucosa and penetrates the gastric wall to various depths.

–may perforate into the lesser sac and erode the pancreas and the splenic artery, causing **fatal hemorrhage.**

B. Duodenal ulcer

–penetrates the wall of the superior (first) part of the duodenum, erodes the gastroduodenal artery, and is commonly located in the **duodenal cap**.

C. Pyloric stenosis

–is narrowing of the gastric pylorus as the result of congenital muscular hypertrophy or an acquired scar from peptic ulceration or pyloric carcinoma.

D. Meckel's diverticulum

–is an **outpouching** (finger-like pouch) of the **ileum** located **2 feet** proximal to the ileocecal junction on the **antimesenteric side**; it is about **2 inches** long and occurs in about **2%** of the population.

–represents persistent portions of the **embryonic yolk stalk** (vitelline or omphalomesenteric duct) and may be free or connected to the umbilicus via a fibrous cord or a fistula.

–may contain **two types** of mucosal (gastric and pancreatic) **tissues** in its wall.

–is clinically important because **bleeding** may occur from an ulcer in its wall.

E. Liver cirrhosis

–is a condition in which liver cells are progressively destroyed and replaced by fibrous tissue that surrounds the intrahepatic blood vessels and biliary radicles, impeding the circulation of blood through the liver.

–causes **portal hypertension,** resulting in esophageal varices, hemorrhoids, and caput medusae.

F. Portal hypertension

–results from **thrombosis of the portal vein** or **liver cirrhosis.**

–causes a dilatation of veins in the lower part of the esophagus, forming **esophageal varices.** Their rupture results in vomiting of blood **(hematemesis).**

–results in **caput medusae** (dilated veins radiating from the umbilicus), which occurs because the paraumbilical veins enclosed in the free margin of the falciform ligament anastomose with branches of the epigastric (superficial and inferior) veins around the umbilicus.

–may result in **hemorrhoids** because of enlargement of veins around the anal canal.

–can be reduced by diverting blood from the portal to the caval system; this is accomplished by anastomosing the splenic vein to the renal vein or by creating a communication between the portal vein and the inferior vena cava.

G. Gallstones (choleliths)

–are formed by solidification of bile constituents, composed chiefly of **cholesterol crystals,** usually mixed with bile pigments and calcium.

–present commonly in **f**at, **f**ertile (multiparous) **f**emales who are over 40 (**f**orty) years of age (**4-F** individuals).

–may become lodged in three sites:

1. Fundus of the gallbladder

–may ulcerate through the wall of the gallbladder into the transverse colon or into the duodenum. In the former case, they are passed naturally to the rectum, but in the latter case they may be held up at the **ileocecal junction,** producing an **intestinal obstruction.**

2. Common bile duct

–obstructs bile flow to the duodenum, leading to **jaundice.**

3. Hepatopancreatic ampulla

–blocks both the biliary and the pancreatic duct systems. In this case, bile may enter the pancreatic duct system, causing aseptic or noninfectious **pancreatitis.**

H. Megacolon (Hirschsprung's disease)

–is caused by the **absence of enteric ganglia in the lower part of the colon,** which leads to dilatation of the colon proximal to the inactive segment.

–is of **congenital** origin and is usually diagnosed during infancy and childhood; symptoms are constipation, abdominal distention, and vomiting.

Retroperitoneal Viscera, Diaphragm, and Posterior Abdominal Wall

I. Kidney, Ureter, and Suprarenal Gland

A. Kidney (Figure 5-15; see Figure 5-20)

–is retroperitoneal and extends from L1–L4 in the erect position. The right kidney lies a little lower than the left, owing to the large size of the right lobe of the liver, and usually is related to rib 12 posteriorly. The left kidney is related to ribs 11 and 12 posteriorly.

–is invested by a firm, fibrous **renal capsule.**

–is surrounded by the **renal fascia,** which divides the fat into two regions. The **perirenal (perinephric) fat** lies in the **perinephric space** between the renal capsule and renal fascia, and the **pararenal (paranephric) fat** lies external to the renal fascia.

–has an indentation, the **hilus,** on its medial border, through which the ureter, renal vessels, and nerves enter or leave the organ.

–consists of the **medulla** and the **cortex,** containing one to two million **nephrons,** which are the anatomical and functional units of the kidney. Each nephron consists of a **renal corpuscle, a proximal convoluted tubule, Henle's loop,** and a **distal convoluted tubule.**

–has arterial segments including the **superior, anterosuperior, anteroinferior, inferior,** and **posterior segments,** which are of surgical importance.

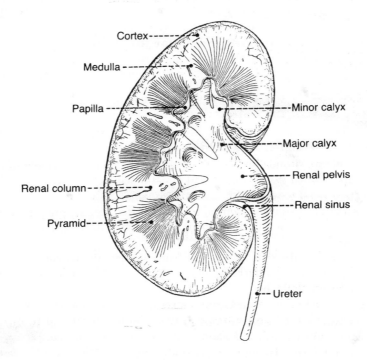

Figure 5-15. Frontal section of the kidney.

–produces and excretes urine, maintains electrolyte (ionic) balance, and produces vasoactive substances that control blood pressure.

1. Cortex

–forms the outer part of the kidney and also projects into the medullary region between the renal pyramids as **renal columns.**

–contains renal corpuscles and proximal and distal convoluted tubules. The **renal corpuscle** consists of a tuft of capillaries, the glomerulus, surrounded by a **glomerular capsule,** which is the invaginated blind end of the nephron.

2. Medulla

–forms the inner part of the kidney and consists of 8 to 12 **renal pyramids** (of Malpighi), which contain straight tubules (**Henle's loops**) and **collecting tubules.** An apex of the renal pyramid, the **renal papilla,** fits into the cup-shaped **minor calyx** on which the collecting tubules open.

3. Minor calyces

–receive urine from the collecting tubules and empty into two or three **major calyces,** which in turn empty into an upper dilated portion of the ureter, the **renal pelvis.**

B. Ureter

–is a **muscular tube** that extends from the kidney to the **urinary bladder.**

–is retroperitoneal, descends on the psoas muscle, is crossed anteriorly by the gonadal vessels, and crosses the bifurcation of the common iliac artery.

–may be obstructed by renal calculi (kidney stones) where it joins the renal pelvis (**ureteropelvic junction**), where it crosses the pelvic brim over the distal end of the common iliac artery, or where it enters the wall of the urinary bladder (**ureterovesicular junction**).

–receives blood from the aorta and from the renal, gonadal, common and internal iliac, umbilical, superior and inferior vesical, and middle rectal arteries.

–is innervated by the lumbar (sympathetic) and pelvic (parasympathetic) splanchnic nerves.

C. Suprarenal (adrenal) gland

–is a retroperitoneal organ lying on the superomedial aspect of the kidney. It is surrounded by a capsule and renal fascia.

–is pyramidal on the right and semilunar on the left.

–has a **cortex** that is essential to life and produces steroid hormones, including mineralocorticoids (aldosterone), glucocorticoids (e.g., cortisone), and sex hormones.

–has a **medulla** that is derived from embryonic neural crest cells, receives preganglionic sympathetic nerve fibers directly, and secretes epinephrine and norepinephrine.

–receives arteries from three sources: the superior suprarenal artery from the **inferior phrenic artery;** the middle suprarenal from the abdominal **aorta;** and the inferior suprarenal artery from the **renal artery.**

–is drained via the suprarenal vein, which empties into the **inferior vena cava** on the right and the **renal vein** on the left.

II. Posterior Abdominal Blood Vessels and Lymphatics

A. Aorta (Figure 5-16)

–passes through the **aortic hiatus** in the diaphragm at the level of T12, descends anterior to the vertebral bodies, and bifurcates into the **right and left common iliac arteries** anterior to L4.

–gives rise to the following:

1. Inferior phrenic arteries

–arise from the aorta immediately below the aortic hiatus, supply the diaphragm, and give rise to the **superior suprarenal arteries.**

–diverge across the crura of the diaphragm, with the left artery passing posterior to the esophagus and the right passing posterior to the inferior vena cava.

2. Middle suprarenal arteries

–arise from the aorta and run laterally on the crura of the diaphragm just superior to the renal arteries.

3. Renal arteries

–arise from the aorta inferior to the origin of the superior mesenteric artery. The right artery is longer and a little lower than the left and passes posterior to the inferior vena cava; the left artery passes posterior to the left renal vein.

–give rise to the **inferior suprarenal and ureteric arteries.**

–divide into the superior, anterosuperior, anteroinferior, inferior, and posterior segmental branches.

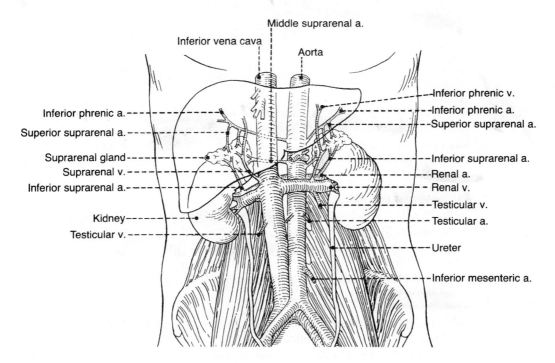

Figure 5-16. Abdominal aorta and its branches.

4. **Testicular or ovarian arteries**

–descend retroperitoneally and run laterally on the psoas major muscle and across the ureter.

a. The **testicular artery** accompanies the ductus deferens into the scrotum, where it supplies the spermatic cord, epididymis, and testis.

b. The **ovarian artery** enters the suspensory ligament of the ovary, supplies the ovary, and anastomoses with the ovarian branch of the uterine artery.

5. **Lumbar arteries**

–consist of four or five pairs that arise from the back of the aorta.

–run posterior to the sympathetic trunk, the inferior vena cava (on the right side), the psoas major muscle, the lumbar plexus, and the quadratus lumborum.

–divide into smaller anterior branches (to supply adjacent muscles) and larger posterior branches, which accompany the dorsal primary rami of the corresponding spinal nerves and divide into spinal and muscular branches.

6. **Middle sacral artery**

–arises from the back of the aorta, just above its bifurcation; descends on the front of the sacrum; and ends in the coccygeal body.

–supplies the rectum and anal canal, and it anastomoses with the lateral sacral and superior and inferior rectal arteries.

B. **Inferior vena cava**

–is formed on the right side of L5 by the union of the two **common iliac veins,** below the bifurcation of the aorta.

–is longer than the abdominal aorta and ascends along the right side of the aorta.

–passes through the **opening for the inferior vena cava** in the central tendon of the diaphragm at the level of T8 and enters the right atrium of the heart.

–receives the right gonadal, suprarenal, and inferior phrenic veins. On the left side, these veins usually drain into the left renal vein.

–also receives the three (left, middle, and right) **hepatic veins.** The middle and left hepatic veins frequently unite for about 1 cm before entering the vena cava.

C. **Cisterna chyli**

–is the lower dilated end of the **thoracic duct** and lies just to the right and posterior to the aorta, usually between two crura of the diaphragm.

–is formed by the **intestinal and lumbar lymph trunks.**

III. Nerves of the Posterior Abdominal Wall

A. **Lumbar plexus** (Figure 5-17)

–is formed by the union of the ventral rami of the first three lumbar nerves and a part of the fourth lumbar nerve.

–lies anterior to the transverse processes of the lumbar vertebrae within the substance of the psoas muscle.

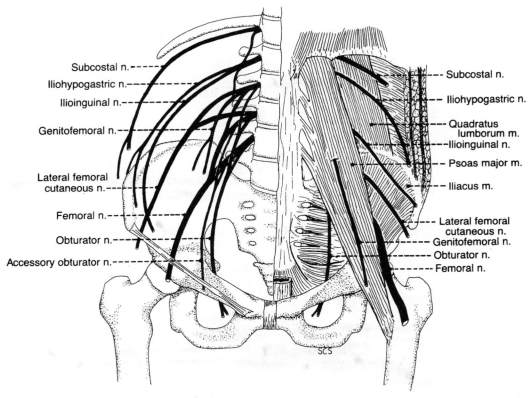

Figure 5-17. Lumbar plexus.

1. **Subcostal nerve (T12)**
   –runs behind the lateral lumbocostal arch and in front of the quadratus lumborum.
   –penetrates the transverse abdominal muscle to run between it and the internal oblique muscle.
   –innervates the **external oblique, internal oblique, transverse, rectus abdominis,** and **pyramidalis muscles.**

2. **Iliohypogastric nerve (L1)**
   –emerges from the lateral border of the psoas muscle and runs in front of the quadratus lumborum.
   –pierces the transverse abdominal muscle near the iliac crest to run between this muscle and the internal oblique muscle.
   –pierces the internal oblique muscle and then continues medially deep to the external oblique muscle.
   –innervates the internal oblique and transverse muscles of the abdomen and divides into an **anterior cutaneous branch,** which innervates the skin above the pubis, and a **lateral cutaneous branch,** which innervates the skin of the gluteal region.

3. **Ilioinguinal nerve (L1)**
   –runs in front of the quadratus lumborum, piercing the transverse and then the internal oblique muscle to run between the internal and external oblique aponeuroses.

–accompanies the **spermatic cord (or the round ligament of the uterus),** continues through the inguinal canal, and emerges through the superficial inguinal ring.

–innervates the internal oblique and transverse muscles and gives off **femoral cutaneous branches** to the upper medial part of the thigh and **anterior scrotal or labial branches.**

4. **Genitofemoral nerve (L1–L2)**

–emerges on the front of the psoas muscle and descends on its anterior surface.

–divides into a **genital branch,** which enters the inguinal canal through the deep inguinal ring to supply the cremaster muscle and the scrotum (or labium majus), and a **femoral branch,** which supplies the skin of the femoral triangle.

5. **Lateral femoral cutaneous nerve (L2–L3)**

–emerges from the lateral side of the psoas muscle and runs in front of the iliacus and behind the inguinal ligament.

–innervates the skin of the anterior and lateral thigh.

6. **Femoral nerve (L2–L4)**

–emerges from the lateral border of the psoas major and descends in the groove between the psoas and iliacus.

–enters the femoral triangle deep to the inguinal ligament and lateral to the femoral vessels, outside the femoral sheath, and divides into numerous branches.

–innervates the skin of the thigh and leg, the muscles of the front of the thigh, and the hip and knee joints.

–innervates the quadriceps femoris, pectineal, and sartorius muscles and gives rise to the **anterior femoral cutaneous nerve** and the **saphenous nerve.**

7. **Obturator nerve (L2–L4)**

–arises from the second, third, and fourth lumbar nerves and descends along the medial border of the psoas muscle. It runs forward on the lateral wall of the pelvis and enters the thigh through the **obturator foramen.**

–divides into **anterior and posterior branches** and innervates the adductor group of muscles, the hip and knee joints, and the skin of the medial side of the thigh.

8. **Accessory obturator nerve (L3–L4)**

–is present in about 9% of the population.

–descends medial to the psoas muscle, passes over the superior pubic ramus, and supplies the hip joint and the pectineal muscle.

9. **Lumbosacral trunk**

–is formed by the lower part of the fourth lumbar nerve and all of the fifth lumbar nerve, which enters into the formation of the sacral plexus.

B. **Autonomic nerves in the abdomen** (Figure 5-18; see Figure 4-16)

1. **Autonomic ganglia**

a. **Sympathetic chain (paravertebral) ganglia**

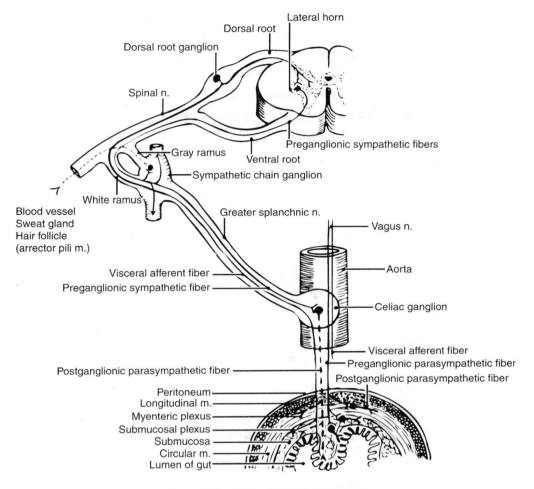

Figure 5-18. Nerve supply to the viscera.

–are composed primarily of ascending and descending preganglionic sympathetic [general visceral efferent (GVE)] fibers and (general) visceral afferent (GVA) fibers.

–also contain cell bodies of the postganglionic sympathetic fibers.

b. Collateral (prevertebral) ganglia

–include the celiac, superior mesenteric, aorticorenal, and inferior mesenteric ganglia, usually located near the origin of the respective arteries.

–are formed by cell bodies of the postganglionic sympathetic fibers.

–receive preganglionic sympathetic fibers by way of the **greater, lesser,** and **least splanchnic nerves.**

2. Splanchnic nerves

a. Thoracic splanchnic nerves

–contain preganglionic sympathetic (GVE) fibers with cell bodies located in the lateral horn (intermediolateral cell column) of the spinal cord as well as GVA fibers with cell bodies located in the dorsal root ganglia.

–The greater splanchnic nerve enters the celiac ganglion, the lesser splanchnic nerve enters the aorticorenal ganglion, and the least splanchnic nerve joins the renal plexus.

b. Lumbar splanchnic nerves

–arise from the lumbar sympathetic trunks and join the celiac, mesenteric, aortic, and superior hypogastric plexuses.
–contain preganglionic sympathetic and GVA fibers.

3. Autonomic plexuses

a. Celiac plexus

–is formed by splanchnic nerves and branches from the vagus nerves.
–also contains the **celiac ganglia,** which receive the greater splanchnic nerves.
–lies on the front of the crura of the diaphragm and on the abdominal aorta at the origins of the celiac trunk and the superior mesenteric and renal arteries.
–extends along the branches of the celiac trunk and forms the **subsidiary plexuses,** which are named according to the arteries along which they pass, such as gastric, splenic, hepatic, suprarenal, and renal plexuses.

b. Aortic plexus

–extends from the celiac plexus along the front of the aorta.
–extends its branches along the arteries and forms plexuses that are named accordingly—superior mesenteric, testicular (or ovarian), and inferior mesenteric.
–continues along the aorta and forms the **superior hypogastric plexus** just below the bifurcation of the aorta.

c. Superior and inferior hypogastric plexuses

4. Enteric division

–consists of the **myenteric (Auerbach's) plexus,** which is located chiefly between the longitudinal and circular muscle layers, and the **submucosal (Meissner's) plexus,** which is located in the submucosa. Both parts consist of preganglionic and postganglionic parasympathetic fibers, postganglionic sympathetic fibers, GVA fibers, and cell bodies of postganglionic parasympathetic fibers.
–have sympathetic nerves that inhibit gastrointestinal (GI) motility and secretion; parasympathetic nerves stimulate GI motility and secretion.

IV. The Diaphragm and its Openings

A. Diaphragm (Figures 5-19 and 5-20)

–arises from the xiphoid process (sternal part), lower six costal cartilages (costal part), medial and lateral lumbocostal arches (lumbar part), vertebrae L1–L3 for the right crus, and vertebrae L1–L2 for the left crus.
–inserts into the **central tendon** and is the principal muscle of inspiration.
–receives somatic motor fibers solely from the phrenic nerve; its central part receives sensory fibers from the phrenic nerve, whereas the peripheral part receives sensory fibers from the intercostal nerves.

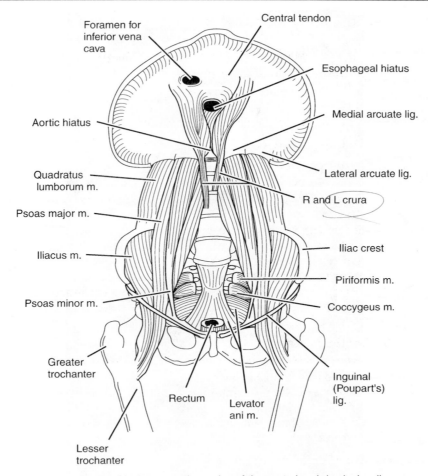

Figure 5-19. Diaphragm and muscles of the posterior abdominal wall.

–receives blood from the musculophrenic, pericardiophrenic, superior phrenic, and inferior phrenic arteries.

–descends when it contracts, causing an increase in thoracic volume by increasing the vertical diameter of the thoracic cavity and thus resulting in a decreased intrathoracic pressure.

–ascends when it relaxes, causing a decrease in thoracic volume with an increased thoracic pressure.

1. **Right crus**

   –is larger and longer than the left crus.
   –originates from vertebrae L1–L3 (the left crus originates from L1–L2).
   –splits to enclose the esophagus.

2. **Medial arcuate ligament (medial lumbocostal arch)**

   –extends from the body of L1 to the transverse process of L1 and passes over the psoas muscle and the sympathetic trunk.

3. **Lateral arcuate ligament (lateral lumbocostal arch)**

   –extends from the transverse process of L1 to rib 12 and passes over the quadratus lumborum.

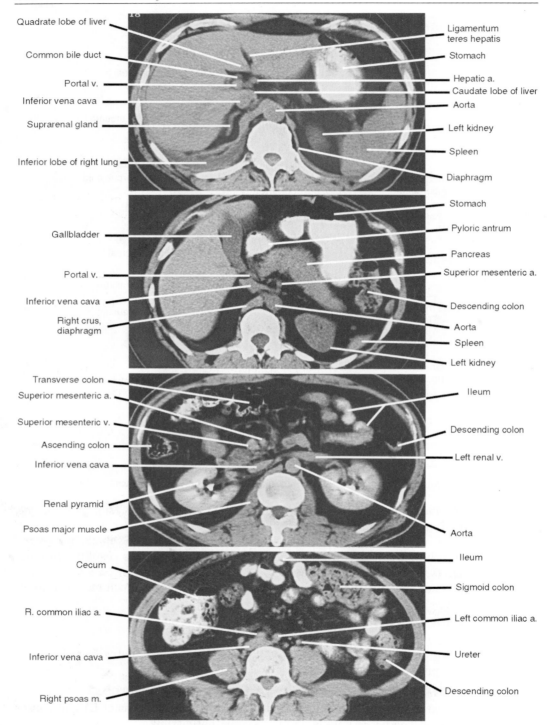

Quadrate lobe of liver
Common bile duct
Portal v.
Inferior vena cava
Suprarenal gland
Inferior lobe of right lung

Ligamentum teres hepatis
Stomach
Hepatic a.
Caudate lobe of liver
Aorta
Left kidney
Spleen
Diaphragm

Stomach
Pyloric antrum
Gallbladder
Pancreas
Portal v.
Superior mesenteric a.
Inferior vena cava
Descending colon
Right crus, diaphragm
Aorta
Spleen
Left kidney

Transverse colon
Superior mesenteric a.
Ileum
Superior mesenteric v.
Descending colon
Ascending colon
Inferior vena cava
Left renal v.
Renal pyramid
Psoas major muscle
Aorta

Ileum
Cecum
Sigmoid colon
R. common iliac a.
Left common iliac a.
Inferior vena cava
Ureter
Right psoas m.
Descending colon

Figure 5-20. Computed tomography (CT) scans of the abdomen at different levels.

B. Apertures through the diaphragm

1. Vena caval hiatus (vena caval foramen)

–lies in the central tendon of the diaphragm at the level of T8 and transmits the inferior vena cava and the right phrenic nerve.

2. Esophageal hiatus

–lies in the muscular part of the diaphragm (right crus) at the level of T10 and transmits the esophagus and anterior and posterior trunks of the vagus nerves.

3. Aortic hiatus

–lies behind or between two crura at the level of T12 and transmits the aorta, thoracic duct, greater splanchnic nerve, and azygos vein.

V. Muscles of the Posterior Abdominal Wall (Table 5-2)

Table 5–2. Muscles of the Posterior Abdominal Wall

Muscle	Origin	Insertion	Nerve	Action
Quadratus lumborum	Transverse processes of L3–L5; iliolumbar ligament; iliac crest	Lower border of last rib; transverse processes of L1–L3	Subcostal n.; L1–L3	Depresses rib 12; flexes trunk laterally
Psoas major	Transverse processes, intervertebral disks and bodies of T12–L5	Lesser trochanter	L2–L3	Flexes thigh and trunk
Psoas minor	Bodies and intervertebral disks of T12–L1	Pectineal line; iliopectineal eminence	L1	Aids in flexing of trunk

VI. Clinical Considerations

A. Renal disorders

1. Horseshoe kidney

–develops as a result of **fusion of the lower poles of two kidneys.**
–may obstruct the urinary tract by its **impingement on the ureters.**

2. Congenital polycystic disease of kidneys

–is a heritable disorder characterized by **numerous cysts** scattered throughout the kidneys.
–is caused by a failure of the collecting tubules to join a calyx, which causes **dilations of the loops of Henle**, resulting in progressive renal dysfunction.
–may be treated by hemodialysis and kidney transplant.

3. Pelvic kidney

–is an **ectopic kidney** that occurs when kidneys fail to ascend and thus remain in the pelvis. Two pelvic kidneys may fuse to form a solid lobed organ due to fusion of the renal anlagen, called a **cake (rosette) kidney.**

4. **Nephroptosis**

   –is downward displacement or **floating of the kidney** caused by loss of supporting fat.

   –occurs frequently among truck drivers, horseback riders, and motorcyclists.

   –may cause a **kink in the ureter** or **compression of the ureter** by an aberrant inferior polar artery, resulting in hydronephrosis.

5. **Hydronephrosis**

   –is **distention of the renal pelvis and calyces** with accumulating urine as a result of obstruction of the ureter.

   –is caused by **renal calculi,** which may lodge within and obstruct a ureter or occlude a renal calyx.

   –may occur in a pregnant woman because the **developing fetus exerts pressure on the ureter** as it crosses the pelvic brim, obstructing urine flow.

B. **Renal transplantation**

   –is performed through a transabdominal (traditionally retroperitoneal) approach to the kidney by connecting the donor renal vessels to the recipient's external iliac vessels and suturing the donor ureter into the urinary bladder.

C. **Esophageal (hiatal) hernia**

   –is a herniation of a part of the stomach through the esophageal hiatus of the diaphragm into the pleural cavity.

   –is caused by an abnormally large esophageal hiatus.

   –may cause vomiting in an infant when it is laid on its back after feeding.

Review Test

Directions: Each of the numbered items or incomplete statements in this section is followed by answers or by completions of the statement. Select the **one** lettered answer or completion that is **best** in each case.

1. An aneurysm of the abdominal aorta at the aortic hiatus of the diaphragm is most likely to result in compression of which of the following pairs of structures?

(A) Vagus nerve and azygos vein
(B) Esophagus and vagus nerve
(C) Azygos vein and thoracic duct
(D) Thoracic duct and vagus nerve
(E) Inferior vena cava and phrenic nerve

2. A 36-year-old woman with yellow pigmentation of the skin and sclerae presents at the outpatient clinic. Which of the following conditions most likely causes obstructive jaundice?

(A) Aneurysm of the splenic artery
(B) Perforated ulcer of the stomach
(C) Damage to the pancreas during splenectomy
(D) Cancer in the head of the pancreas
(E) Cancer in the body of the pancreas

3. If the transversalis fascia has been damaged during development, which of the following structures on the anterior abdominal wall is defective?

(A) Superficial inguinal ring
(B) Deep inguinal ring
(C) Inguinal ligament
(D) Sac of a direct inguinal hernia
(E) Anterior wall of the inguinal canal

4. Lack of preganglionic parasympathetic fibers in the liver may result from a lesion in which of the following nerves?

(A) Phrenic nerve
(B) Lumbar splanchnic nerve
(C) Intercostal nerve
(D) Vagus nerve
(E) Greater splanchnic nerve

5. Destruction of cell bodies of efferent and afferent nerve fibers in visceral branches (splanchnic nerves) of the sympathetic trunk affects which of the following locations?

(A) Ventral horn of the spinal cord; collateral ganglia
(B) Lateral horn of the spinal cord; dorsal root ganglia
(C) Ventral horn of the spinal cord; dorsal root ganglia
(D) Dorsal horn of the spinal cord; sympathetic chain ganglia
(E) Lateral horn of the spinal cord; sympathetic chain ganglia

6. If an abdominal infection spreads retroperitoneally, which of the following structures is most likely affected?

(A) Stomach
(B) Transverse colon
(C) Jejunum
(D) Descending colon
(E) Spleen

7. Which of the following types of nerve fibers stimulates the suprarenal medulla to secrete norepinephrine?

(A) Preganglionic sympathetic fibers
(B) Postganglionic sympathetic fibers
(C) Somatic motor fibers
(D) Postganglionic parasympathetic fibers
(E) Preganglionic parasympathetic fibers

8. Hirschsprung's disease (aganglionic megacolon) is a congenital disease characterized by a dysfunctional distal portion of the colon, which results in an inability to evacuate the bowels. This condition is caused by an absence of which of the following kinds of neural cell bodies?

(A) Sympathetic preganglionic neuron cell bodies
(B) Sympathetic postganglionic neuron cell bodies
(C) Parasympathetic preganglionic neuron cell bodies
(D) Parasympathetic postganglionic neuron cell bodies
(E) Sensory neuron cell bodies

9. Which of the following fetal vessels becomes the round ligament of the liver after birth?

(A) Ductus venosus
(B) Paraumbilical vein
(C) Umbilical artery
(D) Ductus arteriosus
(E) Umbilical vein (left)

10. Which of the following pairs of veins typically terminates in the same vein?

(A) Left and right ovarian veins
(B) Left and right gastroepiploic veins
(C) Left and right colic veins
(D) Left and right suprarenal veins
(E) Left and right hepatic veins

11. A small tumor located anterior to the inferior vena cava would most likely damage which of the following structures?

(A) Right sympathetic trunk
(B) Left third lumbar artery
(C) Third part of the duodenum
(D) Left renal artery
(E) Cisterna chyli

12. A male patient with a perforated gastric ulcer complains of excruciating pain in his epigastrium. If the pain comes from peritoneal irritation by gastric contents in the lesser sac, which of the following nerves contains the fibers that convey this sharp, stabbing pain?

(A) Vagus nerve
(B) Greater splanchnic nerve
(C) Lower intercostal nerve
(D) White rami communicantes
(E) Gray rami communicantes

13. Which of the following nerves would carry afferent impulses of the cremasteric reflex?

(A) Subcostal nerve
(B) Lateral femoral cutaneous nerve
(C) Genitofemoral nerve
(D) Iliohypogastric nerve
(E) Femoral nerve

14. Injury to both the superior mesenteric artery and the vagus nerve affects which portion of the colon?

(A) Ascending and descending segments
(B) Transverse and sigmoid segments
(C) Descending and sigmoid segments
(D) Ascending and transverse segments
(E) Transverse and descending segments

15. A 42-year-old man with portal hypertension resulting from cirrhosis of the liver presents to the emergency department. The most practical method of shunting portal blood around the liver involves which of the following surgical connections?

(A) Superior mesenteric vein to the inferior mesenteric vein
(B) Portal vein to the superior vena cava
(C) Portal vein to the left renal vein
(D) Splenic vein to the left renal vein
(E) Superior rectal vein to the left colic vein

16. Rapid occlusion of direct branches of which of the following arteries results in ischemia of the suprarenal glands?

(A) Aorta; splenic and inferior phrenic arteries
(B) Renal, splenic, and inferior mesenteric arteries
(C) Aorta; inferior phrenic and renal arteries
(D) Superior mesenteric, inferior mesenteric, and renal arteries
(E) Aorta; hepatic and renal arteries

17. A radiograph of a 32-year-old woman reveals a perforation in the posterior wall of the stomach in which the gastric contents have spilled into the lesser sac. The abdominal surgeon who opened the lienogastric (gastrosplenic) ligament to reach the lesser sac cut an artery accidentally. Which of the following vessels is most likely to be injured?

(A) Splenic artery
(B) Gastroduodenal artery
(C) Left gastric artery
(D) Right gastric artery
(E) Left gastroepiploic artery

18. Which of following nerves carries pain sensation caused by irritation of the peritoneum on the central portion of the inferior surface of the diaphragm?

(A) Vagus nerve
(B) Lower intercostal nerve
(C) Phrenic nerve
(D) Greater splanchnic nerve
(E) Subcostal nerve

19. Soon after ligation of the splenic artery just distal to its origin, a surgical resident observes normal blood flow in which of the following arteries?

(A) Short gastric arteries
(B) Dorsal pancreatic artery
(C) Inferior pancreaticoduodenal artery
(D) Left gastroduodenal artery
(E) Artery in the lienorenal ligament

20. During an appendectomy performed at Mc-Burney's point, which of the following structures is most likely to be injured?

(A) Deep circumflex femoral artery
(B) Inferior epigastric artery
(C) Iliohypogastric nerve
(D) Genitofemoral nerve
(E) Spermatic cord

21. Which of the following characteristics is associated with the portal vein or the portal venous system?

(A) Lower blood pressure than in the inferior vena cava
(B) Least risk of venous varices at the lower end of the esophagus as a result of portal hypertension
(C) Distention of the portal vein due to its numerous valves
(D) Caput medusae and hemorrhoids caused by portal hypertension
(E) Less blood flow than in the hepatic artery

22. A physician who is trying to distinguish the jejunum from the ileum has observed that the jejunum has

(A) fewer plicae circulares
(B) fewer mesenteric arterial arcades
(C) less digestion and absorption of nutrients
(D) shorter vasa recta
(E) more fat in its mesentery

23. In a patient with portal hypertension, which of the following veins is most likely to be dilated?

(A) Right colic vein
(B) Inferior epigastric vein
(C) Inferior phrenic vein
(D) Suprarenal vein
(E) Ovarian vein

24. A 26-year-old patient is admitted to the university hospital with a retroperitoneal infection. Which of the following arteries is most likely to be infected?

(A) Left gastric artery
(B) Proper hepatic artery
(C) Middle colic artery
(D) Sigmoid arteries
(E) Dorsal pancreatic artery

25. A pediatric surgeon has cut a structure that is not related to embryonic or fetal blood vessels in a 5-year-old child. Which of the following structures is most likely to be divided?

(A) Lateral umbilical fold
(B) Medial umbilical fold
(C) Ligamentum venosum
(D) Ligamentum teres hepatis
(E) Ligamentum arteriosum

26. An obstruction of the inferior mesenteric vein just before joining the splenic vein is most likely to enlarge which of the following veins?

(A) Middle colic vein
(B) Right colic vein
(C) Inferior pancreaticoduodenal vein
(D) Ileocolic vein
(E) Left colic vein

27. An acute infection involving the dartos muscle most likely leads to an enlargement of which of the following lymph nodes?

(A) Preaortic nodes
(B) Lumbar nodes
(C) External iliac nodes
(D) Superficial inguinal nodes
(E) Common iliac nodes

28. The liver

(A) receives blood only from the hepatic arteries
(B) manufactures red blood cells in an adult
(C) drains bile from the quadrate lobe into the right hepatic duct
(D) drains venous blood into the hepatic veins
(E) functions to concentrate and store bile

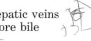

29. The common bile duct

(A) drains bile into the second part of the duodenum
(B) can be blocked by cancer in the body of the pancreas
(C) joins the main pancreatic duct, which carries hormones
(D) is formed by union of the right and left hepatic duct
(E) lies posterior to the portal vein in the right free edge of the lesser omentum

30. The sigmoid colon

(A) is drained by systemic veins
(B) is a retroperitoneal organ
(C) receives parasympathetic preganglionic fibers from the vagus nerve
(D) receives its blood from the superior mesenteric artery
(E) has teniae coli and epiploic appendages

31. To cut off the blood supply to the appendix (if collateral circulation is discounted), a surgeon ligates which of the following arteries?

(A) Middle colic artery
(B) Right colic artery
(C) Ileocolic colic artery
(D) Inferior mesenteric artery
(E) Common iliac artery

32. During gastrocolostomy, a surgeon is ligating all arteries that send branches to the stomach. Which of the following arteries may be spared?

(A) Splenic artery
(B) Gastroduodenal artery
(C) Inferior pancreaticoduodenal artery
(D) Left gastroepiploic artery
(E) Proper hepatic artery

33. Loss of pain sensation from the abdominal viscera may result from a lesion of which of the following structures?

(A) Greater splanchnic nerve
(B) Ventral roots of the spinal nerve
(C) Lower intercostal nerve
(D) Vagus nerve
(E) Gray ramus communicans

34. The aponeurosis of the transverse abdominal muscle most likely contributes to the formation of which of the following?

(A) Linea alba
(B) Anterior layer of rectus sheath above the umbilicus
(C) Posterior layer of rectus sheath below the arcuate line
(D) Lacunar ligament
(E) Internal spermatic fascia

35. A tumor located at the porta hepatis most likely compresses which of the following structures?

(A) Cystic duct
(B) Hepatic veins
(C) Common hepatic artery
(D) Left gastric artery
(E) Branches of the portal vein

36. Which of the following pairs of veins is considered a portal-caval anastomosis?

(A) Hepatic veins and inferior vena cava
(B) Superior and middle rectal vein
(C) Left and right gastric veins
(D) Inferior and superficial epigastric veins
(E) Suprarenal and renal veins

37. The Meckel's diverticulum

(A) is found 2 feet distal to the ileocecal junction
(B) is located on the mesenteric side of the ileum
(C) occurs in about 10% of the population
(D) is a persistent remnant of the embryonic yolk sac
(E) may contain renal and suprarenal tissues

38. A slowly growing tumor in the uncinate process of the pancreas most likely compresses which of the following structures?

(A) Main pancreatic duct
(B) Splenic artery
(C) Portal vein
(D) Superior mesenteric artery
(E) Superior pancreaticoduodenal artery

39. Diagnosis of a direct inguinal hernia requires that the herniated tissue

(A) enters the deep inguinal ring
(B) lies lateral to the inferior epigastric artery
(C) is covered by spermatic fasciae
(D) descends into the scrotum
(E) develops after birth

40. The genitofemoral nerve

(A) runs in front of the quadratus lumborum
(B) is a branch of the femoral nerve
(C) supplies the testis
(D) passes through the deep inguinal ring
(E) gives rise to an anterior scrotal branch

41. The quadrate lobe of the liver

(A) lies between the inferior vena cava and ligamentum venosum
(B) receives blood from the right and left hepatic arteries
(C) drains bile into the left hepatic duct
(D) is a medial superior segment
(E) is functionally a part of the right lobe

42. Obstruction of the inferior vena cava may result in dilatation of which of the following veins?

(A) Left suprarenal vein
(B) Left ascending lumbar vein
(C) Left hepatic vein
(D) Left gastric vein
(E) Portal vein

43. Which of the following structures defines the lateral margin of the rectus abdominis?

(A) Linea alba
(B) Linea semilunaris
(C) Linea semicircularis
(D) Transversalis fascia
(E) Falx inguinalis

44. Severance of which of the following ligaments may damage the paraumbilical vein?

(A) Lienorenal ligament
(B) Lienogastric ligament
(C) Gastrophrenic ligament
(D) Falciform ligament
(E) Hepatoduodenal ligament

45. A knife wound has cut an artery that runs along the superior border of the pancreas. Which of the following arteries is injured?

(A) Right gastric artery
(B) Left gastroepiploic artery
(C) Splenic artery
(D) Gastroduodenal artery
(E) Dorsal pancreatic artery

46. The vagal parasympathetic innervation of the gastrointestinal (GI) tract terminates approximately at which of the following structures?

(A) Duodenojejunal junction
(B) Ileocecal junction
(C) Right colic flexure
(D) Left colic flexure
(E) Anorectal junction

47. Which of the following structures is located between the celiac trunk and the superior mesenteric artery?

(A) Spleen and body of the stomach
(B) Pyloric canal and neck of the pancreas
(C) Transverse colon and ileum
(D) Kidney and head of the pancreas
(E) Duodenal cap and cecum

48. The internal oblique abdominis muscle contributes to the formation of which of the following structures?

(A) Inguinal ligament
(B) Deep inguinal ring
(C) Falx inguinalis
(D) Internal spermatic fascia
(E) Reflected inguinal ligament

49. Laceration of the superior mesenteric artery immediately inferior to the origin of the middle colic artery may reduce blood supply to the

(A) descending colon
(B) duodenum
(C) pancreas
(D) ascending colon
(E) spleen

50. Which of the following statements concerning the kidney and associated structures is correct?

(A) The left kidney lies a bit lower than the right one
(B) The perirenal fat lies external to the renal fascia
(C) The renal fascia does not surround the suprarenal gland
(D) The left renal vein runs anterior to both the aorta and the left renal artery
(E) The right renal artery is shorter than the left one

Directions: Each set of matching questions in this section consists of a list of four to twenty-six lettered options (some of which may be in figures) followed by several numbered items. For each numbered item, select the ONE lettered option that is most closely associated with it. To avoid spending too much time on matching sets with large numbers of options, it is generally advisable to begin each set by reading the list of options. Then, for each item in the set, try to generate the correct answer and locate it in the option list, rather than evaluating each option individually. Each lettered option may be selected once, more than once, or not at all.

Questions 51–55

Match each of the following descriptions with the most appropriate lettered structure in the computed tomography (CT) scan of the abdomen at the level of the twelfth thoracic vertebra.

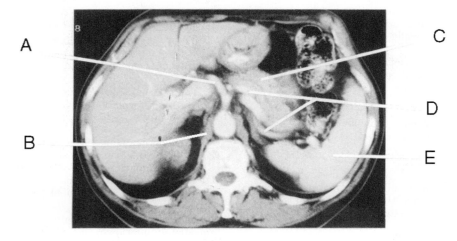

51. Structure that is hematopoietic in early life and later destroys worn-out red blood cells

52. Structure that runs along the superior border of the pancreas and enters the lienorenal ligament

53. Structure that is divided into the proper hepatic and gastroduodenal arteries

54. Structure that provides an attachment of the suspensory muscle of the duodenum (ligament of Treitz)

55. Structure that is retroperitoneal in position and receives blood from the splenic artery

Questions 56–60

Match each of the following descriptions with the most appropriate lettered structure in the computed tomography (CT) scan of the abdomen at the level of the upper lumbar vertebra.

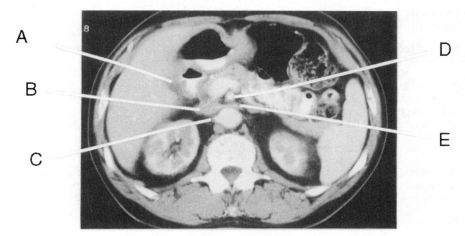

56. Structure that is a direct branch of the aorta and supplies blood to the ascending and transverse colons *D*

57. Structure that receives blood from the liver and kidney and enters the thorax by piercing the central tendon of the diaphragm *C?*

58. Structure that receives bile, concentrates it by absorbing water and salt, and stores it *A*

59. Structure that receives blood from the left gonad and suprarenal gland *E?*

60. Structure that runs behind the inferior vena cava

Answers and Explanations

1-C. The aortic hiatus of the diaphragm transmits the azygos vein and thoracic duct. The vagus nerve passes through the esophageal hiatus, and the right phrenic nerve runs through the vena caval hiatus.

2-D. Because the bile duct traverses the head of the pancreas, cancer in the head of the pancreas obstructs the bile duct, resulting in jaundice.

3-B. The deep inguinal ring lies in the transversalis fascia, just lateral to the inferior epigastric vessels. The superficial inguinal ring is in the aponeurosis of the external oblique muscle. The inguinal ligament and the anterior wall of the inguinal canal are formed by the aponeurosis of the external oblique muscle. The sac of a direct inguinal hernia is formed by the peritoneum.

4-D. The vagus nerves carry preganglionic parasympathetic fibers to the liver.

5-B. The cell bodies of the (general) visceral efferent (GVE) fibers are located in the intermediolateral cell column (or lateral horn) of the spinal cord. The cell bodies of (general) visceral afferent (GVA) fibers are located in the dorsal root ganglia.

6-D. The descending colon is a retroperitoneal organ.

7-A. The suprarenal medulla is the only organ that receives preganglionic sympathetic fibers.

8-D. Aganglionic megacolon (Hirschsprung's disease) is caused by the absence of enteric ganglia (parasympathetic postganglionic neuron cell bodies) in the lower part of the colon, which leads to dilatation of the colon proximal to the inactive segment.

9-E. The left umbilical vein becomes the round ligament of the liver after birth.

10-E. The right and left hepatic veins drain into the inferior vena cava. The right gastroepiploic vein drains into the superior mesenteric vein, but the left one drains into the splenic vein. The right gonadal and suprarenal veins drain into the inferior vena cava, whereas the left ones drain into the left renal vein. The right colic vein ends in the superior mesenteric vein, but the left one terminates in the inferior mesenteric vein.

11-C. The third part of the duodenum (transverse portion) crosses anterior to the inferior vena cava.

12-C. The parietal peritoneum receives pain fibers though the phrenic, lower intercostal, subcostal, iliohypogastric, and ilioinguinal nerves. However, the visceral peritoneum is innervated by visceral nerves and is relatively insensitive to pain. Lower intercostal (somatic) nerves carry an excruciating pain caused by irritation of the parietal peritoneum by gastric contents. The greater splanchnic nerves and white rami communicantes contain pain fibers, which are visceral afferent fibers. The gray rami communicantes contain no sensory fibers.

13-C. Stimulation of the cremaster muscle draws the testis up from the scrotum toward the superficial inguinal ring. The efferent limb of the reflex arc is the genital branch of the genitofemoral nerve, whereas the afferent limb is the femoral branch of the genitofemoral nerve.

14-D. The ascending and transverse colons receive blood from the superior mesenteric artery parasympathetic nerve fibers from the vagus nerve. However, the descending and sigmoid colons receive blood from the inferior mesenteric artery and parasympathetic nerve fibers from the pelvic splanchnic nerve arising from sacral spinal nerves (S2–S4).

15-D. Portal hypertension can be reduced by diverting blood from the portal to the caval system. This is accomplished by connecting the splenic vein to the left renal vein or by creating a communication between the portal vein and the inferior vena cava.

16-C. The suprarenal gland receives arteries from three sources. The superior suprarenal artery arises from the inferior phrenic artery, the middle suprarenal artery arises from the abdominal aorta, and the inferior suprarenal artery arises from the renal artery.

17-E. The left gastroepiploic artery runs through the lienogastric ligament to reach the greater omentum.

18-C. The diaphragm receives somatic motor fibers solely from the phrenic nerves. However, the central part of the diaphragm receives sensory fibers from the phrenic nerve, and the peripheral part of the diaphragm receives such fibers from the intercostal nerves.

19-C. The inferior pancreaticoduodenal artery is a branch of the superior mesenteric artery.

20-C. The iliohypogastric nerve runs medially and inferiorly between the internal oblique and transverse abdominal muscles at McBurney's point, the point midway between the anterior–superior iliac spine and the umbilicus.

21-D. Portal hypertension can cause esophageal varices, caput medusa, and hemorrhoids. The portal vein has higher pressure than systemic veins, the vein and its tributaries have no valves, or, if present, they are insignificant. In addition, the portal vein carries at least twice as much blood as the hepatic artery.

22-B. The ileum has more mesenteric arterial arcades than the jejunum. The plicae circulares (circular folds) in the upper part of the ileum are less prominent than those in the jejunum, but the lower part of the ileum has no plicae circulares. More digestion and absorption of nutrients occurs in the jejunum than in the ileum and longer vasa recta, but less fat is found in its mesentery.

23-A. The right colic vein empties into the superior mesenteric vein, which joins the splenic vein to form the portal vein. The inferior epigastric, inferior phrenic, suprarenal, and ovarian veins belong to the systemic (or caval) venous system and drain directly or indirectly into the inferior vena cava.

24-E. The pancreas is a retroperitoneal organ, except for a small portion of its tail; thus, the dorsal pancreatic artery arising from the splenic artery runs along the superior border of the pancreas behind the peritoneum.

25-A. The lateral umbilical fold (ligament) contains the inferior epigastric artery and vein, which are adult blood vessels. The medial umbilical fold, ligamentum venosum, ligamentum teres hepatis, and ligamentum arteriosum contain fibrous remnants of the umbilical artery, ductus venosus, left umbilical vein, and ductus arteriosus, respectively.

26-E. The left colic vein is a tributary of the inferior mesenteric vein. The middle colic, right colic, inferior pancreaticoduodenal, and ileocolic veins drain into the superior mesenteric vein.

27-D. The superficial inguinal lymph nodes receive lymph from the scrotum, penis, buttocks, and lower part of the anal canal, and their efferent vessels enter primarily to the external iliac nodes and ultimately to the lumbar (aortic) nodes. The dartos muscle forms part of the scrotal layer. The deep inguinal nodes receive lymph from the testis and upper parts of the vagina and anal canal, and their efferent vessels enter the external iliac nodes.

28-D. The liver receives blood from the hepatic artery and portal vein, and drains venous blood into the hepatic veins. The liver plays important roles in bile production and secretion. The quadrate lobe drains bile into the left hepatic duct, not the right hepatic duct, whereas the caudate lobe drains into the right and left hepatic ducts.

29-A. The bile duct is formed by union of the common hepatic and cystic ducts, lies lateral to the proper hepatic artery and anterior to the portal vein in the right free margin of the lesser omentum, and traverses the head of the pancreas. The endocrine part of the pancreas secretes the hormones insulin and glucagon, which are transported through the bloodstream. It drains bile into the second part of the duodenum at the greater papilla.

30-E. The sigmoid colon drains its venous blood through the portal tributaries, has its own mesentery, receives parasympathetic preganglionic fibers from the pelvic splanchnic nerve, and receives blood from the inferior mesenteric artery.

31-C. The appendicular artery is a branch of the ileocolic artery.

32-C. The inferior pancreaticoduodenal artery is the only artery mentioned that does not supply the stomach.

33-A. The greater splanchnic nerve contains pain fibers. Neither the ventral roots of the spinal nerves nor the gray rami communicantes contain sensory nerve fibers. The vagus nerve contains sensory fibers associated with reflexes, but it does not contain pain fibers.

34-A. The linea alba is a tendinous median raphe between the two rectus abdominis muscles. It is formed by the fusion of the aponeuroses of the external oblique, internal oblique, and transverse muscles of the abdomen. The anterior layer of the rectus sheath above the umbilicus is formed by aponeuroses of the external and internal oblique abdominal muscles. The anterior layer of the rectus sheath below the arcuate line is formed by aponeuroses of the external and internal oblique and transverse abdominal muscles, but there is no posterior layer of the rectus sheath below the arcuate line. The lacunar ligament is formed by the external oblique abdominal aponeurosis, whereas the internal spermatic fascia originates from the transversalis fascia.

35-E. The porta hepatis is the transverse fissure (doorway) in the liver and contains the hepatic ducts, proper hepatic artery, and branches of the portal vein.

36-B. Portal-caval anastomoses occur between the left gastric vein and esophageal vein of the azygos, the superior rectal and middle or inferior rectal veins, paraumbilical and superficial epigastric veins, and retrocolic veins and twigs of the renal vein.

37-D. The Meckel's diverticulum, a finger-like pouch of the ileum, is located 2 feet proximal to the ileocecal junction on the antimesenteric border of the ileum. It is about 2 inches long, occurs in about 2% of the population, and contains two types of mucosal (gastric and pancreatic) tissues in its wall. It is a persistent remnant of the yolk stalk (vitelline duct) and may be connected to the umbilicus via a fibrous cord or a fistula.

38-D. The uncinate process of the pancreas is a projection of the lower part of the head to the left behind the superior mesenteric vessels. The superior pancreaticoduodenal artery runs between the duodenum and the head of the pancreas.

39-E. An indirect inguinal hernia is congenital, whereas a direct hernia is acquired (develops after birth).

40-D. The genitofemoral nerve descends on the anterior surface of the psoas muscle and gives rise to a genital branch, which enters the inguinal canal through the deep inguinal ring to supply the cremaster muscle, and a femoral branch, which supplies the skin of the femoral triangle.

41-C. The quadrate lobe of the liver receives blood from the left hepatic artery and drains bile into the left hepatic duct. It is a medial inferior segment and a part of the left lobe. However, the caudate lobe receives blood from the right and left hepatic arteries and drains bile into the right and left hepatic ducts.

42-C. The right and left hepatic veins drain into the inferior vena cava. The left suprarenal vein drains into the left renal vein. The hemiazygos vein, which is formed from the union of the ascending lumbar and subcostal veins, is connected to the left renal vein. The left gastric vein drains into the portal vein, which enters the liver.

43-B. The linea semilunaris is a curved line along the lateral border of the rectus abdominis. The linea alba is a tendinous median raphe between the two rectus abdominis muscles. The linea semicircularis is an arcuate line of the rectus sheath. The falx inguinalis (conjoint tendon) is formed by aponeuroses of the internal oblique and transverse abdominal muscles.

44-D. The free margin of the falciform ligament contains the paraumbilical vein and the ligamentum teres hepatis. The lienorenal ligament contains the splenic vessels and a small portion of the tail of the pancreas. The lienogastric ligament contains the left gastroepiploic and short gastric vessels. The gastrophrenic ligament contains no named structures. The hepatoduodenal ligament, a part of the lesser omentum, contains the bile duct, proper hepatic artery, and portal vein in its free margin.

45-C. The splenic artery arises from the celiac trunk, runs along the superior border of the pancreas, and enters the spleen through the lienorenal ligament and the hilus of the spleen. The right gastric artery runs along the lesser curvature of the stomach, and the left gastroepiploic artery runs along the greater curvature of the stomach. The gastroduodenal artery runs behind the first part of the duodenum. The dorsal pancreatic artery supplies the pancreas.

46-D. Both the vagus nerve and the thoracic splanchnic nerve supply the gastrointestinal (GI) tract and terminate approximately at the left colic flexure (junction of the transverse colon and the descending colon). The descending colon, sigmoid colon, rectum, and anal canal are supplied by the pelvic splanchnic nerve for parasympathetic innervation, and by the lumbar and sacral splanchnic nerves for sympathetic innervation.

47-B. The pyloric canal and the neck of the pancreas are situated anterior to the abdominal aorta between the origin of the celiac trunk and the superior mesenteric artery.

48-C. The falx inguinalis (conjoint tendon) is formed by the aponeuroses of the internal oblique and transverse muscles of the abdomen.

49-D. The right colic artery arises from the superior mesenteric or the ileocolic artery and supplies the ascending colon. The duodenum and pancreas receive blood from the inferior pancreaticoduodenal artery, which arises from the superior mesenteric artery proximal to the origin of the middle colic artery. The spleen receives blood from the splenic artery.

50-D. The renal fascia lies external to the perirenal fat and internal to the pararenal fat, and it also surrounds the suprarenal gland. The right renal artery runs behind the inferior vena cava and is longer than the left renal artery.

51-E. The spleen lies in the left hypochondriac region, is hematopoietic in early life, and later functions in worn-out red blood cell destruction. It filters blood, stores red blood cells, and produces lymphocytes and antibodies.

52-D. The splenic artery is a branch of the celiac trunk, follows a tortuous course along the superior border of the pancreas, and divides into several branches that run through the lienorenal ligament.

53-A. The common hepatic artery is divided into the proper hepatic and gastroduodenal arteries.

54-B. The duodenojejunal flexure is supported by a fibromuscular band called the suspensory ligament of the duodenum (ligament of Treitz), which is attached to the right crus of the diaphragm.

55-C. The pancreas is an endocrine and exocrine gland; is retroperitoneal in position; and receives blood from the splenic, gastroduodenal, and superior mesenteric arteries.

56-D. The superior mesenteric artery, a direct branch of the aorta, supplies blood to the ascending and transverse colons.

57-B. The inferior vena cava, which receives blood from the liver, kidneys, and other abdominal structures, enters the thorax through the vena caval foramen to empty into the right atrium.

58-A. The gallbladder receives bile, concentrates it by absorbing water and salt, and stores it.

59-E. The left renal vein runs anterior to the aorta but posterior to the superior mesenteric artery, and receives blood from the gonad and suprarenal gland.

60-C. The right renal artery arises from the aorta, is longer than the left one, and runs behind the inferior vena cava and the right renal vein.

6

Perineum and Pelvis

Perineal Region

I. Perineum

–is a **diamond-shaped space** that has the same boundaries as the inferior aperture of the pelvis.

–is bounded by the **pubic symphysis** anteriorly, the **ischiopubic rami** antero-laterally, the **ischial tuberosities** laterally, the **sacrotuberous ligaments** posterolaterally, and the **tip of the coccyx** posteriorly.

–has a floor that is composed of skin and fascia and a roof formed by the **pelvic diaphragm** with its fascial covering.

–is divided into an anterior **urogenital triangle** and a posterior **anal triangle** by a line connecting the two **ischial tuberosities.**

II. Urogenital Triangle (Figures 6-1 and 6-2)

A. Superficial perineal space (pouch)

–lies between the **inferior fascia of the urogenital diaphragm (perineal membrane)** and the membranous layer of the superficial perineal fascia **(Colles' fascia).**

–contains the superficial transverse perineal muscle, the ischiocavernosus muscles and crus of the penis or clitoris, the bulbospongiosus muscles and the bulb of the penis or the vestibular bulbs, the central tendon of the perineum, the greater vestibular glands (in the female), branches of the internal pudendal vessels, and the perineal nerve and its branches.

1. Colles' fascia

–is the **deep membranous layer** of the superficial perineal fascia and forms the inferior boundary of the superficial perineal pouch.

–is continuous with the **dartos tunic** of the scrotum, with the **superficial fascia** of the penis, and with the **Scarpa's fascia** of the anterior abdominal wall.

2. Perineal membrane

–is the **inferior fascia of the urogenital diaphragm** that forms the inferior boundary of the deep perineal pouch and the superior boundary of the superficial pouch.

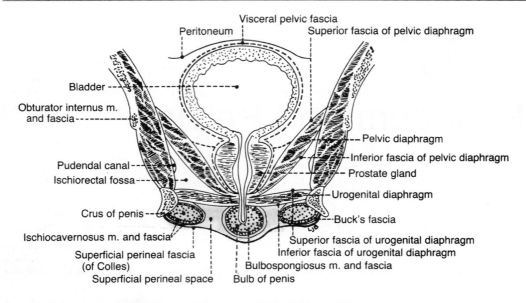

Figure 6-1. Frontal section of the male perineum and pelvis.

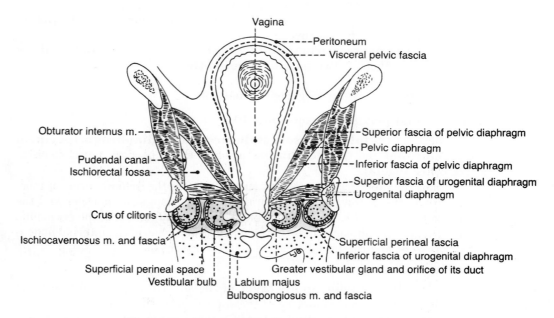

Figure 6-2. Frontal section of the female perineum and pelvis.

–lies between the urogenital diaphragm and the external genitalia, is perforated by the **urethra,** and is attached to the posterior margin of the urogenital diaphragm and the **ischiopubic rami.**

–is thickened anteriorly to form the **transverse ligament of the perineum,** which spans the subpubic angle just behind the deep dorsal vein of the penis.

3. **Muscles of the superficial perineal space** (Figures 6-3 and 6-4)

   a. **Ischiocavernosus muscles**

      –arise from the inner surface of the ischial tuberosities and the ischio-pubic rami.

      –insert into the **corpus cavernosum** (the crus of the penis or clitoris).

      –are innervated by the perineal branch of the pudendal nerve.

      –**maintain erection** of the penis by compressing the crus and the deep dorsal vein of the penis, thereby retarding venous return.

   b. **Bulbospongiosus muscles**

      –arise from the perineal body and fibrous raphe of the bulb of the penis in the male and the perineal body in the female.

      –insert into the **corpus spongiosum** and perineal membrane in the male and the pubic arch and dorsum of the clitoris in the female.

      –are innervated by the perineal branch of the pudendal nerve.

      –**compress the bulb** in the male, impeding venous return from the penis and thereby **maintaining erection.** Contraction (along with contraction of the ischiocavernosus) **constricts the corpus spongiosum,** thereby expelling the last drops of urine or the final semen in ejaculation.

      –**compress the erectile tissue of the vestibular bulbs** in the female and **constrict the vaginal orifice.**

   c. **Superficial transverse perineal muscle**

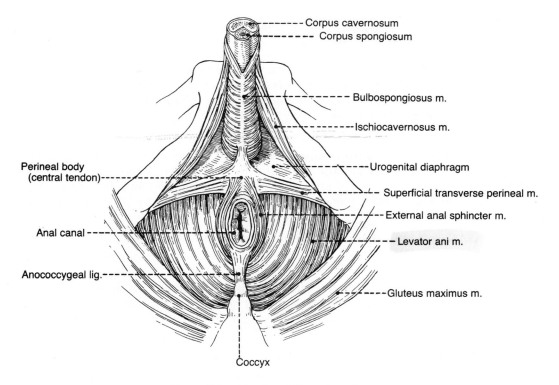

Figure 6-3. Muscles of the male perineum.

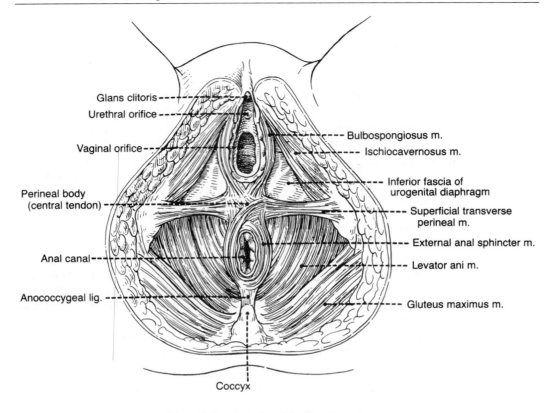

Glans clitoris

Urethral orifice

Vaginal orifice

Perineal body (central tendon)

Anal canal

Anococcygeal lig.

Bulbospongiosus m.

Ischiocavernosus m.

Inferior fascia of urogenital diaphragm

Superficial transverse perineal m.

External anal sphincter m.

Levator ani m.

Gluteus maximus m.

Coccyx

Figure 6-4.   Muscles of the female perineum.

–arises from the ischial rami and tuberosities.
–inserts into the **central tendon (perineal body).**
–is innervated by the perineal branch of the **pudendal nerve.**
–**stabilizes the central tendon.**

4. Perineal body (central tendon of the perineum)

–is a **fibromuscular mass** located in the center of the perineum between the anal canal and the vagina (or the bulb of the penis).
–serves as a site of attachment for the superficial and deep transverse perineal, bulbospongiosus, levator ani, and external anal sphincter muscles.

5. Greater vestibular (Bartholin's) glands

–lie in the superficial perineal space deep to the vestibular bulbs in the female.
–are homologous to the **bulbourethral glands** in the male.
–are compressed during coitus and secrete mucus that **lubricates the vagina.** Ducts open into the **vestibule** between the **labium minora** below the **hymen.**

B. Deep perineal space (pouch)

–lies between the **superior and inferior fasciae of the urogenital diaphragm.**

–contains the deep transverse perineal muscle and sphincter urethrae, the membranous part of the urethra, the bulbourethral glands (in the male), and branches of the internal pudendal vessels and pudendal nerve.

1. **Muscles of the deep perineal space**

    a. **Deep transverse perineal muscle**

    –arises from the inner surface of the **ischial rami.**
    –inserts into the medial tendinous raphe and the perineal body; in the female, it also inserts into the **wall of the vagina.**
    –is innervated by the perineal branches of the pudendal nerve.
    –stabilizes the perineal body and **supports the prostate gland or the vagina.**

    b. **Sphincter urethrae**

    –arises from the inferior pubic ramus.
    –inserts into the median raphe and perineal body.
    –is innervated by the perineal branch of the pudendal nerve.
    –**encircles** and **constricts the membranous urethra** in the male.
    –has an inferior part that is attached to the anterolateral wall of the vagina in the female, forming a **urethrovaginal sphincter** that compresses both the urethra and vagina.

2. **Urogenital diaphragm**

    –consists of the deep transverse perineal muscle and the sphincter urethrae and is invested by superior and inferior fasciae.
    –stretches between the two pubic rami and ischial rami.
    –has inferior fascia that provide attachment to the **bulb of the penis.**
    –is pierced by the membranous urethra (in the male) and by the urethra and the vagina (in the female).
    –does not reach the pubic symphysis anteriorly.

3. **Bulbourethral (Cowper's) glands**

    –lie among the fibers of the sphincter urethrae in the deep perineal pouch in the male, on the posterolateral sides of the membranous urethra. Ducts pass through the inferior fascia of the urogenital diaphragm to open into the bulbous portion of the **spongy (penile) urethra.**

III. Anal Triangle

A. **Ischiorectal (ischioanal) fossa** (see Figures 6-1 and 6-2)

–is the potential space on either side of the anorectum and is separated from the pelvis by the levator ani and its fasciae.
–contains **ischioanal fat,** which allows distention of the anal canal during defecation; the **inferior rectal nerves and vessels,** which are branches of the internal pudendal vessels and the pudendal nerve; and **perineal branches** of the posterior femoral cutaneous nerve.
–contains the **pudendal (Alcock's) canal** on its lateral wall. This is a fascial canal formed by a split in the obturator internus fascia and transmits the pudendal nerve and internal pudendal vessels.
–has the following **boundaries:**

1. **Anterior:** the posterior borders of the superficial and deep transve perineal muscles

2. **Posterior:** the gluteus maximus muscle and the sacrotuberous ligament

3. **Superomedial:** the sphincter ani externus and levator ani muscles

4. **Lateral:** the obturator fascia covering the obturator internus muscle

5. **Floor:** the skin over the anal triangle

B. **Muscles of the anal triangle** (Figure 6-5)

1. **Obturator internus**

   –arises from the inner surface of the **obturator membrane.**
   –has a tendon that passes around the lesser sciatic notch to insert into the medial surface of the greater trochanter of the femur.
   –is innervated by the nerve to the obturator.
   –<u>**laterally rotates the thigh.**</u>

2. **Sphincter ani externus**

   –arises from the tip of the coccyx and the anococcygeal ligament.
   –inserts into the central tendon of the perineum.
   –is innervated by the inferior rectal nerve.
   –**closes the anus.**

3. **Levator ani muscle**

   –arises from the body of the pubis, the arcus tendineus of the levator ani (a thickened part of the obturator fascia), and the ischial spine.
   –inserts into the coccyx and the anococcygeal raphe or ligament.
   –is innervated by the branches of the anterior rami of sacral nerves S3 and S4 and the perineal branch of the pudendal nerve.
   –<u>**supports and raises the pelvic floor.**</u>
   –consists of the **puborectalis, pubococcygeus,** and **iliococcygeus.**
   –has as its most anterior fibers, which are also the most medial, the levator prostatae or pubovaginalis.

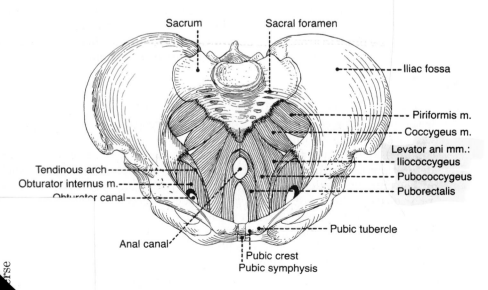

Figure 6-5. Muscles of the perineum and pelvis.

4. **Coccygeus**

–arises from the ischial spine and the sacrospinous ligament.

–inserts into the coccyx and the lower part of the sacrum.

–is innervated by branches of the fourth and fifth sacral nerves.

–**supports and raises the pelvic floor.**

C. **Anal canal** (see Pelvis: VIII B)

IV. External Genitalia and Associated Structures

A. Fasciae and ligaments

1. Fundiform ligament of the penis

–arises from the linea alba and the membranous layer of the superficial fascia of the abdomen.

–splits into left and right parts, **encircles the body of the penis,** and blends with the superficial penile fascia.

–enters the septum of the scrotum.

2. Suspensory ligament of the penis (or the clitoris)

–arises from the pubic symphysis and the arcuate pubic ligament and inserts into the deep fascia of the penis or to the body of the clitoris.

–lies deep to the fundiform ligaments.

3. Deep fascia of the penis (Buck's fascia)

–is a continuation of the deep perineal fascia.

–is continuous with the fascia covering the external oblique muscle and the rectus sheath.

4. Tunica albuginea

–is a **dense fibrous layer** that envelops both the corpora cavernosa and the corpus spongiosum.

–is **very dense** around the **corpora cavernosa,** thereby greatly impeding venous return and resulting in the extreme turgidity of these structures when the erectile tissue becomes engorged with blood.

–is **more elastic** around the **corpus spongiosum,** which, therefore, does not become excessively turgid during erection and permits passage of the ejaculate.

5. Tunica vaginalis

–is a **double serous membrane,** a peritoneal sac on the end of the processus vaginalis that covers the front and sides of the testis and epididymis.

–is a closed sac that is derived from the abdominal peritoneum, forming the **innermost layer of the scrotum.**

–consists of a parietal layer adjacent to the internal spermatic fascia and a visceral layer adherent to the testis and epididymis.

B. Male external genitalia

1. Scrotum

–is a cutaneous pouch consisting of **thin skin** and the underlying **dartos,** which is continuous with the superficial penile fascia and superficial perineal fascia.

–has **no fat,** which is important in maintaining a temperature lower than the rest of the body.

–contains the **testis** and its covering and the **epididymis.**

–is contracted and wrinkled when cold (or sexually stimulated), bringing the testis into close contact with the body to conserve heat; is relaxed when warm and hence is flaccid and distended to dissipate heat.

–receives blood from the external pudendal arteries and the posterior scrotal branches of the internal pudendal arteries.

–is innervated by the anterior scrotal branch of the **ilioinguinal nerve,** the genital branch of the **genitofemoral nerve,** the posterior scrotal branch of the perineal branch of the **pudendal nerve,** and the perineal branch of the **posterior femoral cutaneous nerve.**

2. **Penis** (Figure 6-6)

–consists of three masses of **vascular erectile tissue;** these are the paired corpora cavernosa and the midline corpus spongiosum, which are bounded by tunica albuginea.

–consists of a **root,** which includes two crura and the bulb of the penis; the **body** contains the single corpus spongiosum and the paired corpora cavernosa.

–has a head called the **glans penis,** which is formed by the terminal part of the **corpus spongiosum** and is covered by a free fold of skin, the **prepuce.** The **frenulum** of the prepuce is a median ventral fold passing from the deep surface of the prepuce. The prominent margin of the glans penis is the **corona,** the median slit near the tip of the glans is the **external urethral orifice,** and the terminal dilated part of the urethra in the glans is the **fossa navicularis.**

C. **Female external genitalia**

1. **Labia majora**

–are two **longitudinal folds of skin** that run downward and backward from the **mons pubis** and are joined anteriorly by the **anterior labial commissure.**

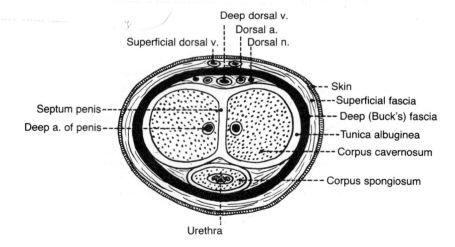

Figure 6-6. Cross-section of the penis.

sympathetic – grey rami

–are homologous to the **scrotum** of the male. Their outer surfaces are covered with pigmented skin, and after puberty, the labia majora are covered with hair.

–contain the terminations of the round ligaments of the uterus.

2. Labia minora

–are hairless and contain no fat, unlike the labia majora.

–are divided into **upper (lateral)** parts, which above the clitoris fuse to form the **prepuce of the clitoris,** and **lower (medial)** parts, which fuse below the clitoris to form the **frenulum of the clitoris.**

3. Vestibule of the vagina (urogenital sinus)

–is the space or cleft between the labia minora.

–has the **openings** for the urethra, the vagina, and the ducts of the greater vestibular glands in its floor.

4. Clitoris

–is homologous to the **penis** in the male; consists of **erectile tissue** and is enlarged as a result of engorgement with blood.

–consists of two crura, two corpora cavernosa, and a glans, but **no corpus spongiosum.** The **glans clitoris** is derived from the **corpora cavernosa** and is covered by a sensitive epithelium.

V. Nerve Supply of the Perineal Region (Figure 6-7)

A. Pudendal nerve (S2–S4)

–passes through the greater sciatic foramen between the piriformis and coccygeus muscles.

–crosses the ischial spine and enters the perineum with the internal pudendal artery through the lesser sciatic foramen.

–enters the **pudendal canal,** gives rise to the inferior rectal nerve and the perineal nerve, and terminates as the **dorsal nerve of the penis (or clitoris).**

B. Inferior rectal nerve

–arises within the pudendal canal, divides into several branches, crosses the ischiorectal fossa, and innervates the sphincter ani externus and the skin around the anus.

C. Perineal nerve

–arises within the pudendal canal and divides into a **deep branch,** which supplies all of the perineal muscles, and a **superficial (posterior scrotal or labial) branch,** which, in turn, divides into two branches to supply the scrotum or labia majora.

D. Dorsal nerve of the penis (or clitoris)

–pierces the perineal membrane, runs between the two layers of the suspensory ligament of the penis or clitoris, and runs deep to the deep fascia on the dorsum of the penis or clitoris to innervate the skin, prepuce, and glans.

VI. Blood Supply of the Perineal Region (see Figure 6-7)

A. Internal pudendal artery

–arises from the internal iliac artery.

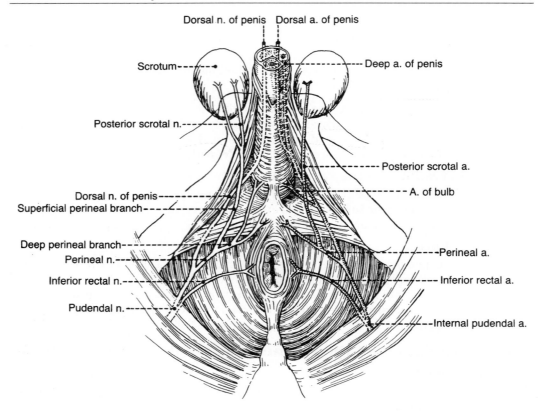

Figure 6-7. Internal pudendal artery and pudendal nerve and branches.

–leaves the pelvis by way of the greater sciatic foramen below the piriformis and coccygeus and immediately enters the perineum through the lesser sciatic foramen by hooking around the ischial spine.

–is accompanied by the pudendal nerve during its course.

–passes along the lateral wall of the ischiorectal fossa in the pudendal canal.

–gives rise to the following:

1. **Inferior rectal artery**

    –arises within the pudendal canal, pierces the wall of the pudendal canal, and breaks into several branches, which cross the ischiorectal fossa to **muscles and skin around the anal canal.**

2. **Perineal arteries**

    –supply the superficial perineal muscles and give rise to **transverse perineal branches** and **posterior scrotal (or labial) branches.**

3. **Artery of the bulb**

    –arises within the deep perineal space, pierces the perineal membrane, and supplies the bulb of the penis and the bulbourethral glands (in the male) and the vestibular bulbs and the greater vestibular gland (in the female).

4. **Urethral artery**

    –pierces the perineal membrane, enters the corpus spongiosum of the penis, and continues to the **glans penis.**

5. Deep arteries of the penis or clitoris

–are terminal branches of the internal pudendal artery.

–pierce the perineal membrane, run through the center of the **corpus cavernosum** of the penis or clitoris, and supply its erectile tissue.

6. Dorsal arteries of the penis or clitoris

–pierce the perineal membrane and pass through the suspensory ligament of the penis or clitoris.

–run along its dorsum on each side of the deep dorsal vein and deep to the deep fascia (Buck's fascia) and superficial to the tunica albuginea to supply the **glans** and prepuce.

B. External pudendal artery

–arises from the femoral artery, emerges through the saphenous ring, and passes medially over the spermatic cord or the round ligament of the uterus to supply the **skin above the pubis, penis, and scrotum or labium majus.**

C. Veins of the penis

1. Deep dorsal vein of the penis

–is an unpaired vein that begins in the sulcus behind the glans and lies in the dorsal midline deep to the deep fascia and superficial to the tunica albuginea.

–leaves the perineum through the gap between the **arcuate pubic ligament** and the **transverse perineal ligament.**

–passes through the suspensory ligament of the penis below the arcuate pubic ligament and drains into the prostatic and pelvic venous plexuses.

2. Superficial dorsal vein of the penis

–runs toward the pubic symphysis between the superficial and deep fasciae on the dorsum of the penis and divides into the right and left branches, which terminate in the **external (superficial) pudendal veins.** The external pudendal vein drains into the greater saphenous vein.

D. Lymph nodes and vessels (Figure 6-8)

1. Lymphatic drainage of the perineum

–occurs via the superficial inguinal lymph nodes, which receive lymph from the lower abdominal wall, buttocks, penis, scrotum, labium majus, and lower parts of the vagina and anal canal. These nodes have efferent vessels that drain primarily into the **external iliac nodes** and ultimately to the **lumbar (aortic) nodes.**

2. Lymphatic drainage of the pelvis

–follows the internal iliac vessels to the internal iliac nodes and subsequently to the **lumbar (aortic) nodes.**

a. Internal iliac nodes receive lymph from the upper part of the rectum and vagina and other pelvic organs, and they drain into the common iliac and then to the lumbar (aortic) nodes. However, lymph from the uppermost part of the rectum drains into the inferior mesenteric nodes and then to the aortic nodes.

b. Lymph from the testis or ovary drains along the gonadal vessels directly into the aortic nodes.

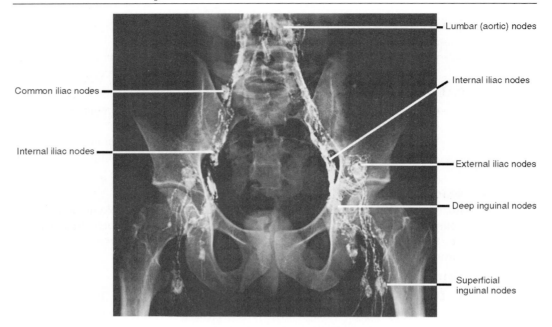

Common iliac nodes

Internal iliac nodes

Lumbar (aortic) nodes

Internal iliac nodes

External iliac nodes

Deep inguinal nodes

Superficial inguinal nodes

Figure 6-8. Lymphograph of the pelvis and lumbar region.

VII. Clinical Considerations

A. Extravasated urine

–may result from **rupture of the spongy urethra** below the urogenital diaphragm; urine may pass into the superficial perineal space.

–spreads inferiorly into the scrotum, anteriorly around the penis, and superiorly into the abdominal wall.

–cannot spread laterally into the thigh, because the inferior fascia of the urogenital diaphragm (the perineal membrane) and the superficial fascia of the perineum are firmly attached to the ischiopubic rami and are connected with the deep fascia of the thigh (fascia lata).

–cannot spread posteriorly into the anal region, because the perineal membrane and Colles' fascia are continuous with each other around the superficial transverse perineal muscles.

B. Hydrocele

–is an **accumulation of fluid in the cavity of the tunica vaginalis of the testis** or along the spermatic cord.

C. Varicocele

–occurs when **enlargement (varicosity) of the veins of the spermatic cord** appears like a "bag of worms," accompanied by a constant pulling and dragging, frequently causing oligospermia.

–is more common on the left side, probably as a result of a malignant tumor of the left kidney, which blocks the exit of the testicular vein.

D. Vasectomy

–is **surgical excision of a portion of the vas deferens** (ductus deferens) through the scrotum.

–stops the passage of spermatozoa, but neither reduces the amount of ejaculate greatly nor diminishes sexual desire.

E. Mediolateral episiotomy

–is a **surgical incision through the posterolateral vaginal wall,** just lateral to the perineal body, to enlarge the birth canal and thus prevent uncontrolled tearing during parturition. In a **median episiotomy,** the incision is carried posteriorly in the midline through the posterior vaginal wall and the central tendon (perineal body).

F. Pudendal block

–is performed by injecting a local anesthetic in the vicinity of the pudendal nerve.

–is accomplished by inserting a needle through the posterolateral vaginal wall, just beneath the pelvic diaphragm and angled toward the ischial tuberosity, thus placing the needle in the vicinity of the pudendal canal.

Pelvis

I. Bony Pelvis (Figures 6-9, 6-10, and 6-11)

A. Pelvis

–is the **basin-shaped ring of bone** formed by the two **hip bones,** the **sacrum,** and the **coccyx.** (The hip, or coxal bone, consists of the ilium, ischium, and pubis.)

–is divided by the **pelvic brim** or iliopectineal line into the **pelvis major (false pelvis)** above and the **pelvis minor (true pelvis)** below.

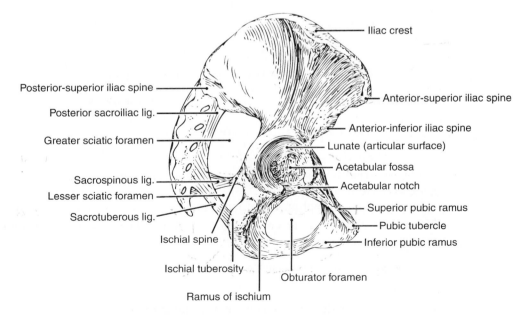

Figure 6-9. Lateral view of the hip bone.

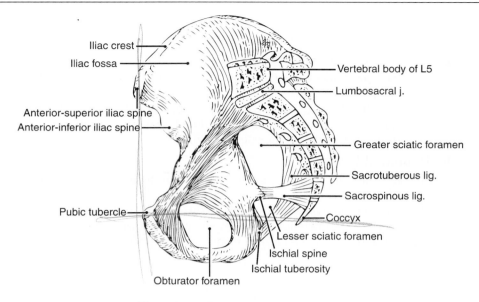

Figure 6-10. Medial view of the hip bone.

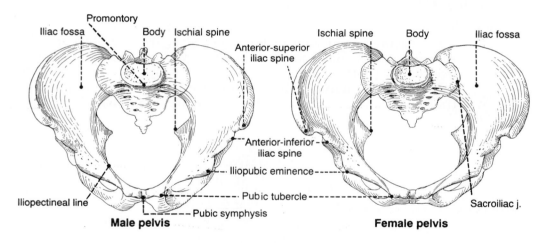

Figure 6-11. Male and female pelvic bones.

–has an outlet that is closed by the coccygeus and levator ani muscles, which form the **floor of the pelvis.**

–is normally tilted in anatomic position. Thus:

1. The anterior–superior iliac spine and the pubic tubercles are in the same vertical plane.

2. The coccyx is in the same horizontal plane as the upper margin of the pubic symphysis.

3. The axis of the pelvic cavity running through the central point of the inlet and the outlet almost parallels the curvature of the sacrum.

B. Upper pelvic aperture (pelvic inlet or pelvic brim)

–is the **superior rim of the pelvic cavity;** is bounded posteriorly by the promontory of the sacrum and the anterior border of the ala of the sacrum **(sacral part),** laterally by the arcuate or iliopectineal line of the ilium **(iliac part),** and anteriorly by the pectineal line, the pubic crest, and the superior margin of the pubic symphysis **(pubic part).**

–is measured using transverse, oblique, and anteroposterior (conjugate) diameters.

C. Lower pelvic aperture (pelvic outlet)

–is a **diamond-shaped aperture** bounded posteriorly by the sacrum and coccyx; laterally by the ischial tuberosities and sacrotuberous ligaments; and anteriorly by the pubic symphysis, arcuate ligament, and rami of the pubis and ischium.

–is closed by the pelvic and urogenital diaphragms.

D. Pelvis major (false pelvis)

–is the expanded portion of the bony pelvis above the pelvic brim.

E. Pelvis minor (true pelvis)

–is the **cavity of the pelvis** below the pelvic brim (or superior aperture) and above the pelvic outlet (or inferior aperture).

–has an outlet that is closed by the coccygeus and levator ani muscles and the perineal fascia, which form the floor of the pelvis.

F. Differences between the female and male pelvis

1. The **bones** of the female pelvis are usually **smaller,** lighter, and thinner than those of the male.

2. The **inlet** is transversely **oval** in the female and heart-shaped in the male.

3. The **outlet** is **larger** in the female than in the male because of the everted ischial tuberosities in the female.

4. The **cavity** is **wider** and **shallower** in the female than in the male.

5. The **subpubic angle** or pubic arch is **larger** and the **greater sciatic notch** is **wider** in the female than in the male.

6. The female sacrum is shorter and wider than the male sacrum.

7. The **obturator foramen** is **oval** or triangular in the female and round in the male.

II. Joints of the Pelvis (see Figures 6-10 and 6-11)

A. Lumbosacral joint

–is the joint between vertebra L5 and the base of the sacrum, joined by an intervertebral disk and supported by the iliolumbar ligaments.

B. Sacroiliac joint

–is a **synovial joint** of an irregular plane type between the articular surfaces of the sacrum and ilium.

–is covered by cartilage and is supported by the anterior, posterior, and interosseous sacroiliac ligaments.

–**transmits the weight of the body to the hip bone.**

C. Sacrococcygeal joint

–is a **cartilaginous joint** between the sacrum and coccyx, reinforced by the anterior, posterior, and lateral sacrococcygeal ligaments.

D. Pubic symphysis

–is a **cartilaginous or fibrocartilaginous joint** between the pubic bones in the median plane.

III. Pelvic Diaphragm (see Figure 6-5)

–forms the **pelvic floor** and **supports all of the pelvic viscerae.**
–is formed by the **levator ani and coccygeus** muscles and their fascial coverings.
–lies posterior and deep to the urogenital diaphragm as well as medial and deep to the ischiorectal fossa.
–on contraction, **raises the entire pelvic floor.**
–flexes the anorectal canal during **defecation** and helps the voluntary control of **micturition.**
–helps direct the fetal head toward the birth canal at **parturition.**

IV. Ligaments of the Female Pelvis

A. Broad ligament of the uterus (Figures 6-12 and 6-13)

–consists of **two layers of peritoneum,** extends from the lateral margin of the uterus to the lateral pelvic wall, and serves to hold the uterus in position.
–contains the uterine tube, uterine vessels, round ligament of the uterus, ovarian ligament, ureter, uterovaginal nerve plexus, and lymphatic vessels.
–does not contain the ovary but gives attachment to the ovary through the **mesovarium.**
–has a posterior layer that curves from the isthmus of the uterus (the **recto-uterine fold)** to the posterior wall of the pelvis alongside the rectum.

1. Mesovarium

–is a fold of peritoneum that connects the anterior surface of the **ovary** with the posterior layer of the broad ligament.

2. Mesosalpinx

–is a fold of the broad ligament that suspends the **uterine tube.**

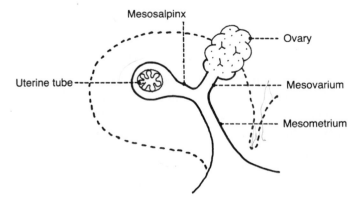

Figure 6-12. Sagittal section of the broad ligament.

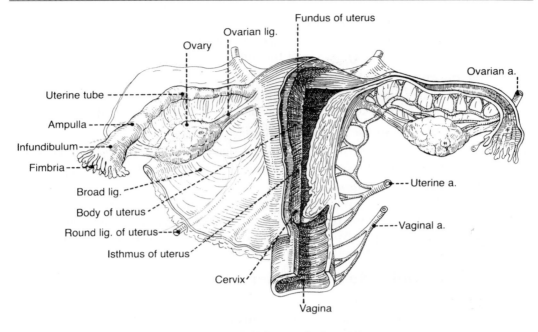

Uterine tube
Ampulla
Infundibulum
Fimbria
Broad lig.
Body of uterus
Round lig. of uterus
Isthmus of uterus
Ovary
Ovarian lig.
Fundus of uterus
Ovarian a.
Uterine a.
Vaginal a.
Cervix
Vagina

Figure 6-13. Female reproductive organs.

3. Mesometrium
　　–is a major part of the broad ligament below the mesosalpinx and meso-varium.

B. Round ligament of the uterus
　　–is attached to the uterus in front of and below the attachment of the uterine tube and represents the remains of the lower part of the **gubernaculum.**
　　–runs within the layers of the broad ligament, contains smooth muscle fibers, and holds the fundus of the uterus forward, keeping the uterus anteverted and anteflexed.
　　–enters the inguinal canal at the deep inguinal ring, emerges from the superficial inguinal ring, and becomes lost in the subcutaneous tissue of the labium majus.

C. Ovarian ligament
　　–is a **fibromuscular cord** that extends from the uterine end of the ovary to the side of the uterus below the uterine tube through the broad ligament.
　　–runs within the layers of the broad ligament.

D. Suspensory ligament of the ovary
　　–is a **band of peritoneum** that extends upward from the ovary to the pelvic wall and transmits the ovarian vessels, nerves, and lymphatics.

E. Lateral or transverse cervical (cardinal or Mackenrodt's) ligaments of the uterus
　　–are **fibromuscular condensations of pelvic fascia** from the cervix and the lateral fornices of the vagina to the pelvic walls.
　　–extend laterally below the base of the broad ligament.
　　–contain smooth muscle fibers and **support the uterus.**

F. Pubocervical ligaments

–are firm bands of connective tissue that extend from the posterior surface of the pubis to the cervix of the uterus.

G. Sacrocervical ligaments

–are firm fibromuscular bands of pelvic fascia that extend from the lower end of the sacrum to the cervix and the upper end of the vagina.

H. Pubovesical (or puboprostatic) ligaments

–are condensations of the pelvic fascia that extend from the neck of the bladder (or the prostate gland in the male) to the pelvic bone.

I. Rectouterine ligaments

–**hold the cervix back and upward** and sometimes elevate a shelf-like fold of peritoneum (**rectouterine fold**), which passes from the isthmus of the uterus to the posterior wall of the pelvis lateral to the rectum. It corresponds to the **sacrogenital fold** in the male.

V. Ureter and Urinary Bladder (Figures 6-14 and 6-15)

A. Ureter

–is a **muscular tube** that **transmits urine** by peristaltic waves.

–has **three constrictions** along its course: at its origin where the pelvis of the ureter joins the ureter, where it crosses the pelvic brim, and at its junction with the bladder.

–crosses the **pelvic brim** in front of the bifurcation of the common iliac artery, descends retroperitoneally on the lateral pelvic wall, runs medial to the umbilical artery and the obturator vessels and posterior to the ovary, forming the posterior boundary of the ovarian fossa.

–lies 1 to 2 cm lateral to the cervix of the uterus in the female. It is accompanied in its course by the uterine artery, which runs above and anterior to it in the base of the broad ligament of the uterus. Because of its location, it is sometimes injured by a clamp during surgical procedures, and may be ligated and sectioned by mistake during a hysterectomy. It can be remembered by the mnemonic device, "water (ureter) runs under the bridge (uterine artery)."

–passes posterior and inferior to the ductus deferens and lies in front of the seminal vesicle before entering the posterolateral aspect of the bladder in the male.

–receives blood from the aorta, the renal, gonadal, common and internal iliac, umbilical, superior and inferior vesical, and middle rectal arteries.

B. Urinary bladder

–is situated below the peritoneum and is slightly lower in the female than in the male.

–extends upward above the pelvic brim as it fills; may reach as high as the umbilicus if fully distended.

–has the **apex** at the anterior end, and the **fundus or base** as its posteroinferior triangular portion.

–has a **neck,** which is the area where the fundus and the inferolateral surfaces come together, leading into the **urethra.**

–has an **uvula,** which is a small eminence at the apex of its trigone, projecting into the orifice of the urethra. The **trigone** is bounded by the two orifices

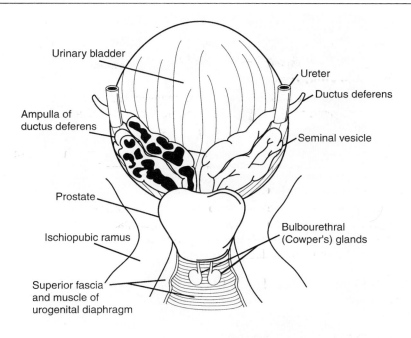

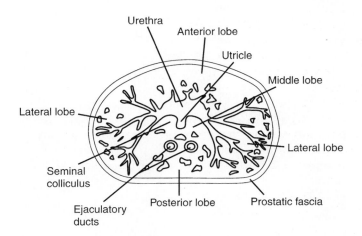

Figure 6-14. Male urogenital organs.

of the ureters and the internal urethral orifice, around which is a thick circular layer called the **internal sphincter** (sphincter vesicae).

—has associated musculature (bundles of smooth muscle fibers) that as a whole is known as the **detrusor muscle of the bladder.**

—receives blood from the superior and inferior vesical arteries (and from the vaginal artery in the female). Its venous blood is drained by the **prostatic (or vesical) plexus** of veins, which empties into the internal iliac vein.

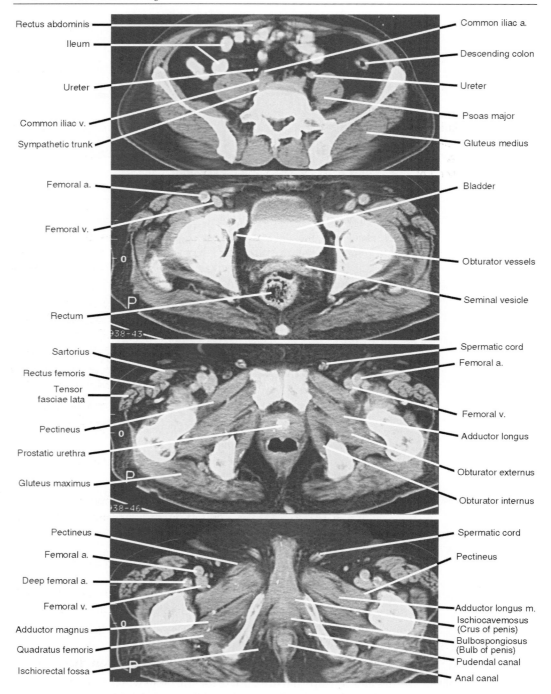

Rectus abdominis
Ileum
Ureter
Common iliac v.
Sympathetic trunk

Common iliac a.
Descending colon
Ureter
Psoas major
Gluteus medius

Femoral a.
Femoral v.

Rectum

Bladder

Obturator vessels

Seminal vesicle

Sartorius
Rectus femoris
Tensor fasciae lata
Pectineus
Prostatic urethra
Gluteus maximus

Spermatic cord
Femoral a.

Femoral v.
Adductor longus

Obturator externus
Obturator internus

Pectineus
Femoral a.
Deep femoral a.
Femoral v.
Adductor magnus
Quadratus femoris
Ischiorectal fossa

Spermatic cord
Pectineus

Adductor longus m.
Ischiocavemosus
(Crus of penis)
Bulbospongiosus
(Bulb of penis)
Pudendal canal
Anal canal

Figure 6-15. Computed tomography (CT) scans of the pelvis and perineum.

–is innervated by nerve fibers from the vesical and prostatic plexuses, which are extensions from the inferior hypogastric plexuses. The parasympathetic nerve originating from the cord segment S2–S4 causes the musculature (detrusor) of the bladder wall to contract, relaxes the internal sphincter, and promotes emptying.

C. Micturition (urination)

–is initiated by stimulating **stretch receptors in the detrusor muscle** in the bladder wall by the increasing volume (about 300 ml for adults) of urine. **Afferent** impulses arise from these receptors in the bladder wall and enter the spinal cord (S2–S4) via the pelvic splanchnic nerves.

–can be assisted by contraction of the abdominal muscles, which increases the intra-abdominal and pelvic pressures.

–involves the following processes:

1. **Sympathetic** fibers induce **relaxation of the bladder wall** and constrict the internal sphincter, inhibiting emptying. (They may also activate the detrusor to prevent the reflux of semen into the bladder during ejaculation.)

2. **Parasympathetic** preganglionic fibers in the pelvic splanchnic nerves synapse in the pelvic (inferior hypogastric) plexus; postganglionic fibers to the bladder musculature induce a reflex **contraction of the detrusor muscle** and relaxation of the internal sphincter, enhancing the urge to void.

3. **Somatic motor** fibers in the pudendal nerve cause voluntary **relaxation** of the **external urethral sphincter,** and the bladder begins to void.

4. At the end of micturition, the external urethral sphincter contracts and **bulbospongiosus muscles** in the male expel the last few drops of urine from the urethra.

VI. Male Genital Organs (Figures 6-16 and 6-17; see Figure 6-14)

A. Testis

–develops retroperitoneally and descends into the scrotum retroperitoneally.

–is covered by the **tunica albuginea,** which lies beneath the visceral layer of the **tunica vaginalis.**

–**produces spermatozoa** and **secretes sex hormones.**

–is supplied by the testicular artery from the abdominal aorta and is drained by veins of the pampiniform plexus.

–has lymph vessels that ascend with the testicular vessels and drain into the lumbar (aortic) nodes; lymphatic vessels in the scrotum drain into the superficial inguinal nodes.

B. Epididymis

–consists of a head, body, and tail, and contains a **convoluted duct** about 6 m (20 feet) long.

–functions in the **maturation and storage of spermatozoa** in the head and body, as well as **propulsion of the spermatozoa** into the ductus deferens.

C. Ductus deferens

–is a thick-walled tube, which enters the pelvis at the deep inguinal ring at the lateral side of the inferior epigastric artery.

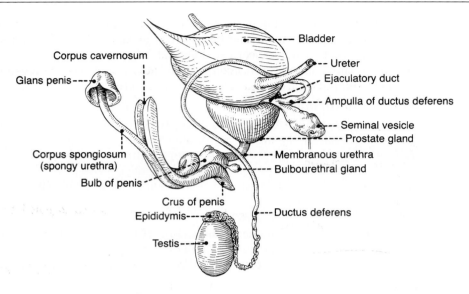

Figure 6-16. Male reproductive organs.

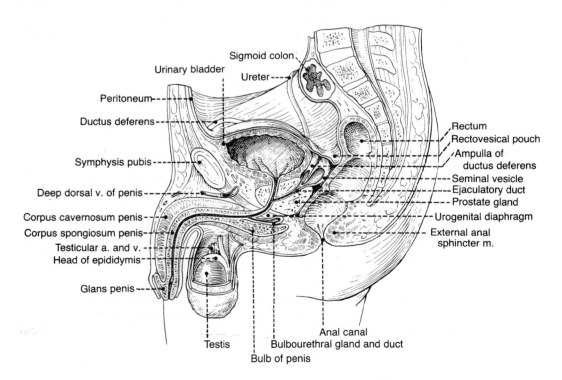

Figure 6-17. Sagittal section of the male pelvis.

–crosses the medial side of the umbilical artery and obturator nerve and vessels, passes superior to the ureter near the wall of the bladder, and is dilated to become the **ampulla** at its terminal part.

–contains fructose, which is nutritive to spermatozoa, and receives innervation primarily from sympathetic nerves of the hypogastric plexus and parasympathetic nerves of the pelvic plexus.

D. Ejaculatory ducts

–are formed by the union of the ductus deferens with the ducts of the seminal vesicles. Peristaltic contractions of the muscular layer of the ductus deferens and the ejaculatory ducts propel spermatozoa with seminal fluid into the urethra.

–open into the prostatic urethra on the **seminal colliculus** just lateral to the blind **prostatic utricle** (see VI G).

E. Seminal vesicles

–are enclosed by dense endopelvic fascia and are **lobulated glandular structures** that are diverticula of the ductus deferens.

–lie inferior and lateral to the ampullae of the ductus deferens against the fundus (base) of the bladder.

–produce the alkaline constituent of the **seminal fluid,** which contains fructose and choline. **Fructose** provides a **forensic determination** for occurrence of **rape,** whereas **choline** crystals provides the basis for the determination of the **presence of semen (Florence's test).**

–have lower ends that become narrow and form ducts, which join the ampullae of the ductus deferens to form the **ejaculatory ducts.**

–do not store spermatozoa, as was once thought; this is done by the epididymis, the ductus deferens, and its ampulla.

F. Prostate gland

–is located at the base of the urinary bladder and consists chiefly of glandular tissue mixed with smooth muscle and fibrous tissue.

–has five lobes: the **anterior lobe** (or isthmus), which lies in front of the urethra and is devoid of glandular substance; the **middle (median) lobe,** which lies between the urethra and the ejaculatory ducts and is prone to **benign hypertrophy** obstructing the internal urethral orifice; the **posterior lobe,** which lies behind the urethra and below the ejaculatory ducts, contains glandular tissue and is prone to **carcinomatous transformation**; and the **right and left lateral lobes,** which are situated on either side of the urethra and form the main mass of the gland.

–secretes a fluid that produces the characteristic **odor of semen.** This fluid, together with the secretion from the seminal vesicles and the bulbourethral glands, and the spermatozoa, constitute the **semen or seminal fluid.**

–secretes **prostate-specific antigen (PSA),** prostaglandins, citric acid and acid phosphatase, and proteolytic enzymes.

–has ducts that open into the **prostatic sinus,** a groove on either side of the **urethral crest.**

–receives the **ejaculatory duct,** which opens into the urethra on the **seminal colliculus** just lateral to the blind **prostatic utricle.**

G. Urethral crest

–is located on the posterior wall of the **prostatic urethra** and has numerous openings for the prostatic ducts on either side.

–has an ovoid-shaped enlargement called the **seminal colliculus (verumontanum),** on which the two ejaculatory ducts and the prostatic utricle open. At the summit of the colliculus is the **prostatic utricle,** which is an invagination (a blind pouch) about 5 mm deep; it is analogous to the uterus and vagina in the female.

H. Prostatic sinus

–is a groove between the urethral crest and the wall of the prostatic urethra and receives the ducts of the prostate gland.

I. Erection

–depends on **stimulation of parasympathetics** from the pelvic splanchnic nerves, which dilates the arteries supplying the erectile tissue, and thus causes engorgement of the corpora cavernosa and corpus spongiosum, compressing the veins and thus impeding venous return and causing full erection.

–is also maintained by **contraction of the bulbospongiosus and ischiocavernosus muscles,** which compresses the erectile tissues of the bulb and the crus.

–is often described using a popular mnemonic device: **p**oint (erection by **p**arasympathetic) and **s**hoot (ejaculation by **s**ympathetic).

J. Ejaculation

–begins with nervous stimulation. Friction to the glans penis and other sexual stimuli result in **excitation of sympathetic fibers,** leading to contraction of the smooth muscle of the epididymal ducts, the ductus deferens, the seminal vesicles, and the prostate in turn.

–occurs as a result of contraction of the smooth muscle, thus pushing spermatozoa and the secretions of both the seminal vesicles and prostate into the prostatic urethra, where they join secretions from the bulbourethral and penile urethral glands. All of these secretions are **ejected** together from the penile urethra as a result of the rhythmic contractions of the bulbospongiosus, which compresses the urethra.

–involves contraction of the sphincter of the bladder. This prevents the entry of urine into the prostatic urethra and the reflux of the semen into the bladder.

VII. Female Genital Organs (Figure 6-18; see Figure 6-13)

A. Ovaries

–lie on the posterior aspect of the **broad ligament** on the side wall of the pelvic minor and are bounded by the external and internal iliac vessels.

–are not covered by the peritoneum, and thus the ovum or oocyte is expelled into the peritoneal cavity and then into the uterine tube.

–are not enclosed in the broad ligament, but their anterior surface is attached to the posterior surface of the broad ligament by the **mesovarium.**

–have a surface that is covered by **germinal (columnar) epithelium,** which is modified from the developmental peritoneal covering of the ovary.

–are supplied primarily by the ovarian arteries, which are contained in the suspensory ligament and anastomose with branches of the uterine artery.

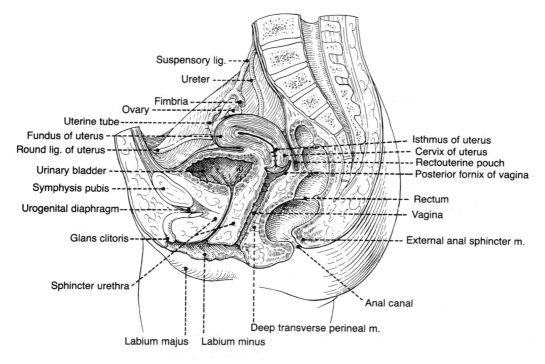

Suspensory lig.
Ureter
Fimbria
Ovary
Uterine tube
Fundus of uterus
Round lig. of uterus
Urinary bladder
Symphysis pubis
Urogenital diaphragm
Glans clitoris
Sphincter urethra
Labium majus   Labium minus
Deep transverse perineal m.
Anal canal
External anal sphincter m.
Vagina
Rectum
Posterior fornix of vagina
Rectouterine pouch
Cervix of uterus
Isthmus of uterus

Figure 6-18.   Sagittal section of the female pelvis.

–are drained by the ovarian veins; the right ovarian vein joins the inferior vena cava, and the left ovarian vein joins the left renal vein.

B. Uterine tubes

–extend from the uterus to the uterine end of the ovaries and **connect the uterine cavity to the peritoneal cavity.**

–are each subdivided into four parts: the **uterine part,** the **isthmus,** the **ampulla** (the longest and widest part), and the **infundibulum** (the funnel-shaped termination formed of **fimbriae).**

–**convey the fertilized or unfertilized oocytes to the uterus** by ciliary action and muscular contraction, which takes 3 to 4 days.

–transport spermatozoa in the opposite direction; **fertilization** takes place within the tube, usually in the **infundibulum or ampulla.**

C. Uterus

–is the organ of gestation, in which the fertilized oocyte normally becomes embedded and the developing organism grows until its birth.

–is normally **anteverted** (i.e., angle of 90° at the junction of the vagina and cervical canal) and **anteflexed** (i.e., angle of 160°–170° at the junction of the cervix and body).

–is supported by the pelvic diaphragm; the urogenital diaphragm; the round, broad, lateral, or transverse cervical (cardinal) ligaments; and the pubocervical, sacrocervical, and rectouterine ligaments.

–is supplied primarily by the uterine artery and secondarily by the ovarian artery.

–has an anterior surface that rests on the posterosuperior surface of the bladder.

–is divided into four parts for the purpose of description:

1. Fundus

–is the **rounded part** of the uterus located superior and anterior to the plane of the entrance of the uterine tube.

2. Body

–is the main part of the uterus located inferior to the fundus and superior to the isthmus. The uterine cavity is triangular in the **coronal section** and is continuous with the lumina of the uterine tube and with the internal os.

3. Isthmus

–is the **constricted part** of the uterus located between the body and cervix of the uterus. It corresponds to the internal os.

4. Cervix

–is the inferior narrow part of the uterus that projects into the vagina and divides into the following regions:

a. Internal os, the junction of the cervical canal with the uterine body

b. Cervical canal, the cavity of the cervix between the internal and external ostia

c. External os, the opening of the cervical canal into the vagina

D. Vagina

–extends between the vestibule and the cervix of the uterus.

–is located at the lower end of the birth canal.

–serves as the **excretory channel** for the products of menstruation; also serves to receive the penis during coitus.

–has a **fornix** that forms the recess between the cervix and the wall of the vagina.

–opens into the vestibule is partially closed by a membranous crescentic fold, the **hymen.**

–is supported by the levator ani; the transverse cervical, pubocervical, and sacrocervical ligaments (upper part); the urogenital diaphragm (middle part); and the perineal body (lower part).

–receives blood from the vaginal branches of the uterine artery and of the internal iliac artery.

–has lymphatic drainage in two directions: The lymphatics from the upper three-fourths drain into the internal iliac nodes; those from the lower one-fourth, below the hymen, drain downward to the perineum and thus into the superficial inguinal nodes.

VIII. Rectum and Anal Canal

A. Rectum (see Figure 6-15)

–is the part of the **large intestine** that extends from the sigmoid colon to the anal canal and follows the curvature of the sacrum and coccyx.

–has a lower dilated part called the **ampulla,** which lies immediately above the pelvic diaphragm and **stores the feces.**

–has a peritoneal covering on its anterior, right, and left sides for the proximal third; only on its front for the middle third; and no covering for the distal third.

–has a mucous membrane and a circular muscle layer that forms three permanent transverse folds **(Houston's valves),** which appear to support the fecal mass.

–receives blood from the superior, middle, and inferior rectal arteries and the middle sacral artery. (The superior rectal artery pierces the muscular wall and courses in the submucosal layer and anastomoses with branches of the inferior rectal artery. The middle rectal artery supplies the posterior part of the rectum.)

–has venous blood that returns to the portal venous system via the superior rectal vein and to the caval (systemic) system via the middle and inferior rectal veins. (The middle rectal vein drains primarily the muscular layer of the lower part of the rectum and upper part of the anal canal.)

–receives parasympathetic nerve fibers by way of the pelvic splanchnic nerve.

B. Anal canal (see Figure 6-15)

–lies below the pelvic diaphragm and ends at the **anus.**

–is divided into an upper two-thirds **(visceral portion),** which belongs to the intestine, and a lower one-third **(somatic portion),** which belongs to the perineum with respect to mucosa, blood supply, and nerve supply.

–has **anal columns,** which are 5 to 10 longitudinal folds of mucosa in its upper half (each column contains a small artery and a small vein).

–has **anal valves,** which are crescent-shaped mucosal folds that connect the lower ends of the anal columns.

–has **anal sinuses,** which are a series of pouch-like recesses at the lower end of the anal column in which the anal glands open.

–has an **internal anal sphincter,** which is a thickening of the circular smooth muscle in the lower part of the rectum that is separated from the **external anal sphincter** (skeletal muscle has three parts: subcutaneous, superficial, and deep) by the intermuscular groove called **Hilton's white line.**

–has a point of demarcation between visceral and somatic portions called the **pectinate (dendate) line,** which is a serrated line following the anal valves and crossing the bases of the anal columns.

1. The epithelium is **columnar** or **cuboidal** above the pectinate line and **stratified squamous** below it.

2. Venous drainage above the pectinate line goes into the **portal venous system** mainly via the superior rectal vein; below the pectinate line, it goes into the **caval system** via the middle and inferior rectal veins.

3. The lymphatic vessels drain into the **internal iliac nodes** above the line and into the **superficial inguinal nodes** below it.

4. The sensory innervation above the line is through fibers from the pelvic plexus and thus is of the **visceral** type; the sensory innervation below it is by **somatic** nerve fibers of the pudendal nerve (which are very sensitive).

5. **Internal hemorrhoids** occur above the pectinate line, and **external hemorrhoids** occur below it.

C. Defecation

–is initiated by **distention of the rectum,** which has filled from the sigmoid colon, and afferent impulses transmitted to the spinal cord by the pelvic splanchnic nerve. The pelvic splanchnic nerve increases peristalsis (contracts smooth muscles in the rectum), whereas sympathetic nerve causes a decrease in peristalsis, maintains tone in the internal sphincter, and contains vasomotor and sensory (pain) fibers.

–involves the following:

1. The intra-abdominal pressure is increased by holding the breath and contracting the diaphragm, the abdominal muscles, and the levator ani, thus facilitating the expulsion of feces.

2. The **puborectalis** relaxes, so decreasing the angle between the ampulla of the rectum and the upper portion of the anal canal, thus aiding defecation.

3. The smooth muscle in the wall of the rectum contracts, the internal anal sphincter relaxes, and the external anal sphincter relaxes to pass the feces.

4. After evacuation, the contraction of the puborectalis and the anal sphincters closes the anal canal.

IX. Blood Vessels of the Pelvis (Figure 6-19)

A. Internal iliac artery

–arises from the bifurcation of the common iliac artery, in front of the sacroiliac joint, and is crossed in front by the ureter at the pelvic brim.

–is commonly divided into a **posterior division,** which gives rise to the iliolumbar, lateral sacral, and superior gluteal arteries; and an **anterior division,** which gives rise to the inferior gluteal, internal pudendal, umbilical, obturator, inferior vesical, middle rectal, and uterine arteries.

1. Iliolumbar artery

–runs superolaterally to the iliac fossa, deep to the psoas major.

–divides into an **iliac branch** supplying the iliacus muscle and the ilium, and a **lumbar branch** supplying the psoas major and quadratus lumborum muscles.

2. Lateral sacral artery

–passes medially in front of the sacral plexus, giving rise to **spinal branches,** which enter the anterior sacral foramina to supply the spinal meninges and the roots of the sacral nerves, as well as the muscles and skin overlying the sacrum.

3. Superior gluteal artery

–usually runs between the lumbosacral trunk and the first sacral nerve.

–leaves the pelvis through the **greater sciatic foramen** above the piriformis muscle to supply muscles in the buttocks.

4. Inferior gluteal artery

–runs between the first and second or between the second and third sacral nerves.

–leaves the pelvis through the **greater sciatic foramen,** inferior to the piriformis.

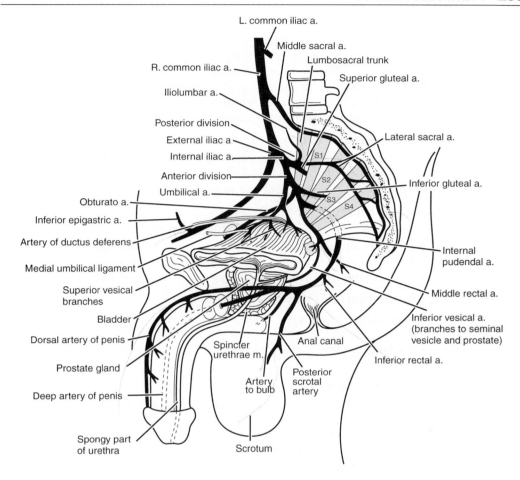

Figure 6-19. Branches of the internal iliac artery.

5. Internal pudendal artery

  –leaves the pelvis through the greater sciatic foramen, passing between the piriformis and coccygeus muscles, and enters the perineum through the **lesser sciatic foramen.**

6. Umbilical artery

  –runs forward along the lateral pelvic wall and along the side of the bladder.

  –has a proximal part that gives rise to the **superior vesical artery** to the superior part of the bladder and, in the male, to the **artery of the ductus deferens,** which supplies the ductus deferens, the seminal vesicles, the lower part of the ureter, and the bladder.

  –has a distal part that is obliterated and continues forward as the **medial umbilical ligament.**

7. Obturator artery

  –usually arises from the internal iliac artery, but in about 20% to 30% of the population it arises from the inferior epigastric artery. It then passes close to or across the femoral canal to reach the obturator foramen and hence is susceptible to damage during hernia operations.

–runs through the upper part of the obturator foramen, divides into **anterior and posterior branches,** and supplies the muscles of the thigh.

–forms a **posterior branch** that gives rise to an acetabular branch, which enters the joint through the acetabular notch and reaches the head of the femur by way of the ligamentum capitis femoris.

8. **Inferior vesical artery**

   –occurs in the male and corresponds to the **vaginal artery** in the female.

   –supplies the fundus of the bladder, prostate gland, seminal vesicles, ductus deferens, and lower part of the ureter.

9. **Vaginal artery**

   –arises from the uterine or internal iliac artery.

   –gives rise to numerous branches to the anterior and posterior wall of the vagina and makes longitudinal anastomoses in the median plane to form the **anterior and posterior azygos arteries of the vagina.**

10. **Middle rectal artery**

    –runs medially to supply mainly the muscular layer of the lower part of the rectum and the upper part of the anal canal.

    –also supplies the prostate gland and seminal vesicles (or vagina) and the ureter.

11. **Uterine artery**

    –is homologous to the **artery of the ductus deferens** in the male.

    –arises from the internal iliac artery or in common with the vaginal or middle rectal artery.

    –runs medially in the base of the broad ligament to reach the junction of the cervix and the body of the uterus and runs in front of and above the ureter near the lateral fornix of the vagina.

    –divides into a large **superior branch,** supplying the body and fundus of the uterus, and a smaller **vaginal branch,** supplying the cervix and vagina.

    –takes a tortuous course along the lateral margin of the uterus and ends by anastomosing with the ovarian artery.

B. **Median sacral artery**

   –is an unpaired artery, arising from the posterior aspect of the abdominal aorta just before its bifurcation.

   –descends in front of the sacrum, supplying the posterior portion of the rectum, and ends in the **coccygeal body,** which is a small cellular and vascular mass located in front of the tip of the coccyx.

C. **Superior rectal artery**

   –is the direct continuation of the inferior mesenteric artery.

D. **Ovarian artery**

   –arises from the abdominal aorta, crosses the proximal end of the external iliac artery to enter the pelvic minor, and reaches the ovary through the suspensory ligament of the ovary.

X. Nerve Supply to the Pelvis

A. Sacral plexus

–is formed by the fourth and fifth lumbar ventral rami (the lumbosacral trunk) and the first four sacral ventral rami.

–lies largely on the internal surface of the piriformis muscle in the pelvis.

1. Superior gluteal nerve (L4–S1)

–leaves the pelvis through the greater sciatic foramen, above the piriformis.

–innervates the gluteus medius, gluteus minimis, and tensor fascia lata muscles.

2. Inferior gluteal nerve (L5–S2)

–leaves the pelvis through the greater sciatic foramen, below the piriformis.

–innervates the gluteus maximus muscle.

[handwritten margin note: Postr div.]

3. Sciatic nerve (L4–S3)

–is the **largest nerve in the body** and is composed of **peroneal** and **tibial** parts.

–leaves the pelvis through the greater sciatic foramen below the piriformis.

–enters the thigh in the hollow between the ischial tuberosity and the greater trochanter of the femur.

4. Nerve to the obturator internus muscle (L5–S2)

–leaves the pelvis through the greater sciatic foramen below the piriformis.

–enters the perineum through the lesser sciatic foramen.

–innervates the obturator internus and superior gemellus muscles.

5. Nerve to the quadratus femoris muscle (L5–S1)

–leaves the pelvis through the greater sciatic foramen, below the piriformis.

–descends deep to the gemelli and obturator internus muscles and ends in the deep surface of the quadratus femoris, supplying the quadratus femoris and the inferior gemellus muscles.

6. Posterior femoral cutaneous nerve (S1–S3)

–leaves the pelvis through the greater sciatic foramen below the piriformis.

–lies alongside the sciatic nerve and descends on the back of the knee.

–gives rise to several **inferior cluneal nerves** and **perineal branches.**

7. Pudendal nerve (S2–S4)

–leaves the pelvis through the greater sciatic foramen below the piriformis.

–enters the perineum through the lesser sciatic foramen and the pudendal canal in the lateral wall of the ischiorectal fossa.

8. Branches distributed to the pelvis

–include the nerve to the piriformis muscle (S1–S2), the nerves to the levator ani and coccygeus muscles (S3–S4), the nerve to the sphincter ani externus muscle, and the pelvic splanchnic nerves (S2–S4).

B. Autonomic nerves

1. Superior hypogastric plexus

–is the continuation of the aortic plexus below the aortic bifurcation and receives the lower two lumbar splanchnic nerves.

–lies behind the peritoneum, descends in front of the fifth lumbar vertebra, and ends by bifurcation into the **right and left hypogastric nerves** in front of the sacrum.

–contains preganglionic and postganglionic sympathetic fibers, visceral afferent fibers, and few, if any, parasympathetic fibers, which may run a recurrent course through the inferior hypogastric plexus.

2. **Hypogastric nerve**

–is the lateral extension of the superior hypogastric plexus and lies in the extraperitoneal connective tissue lateral to the rectum.

–provides branches to the sigmoid colon and the descending colon.

–is joined by the pelvic splanchnic nerves to form the inferior hypogastric or pelvic plexus.

3. **Inferior hypogastric (pelvic) plexus**

–is formed by the union of **hypogastric, pelvic splanchnic, and sacral splanchnic nerves** and lies against the posterolateral pelvic wall, lateral to the rectum, vagina, and base of the bladder.

–contains **pelvic ganglia,** in which both sympathetic and parasympathetic preganglionic fibers synapse. Hence, it consists of preganglionic and postganglionic sympathetic fibers, preganglionic and postganglionic parasympathetic fibers, and visceral afferent fibers.

–gives rise to subsidiary plexuses, including the middle rectal plexus, uterovaginal plexus, vesical plexus, differential plexus, and prostatic plexus.

4. **Sacral splanchnic nerves**

–consist primarily of preganglionic sympathetic fibers that come off the chain and synapse in the inferior hypogastric (pelvic) plexus.

5. **Pelvic splanchnic nerves (nervi erigentes)**

–are the only splanchnic nerves that carry parasympathetic fibers. (All other splanchnic nerves are sympathetic.)

–arise from the sacral segment of the spinal cord (S2–S4).

–contribute to the formation of the pelvic (or inferior hypogastric) plexus, and supply the descending colon, sigmoid colon, and other viscera in the pelvis and perineum.

XI. Clinical Considerations

A. Uterine prolapse

–is the **protrusion of the cervix** of the uterus into the vagina close to the vestibule.

–causes a **bearing-down sensation** in the womb and an increased frequency of and burning sensation on urination.

–occurs as a result of advancing age and is characterized by increased relaxation and loss of tonus of the muscular and fascial structures such as the pelvic and urogenital diaphragmata, the ovarian and cardinal ligaments, and the broad and round ligaments of the uterus that constitute the support of the uterus and other pelvic viscera.

–may be surgically corrected; however, during prolapse surgery, the ureter may be mistaken for the uterine artery and erroneously ligated. (The uterine artery crosses superior and then anterior to the ureter.)

B. Hemorrhoids

–are dilated internal and external venous plexuses around the rectum and anal canal.

1. **Internal hemorrhoids** occur above the pectinate line and are covered by mucous membrane; their pain fibers are carried by autonomic nerves.

2. **External hemorrhoids** are situated below the pectinate line, are covered by skin, and are more painful than internal hemorrhoids because their pain fibers are carried by the **inferior rectal nerves.**

C. Hysterectomy

–is **surgical removal of the uterus,** performed either through the abdominal wall or through the vagina.

–may result in injury to the ureter, which lies in the transverse cardinal ligament beneath the uterine artery.

D. Prostatectomy

–is **surgical removal of a part of the hypertrophied prostate gland.**

–**Hypertrophy** occurs most in the **middle lobe**, obstructing the internal urethral orifice and thus leading to **nocturia** (excessive urination at night), **dysuria** (difficulty or pain in urination), and **urgency** (sudden desire to urinate).

–**Cancer** occurs most in the **posterior lobe**.

–**T**ransurethral **r**esection of the **p**rostate (TURP) is surgical removal of the prostate by means of a cystoscope passed through the urethra.

E. Vaginal examination

–is an examination of pelvic structures through the vagina:

1. **Inspection with a speculum**

–allows observation of the vaginal walls, the posterior fornix as the site of **culdocentesis** (aspiration of fluid from the rectouterine excavation by puncture of the vaginal wall), the **uterine cervix**, and the **cervical os**.

2. **Digital examination**

–allows palpation of the **urethra** and **bladder** through the anterior fornix of the vagina; the **perineal body, rectum, coccyx, and sacrum** through the posterior fornix; and the **ovaries, uterine tubes, ureters, and ischial spines** through the lateral fornices.

3. **Bimanual examination**

–is performed by placing the fingers of one hand in the vagina and exerting pressure on the lower abdomen with the other hand.

–enables physicians to determine the **size** and **position** of the **uterus**, to palpate the **ovaries** and **uterine tubes**, and to detect **pelvic inflammation** or **neoplasms**.

F. Rectal examination

–is used to determine the size and consistency of the **prostate gland.**

–is also used to palpate the **bladder, seminal vesicle**, and **ampulla** of the **ductus deferens** anteriorly; the **coccyx** and **sacrum** posteriorly; and the **ischiorectal fossa (abscess)** laterally.

G. Culdocentesis

–is aspiration of fluid from the cul-de-sac (rectouterine excavation) by puncture of the vaginal vault near the midline between the uterosacral ligaments.

H. Endometriosis

–is a benign disorder in which a mass of endometrial tissue (stroma and glands) occurs aberrantly in various locations, including the uterine wall, ovaries, or other extraendometrial sites.

–frequently forms cysts containing altered blood.

Review Test

Directions: Each of the numbered items or incomplete statements in this section is followed by answers or by completions of the statement. Select the **one** lettered answer or completion that is **best** in each case.

1. Carcinoma of the uterus can spread directly to the labia majora in lymphatics that follow which of the following structures?

(A) Pubic arcuate ligament
(B) Suspensory ligament of the ovary
(C) Cardinal ligament
(D) Suspensory ligament of the clitoris
(E) Round ligament of the uterus

2. Tenderness and swelling of the left testicle may be produced by thrombosis in which of the following veins?

(A) Left internal pudendal vein
(B) Left renal vein
(C) Left internal iliac vein
(D) Left inferior epigastric vein
(E) Left external pudendal vein

3. If a stab wound injures structures that leave the pelvis above the piriformis muscle, which of the following structures is most likely to be damaged?

(A) Sciatic nerve
(B) Internal pudendal artery
(C) Superior gluteal nerve
(D) Inferior gluteal artery
(E) Posterior femoral cutaneous nerve

4. Which of the following ligaments normally is found in the inguinal canal?

(A) Suspensory ligament of the ovary
(B) Ovarian ligament
(C) Mesosalpinx
(D) Round ligament of the uterus
(E) Rectouterine ligament

5. Parasympathetic preganglionic fibers in the pelvic splanchnic nerves synapse in which of the following ganglia?

(A) Ganglia in or near the viscerae or pelvic plexus
(B) Sympathetic chain ganglia
(C) Collateral ganglia
(D) Dorsal root ganglia
(E) Ganglion impar

6. As the uterine artery passes from the internal iliac artery to the uterus, it crosses which of the following structures that is sometimes mistakenly ligated during pelvic surgery?

(A) Ovarian artery
(B) Ovarian ligament
(C) Uterine tube
(D) Ureter
(E) Round ligament of the uterus

7. Tearing of the pelvic diaphragm during childbirth leads to paralysis of which of the following muscles?

(A) Piriformis
(B) Sphincter urethrae
(C) Obturator internus
(D) Levator ani
(E) Sphincter ani externus

8. A lesion on the sacral splanchnic nerves would primarily damage which of the following nerve fibers?

(A) Postganglionic parasympathetic fibers
(B) Postganglionic sympathetic fibers
(C) Preganglionic sympathetic fibers
(D) Preganglionic parasympathetic fibers
(E) Postganglionic sympathetic and parasympathetic fibers

9. Which of the following statements is correct?

(A) The ovary lies within the broad ligament
(B) The glans clitoris is formed from the corpora cavernosa
(C) Erection of the penis is a sympathetic response
(D) Ejaculation follows parasympathetic stimulation
(E) The ureter crosses superior to the uterine artery near the uterine cervix

261

UGdiaphgm=sphincter urethae & trans.perineum

10. Which of the following structures constitutes the superior boundary of the superficial perineal space?

(A) Pelvic diaphragm
(B) Colles' fascia
(C) Superficial layer of the superficial fascia
(D) Deep layer of the superficial fascia
(E) Perineal membrane

11. A slowly growing tumor in the deep perineal space would most likely injure which of the following structures?

(A) Bulbourethral glands
(B) Crus of penis
(C) Bulb of vestibule
(D) Spongy urethra
(E) Great vestibular gland

12. Which of the following lobes of the prostate gland is commonly involved in benign hypertrophy, which obstructs the prostatic urethra?

(A) Anterior lobe
(B) Middle lobe
(C) Right lateral lobe
(D) Left lateral lobe
(E) Posterior lobe

13. The prostatic ducts open into or on which of the following structures?

(A) Membranous part of the urethra
(B) Seminal colliculus
(C) Cavernous urethra
(D) Prostatic sinus
(E) Prostatic utricle

14. The duct of the seminal vesicle

(A) joins the duct of a bulbourethral gland to form the ejaculatory duct
(B) opens into the membranous urethra
(C) transmits spermatozoa into the membranous urethra
(D) widens to form the ampulla of the ductus deferens
(E) unites with the ductus deferens to form an ejaculatory duct

15. Which of the following events occurs during ejaculation?

(A) Opening of the urethral sphincter at the neck of the bladder
(B) Pumping out of secretions of the prostate gland and seminal vesicles
(C) Relaxation of smooth muscles in the ductus deferens
(D) Accumulation of semen in the prostatic urethra
(E) Excretion of urine from the bladder

16. Destruction of the urogenital diaphragm most likely causes paralysis of which of the following muscles?

(A) Sphincter urethrae
(B) Coccygeus
(C) Superficial transversus perinei
(D) Levator ani
(E) Obturator internus

17. A benign tumor located near a gap between the arcuate pubic ligament and the transverse perineal ligament might compress which of the following structures?

(A) Dorsal nerve of the penis
(B) Deep dorsal vein of the penis
(C) Superficial dorsal vein
(D) Dorsal artery of the penis
(E) Deep artery of the penis

18. If an obstetrician performs a median episiotomy that damages the perineal body, the function of which of the following muscles might be impaired?

(A) Ischiocavernosus and sphincter urethrae
(B) Deep transverse perineal and obturator internus
(C) Bulbospongiosus and superficial transverse perineal
(D) External anal sphincter and sphincter urethrae
(E) Bulbospongiosus and ischiocavernosus

19. A 22-year-old man has a gonorrheal infection that has infiltrated the space between the inferior fascia of the urogenital diaphragm and the superficial perineal fascia. Which of the following structures might be inflamed?

(A) Prostate gland
(B) Bulbourethral gland
(C) Membranous part of the male urethra
(D) Superficial transverse perineal muscle
(E) Sphincter urethrae

20. Which of the following ducts opens into the prostatic sinus?

(A) Duct of the seminal vesicle
(B) Ducts of the prostate gland
(C) Ejaculatory duct
(D) Duct of the bulbourethral gland
(E) Ductus deferens

21. The normal position of the uterus is

(A) anteflexed and anteverted
(B) retroflexed and anteverted
(C) anteflexed and retroverted
(D) retroverted and retroflexed
(E) anteverted and retroverted

22. The deep dorsal vein of the penis

(A) lies deep to Buck's fascia
(B) drains into the prostatic venous plexus
(C) lies lateral to the dorsal artery of the penis
(D) is found in the corpus spongiosum
(E) is dilated during erection

23. A 62-year-old man is incapable of penile erection after rectal surgery with prostatectomy. The patient most likely has a lesion of which of the following nerves?

(A) Dorsal nerve of the penis
(B) Perineal nerve
(C) Hypogastric nerve
(D) Sacral splanchnic nerve
(E) Pelvic splanchnic nerve

24. Which of the following structures is drained by the lumbar (aortic) lymph nodes?

(A) Perineum
(B) Lower part of the vagina
(C) External genitalia
(D) Ovary
(E) Lower part of the anterior abdominal wall

25. Infection within the ischiorectal fossa most likely injures which of the following structures?

(A) Vestibular bulb
(B) Seminal vesicle
(C) Greater vestibular gland
(D) Inferior rectal nerve
(E) Internal pudendal artery

26. Which of the following statements concerning structures in the perineum and pelvis is correct?

(A) The dorsal artery of the penis supplies the glans penis
(B) The mesometrium is a fold of peritoneum that suspends the uterine tube
(C) The duct of the bulbourethral gland opens into the membranous urethra
(D) The duct of the greater vestibular gland opens into the vagina
(E) The anterior lobe of the prostate gland is prone to carcinomatous transformation

27. Which of the following structures plays the most important role in the support of the uterus?

(A) Levator ani
(B) Sphincter urethrae
(C) Uterosacral ligament
(D) Ovarian ligament
(E) Arcuate pubic ligament

28. A 16-year-old boy presents to the emergency department with rupture of the penile urethra. Extravasated urine from this injury can spread into which of the following structures?

(A) Scrotum
(B) Ischiorectal fossa
(C) Deep perineal space
(D) Testis
(E) Thigh

29. During vaginal examination, which of the following structures may be palpated?

(A) Apex of the urinary bladder
(B) Fundus of the uterus
(C) Terminal part of the round ligament of the uterus
(D) Body of the clitoris
(E) Uterine cervix

30. Which of the following structures lies in the broad ligament for all or part of its course?

(A) Ovary
(B) Proximal part of the pelvic ureter
(C) Terminal part of the round ligament of the uterus
(D) Uterine tube
(E) Suspensory ligament of the ovary

31. During rectal examination in the male, which of the following structures is most readily palpated?

(A) Prostate gland
(B) Epididymis
(C) Ejaculatory duct
(D) Ureter
(E) Testis

32. Which of the following statements concerning the levator ani is correct?

(A) It is innervated by the pelvic splanchnic nerve
(B) The iliococcygeus is the most anteromedial part of the levator ani
(C) The pubococcygeus may be torn during parturition
(D) It forms the lateral wall of the ischiorectal fossa
(E) It forms the major part of the urogenital diaphragm

33. Part of the boundary of the pelvic inlet is formed by which of the following structures?

(A) Promontory of the sacrum
(B) Anterior–inferior iliac spine
(C) Inguinal ligament
(D) Iliac crest
(E) Pubic tubercle

34. A 32-year-old patient with multiple fractures of the pelvis has no cutaneous sensation in the urogenital triangle. The function of which of the following nerves is most likely to be spared?

(A) Ilioinguinal nerve
(B) Iliohypogastric nerve
(C) Posterior cutaneous nerve of the thigh
(D) Pudendal nerve
(E) Genitofemoral nerve

35. The victim of an automobile accident has received destructive damage to structures that form the boundary of the perineum. Which of the following structures is spared?

(A) Pubic arcuate ligament
(B) Tip of the coccyx
(C) Ischial tuberosities
(D) Sacrospinous ligament
(E) Sacrotuberous ligament

36. Which of the following statements is most applicable to the scrotum?

(A) It is innervated by the ilioinguinal nerve
(B) It receives blood primarily from the testicular artery
(C) Its venous blood drains primarily into the renal vein on the left
(D) Its lymphatic drainage is primarily into upper lumbar nodes
(E) Its dartos tunic is continuous with perineal membrane

37. A 37-year-old woman with uterine prolapse has an intact anal canal. Which of the following structures is most likely to function normally?

(A) External anal sphincter
(B) Broad ligament of the uterus
(C) Cardinal (transverse) cervical ligament
(D) Pelvic diaphragm
(E) Sphincter urethrae

38. When performing a mediolateral episiotomy during breech delivery, an obstetrician should avoid incising which of the following structures?

(A) Vaginal wall
(B) Superficial transverse perineal muscle
(C) Bulbospongiosus
(D) Levator ani
(E) Perineal membrane

39. During pelvic surgery, a surgeon notices severe bleeding from the artery that remains within the true pelvis. Which of the following arteries is most likely to be injured?

(A) Iliolumbar artery
(B) Obturator artery
(C) Uterine artery
(D) Internal pudendal artery
(E) Inferior gluteal artery

40. Which of the following nerves from the lumbosacral plexus remains within the abdominal or pelvic cavity?

(A) Ilioinguinal nerve
(B) Genitofemoral nerve
(C) Lumbosacral trunk
(D) Femoral nerve
(E) Lateral femoral cutaneous nerve

41. Infection in the deep perineal space would most likely damage which of the following structures?

(A) Ischiocavernosus muscles
(B) Superficial transverse perineal muscles
(C) Levator ani
(D) Sphincter urethrae
(E) Bulbospongiosus

42. Upper lumbar nodes most likely receive lymph from which of the following structures?

(A) Lower part of the anal canal
(B) Labium majus
(C) Clitoris
(D) Testis
(E) Scrotum

43. Which of the following structures most likely crosses the pelvic brim?

(A) Deep dorsal vein of the penis
(B) Uterine tube
(C) Ovarian ligament
(D) Uterine artery
(E) Lumbosacral trunk

44. Which of the following statements is most applicable to the bulbourethral (Cowper's) gland?

(A) It lies in the superficial perineal space
(B) It is embedded in the sphincter urethrae
(C) It produces sperm
(D) Its duct opens into the membranous portion of the penile urethra
(E) It lies on either side of the bulb of the penis

45. Which of the following statements best explains the sphincter urethrae?

(A) Smooth muscle
(B) Innervated by the perineal nerve
(C) Lying between the perineal membrane and Colles' fascia
(D) Enclosed in the pelvic fascia
(E) Part of the pelvic diaphragm

46. The pudendal nerve

(A) passes superficial to the sacrotuberous ligament
(B) innervates the testis and epididymis
(C) provides motor fibers to the coccygeus
(D) can be blocked by injecting an anesthetic near the inferior margin of the ischial spine
(E) arises from the lumbar plexus

47. Which of the following statements concerning the ischiorectal fossa is correct?

(A) It accumulates urine leaking from rupture of the bulb of the penis
(B) It contains the inferior rectal vessels
(C) It has a pudendal canal along its medial wall
(D) It is bounded anteriorly by the sacrotuberous ligament
(E) It contains a perineal branch of the fifth lumbar nerve

48. The seminal colliculus of the prostate gland is infected, and its fine openings are closed. Which of the following structures is most likely to be disturbed?

(A) Ducts of the prostate gland
(B) Prostatic utricle
(C) Ducts of the bulbourethral glands
(D) Ejaculatory ducts
(E) Duct of the seminal vesicles

49. Which of the following best describes characteristics of structures above the pectinate line of the anal canal?

(A) Stratified squamous epithelium
(B) Venous drainage into the caval system
(C) Lymphatic drainage into the superficial inguinal nodes
(D) Visceral sensory innervation
(E) External hemorrhoids

50. Which of the following best describes characteristics of the male pelvis compared to the female?

(A) Smaller and lighter
(B) Transversely oval inlet
(C) Smaller outlet
(D) Wider and shallower cavity
(E) Larger subpubic angle

Directions: Each set of matching questions in this section consists of a list of four to twenty-six lettered options (some of which may be in figures) followed by several numbered items. For each numbered item, select the ONE lettered option that is most closely associated with it. To avoid spending too much time on matching sets with large numbers of options, it is generally advisable to begin each set by reading the list of options. Then, for each item in the set, try to generate the correct answer and locate it in the option list, rather than evaluating each option individually. Each lettered option may be selected once, more than once, or not at all.

Questions 51–55

Answer questions 51–55 using the diagram below.

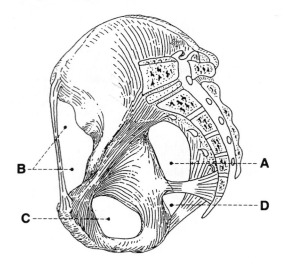

51. Which of the following structures passes through C?

(A) Iliolumbar artery
(B) Umbilical artery
(C) Ilioinguinal nerve
(D) Obturator nerve
(E) Nerve to the obturator internus muscle

52. Which of the following structures passes through D?

(A) Pudendal nerve
(B) Posterior cutaneous nerve of the thigh
(C) Tendon of the obturator externus muscle
(D) Inferior gluteal artery
(E) Piriformis muscle

53. Which of the following structures passes through A?

(A) Quadratus femoris muscle
(B) Lumbosacral trunk
(C) Internal pudendal artery
(D) Obturator nerve
(E) Tendon of the obturator internus muscle

54. Which of the following structures passes through B?

(A) Greater saphenous vein
(B) Saphenous nerve
(C) External pudendal artery
(D) Femoral vein
(E) Genitofemoral nerve

55. Which of the following structures passes through both A and D?

(A) External pudendal artery
(B) Nerve to quadratus femoris
(C) Obturator nerve
(D) Tendon of the obturator internus
(E) Pudendal nerve

Questions 56–60

Match each of the following descriptions with the appropriate lettered structure in the magnetic resonance image (MRI) of the perineum and pelvis in the female.

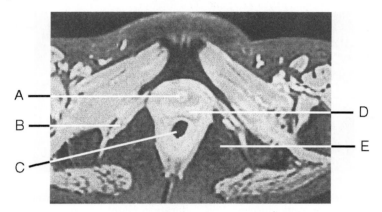

56. Structure that extends between the vestibule and the cervix of the uterus and serves as the excretory channel for the products of menstruation   *A ? D*

57. Structure in the female that is much shorter than that in the male   *A.*

58. Structure into which hemorrhage occurs following injury to the inferior rectal vessels   */C 4*

59. Structure that has Houston's valve or fold, with its venous blood drained by the portal venous system   *C ,*

60. Structure that is innervated by the nerve passing through both the greater and lesser sciatic foramina

Questions 61–65

Match each of the following descriptions with the appropriate lettered structure in the computed tomography (CT) scan of the perineum and pelvis in the male.

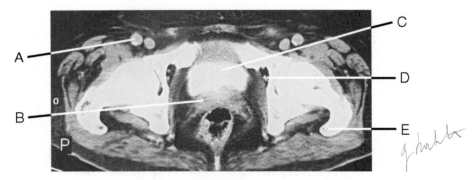

61. Structure that when fractured results in paralysis of the obturator internus muscles

62. Structure that secretes fluid containing fructose, which allows for forensic determination of rape

63. Structure in which ligation of the external iliac artery reduces blood pressure

64. Structure that a knife wound in the obturator foramen might injure

65. Visceral organ that a stab wound immediately superior to the pubic symphysis on the anterior pelvic wall would most likely injure first

Answers and Explanations

1-E. The round ligament of the uterus runs laterally from the uterus through the deep inguinal ring, inguinal canal, and superficial inguinal ring and becomes lost in the subcutaneous tissues of the labium majus. Thus, carcinoma of the uterus can spread directly to the labium majus by traveling in lymphatics that follow the ligament.

2-B. A tender swollen left testis may be produced by thrombosis in the left renal vein, because the left testicular vein drains into the left renal vein.

3-C. The superior gluteal nerve leaves the pelvis through the greater sciatic foramen, above the piriformis. The sciatic nerve, internal pudendal vessels, inferior gluteal vessels and nerve, and posterior femoral cutaneous nerve leave the pelvis below the piriformis.

4-D. The round ligament of the uterus is found in the inguinal canal along its course.

5-A. The pelvic splanchnic nerves carry preganglionic parasympathetic [general visceral efferent (GVE)] fibers that synapse in the ganglia of the inferior hypogastric plexus and in terminal ganglia in the muscular walls of the pelvic organs.

6-D. The ureter runs under the uterine artery near the cervix; thus, the ureter is sometimes mistakenly ligated during pelvic surgery.

7-D. The pelvic diaphragm is formed by the levator ani and coccygeus, whereas the urogenital diaphragm consists of the sphincter urethrae and deep transverse perinei muscles.

8-C. The sacral splanchnic nerves consist primarily of preganglionic sympathetic neurons.

9-B. The glans clitoris is derived from the corpora cavernosa, whereas the glans penis is the expanded terminal part of the corpus spongiosum. Erection of the penis is caused by parasympathetic stimulation, whereas ejaculation is mediated via the sympathetic nerve.

10-E. The superior (deep) boundary of the superficial perineal space is the perineal membrane (inferior fascia of the urogenital diaphragm). Colles' fascia is the deep membranous layer of the superficial perineal fascia.

11-A. The deep perineal space contains the bulbourethral (Cowper's) glands. The spongy urethra, great vestibular gland, crus of the penis, and bulb of the vestibule are found in the superficial perineal space.

12-B. The middle lobe of the prostate gland is commonly involved in benign prostatic hypertrophy, resulting in obstruction of the prostatic urethra, whereas the posterior lobe is commonly involved in carcinomatous transformation. The anterior lobe contains little glandular tissue, and two lateral lobes on either side of the urethra form the major part of the gland.

13-D. Ducts from the prostate gland open into the prostatic sinus, which is a groove on either side of the urethral crest. The prostate gland receives the ejaculatory duct, which opens into the prostatic urethra on the seminal colliculus just lateral to the prostatic utricle.

14-E. A duct from a seminal vesicle joins the ductus deferens to form an ejaculatory duct.

15-B. Ejaculation occurs with the contraction of smooth muscle of the epididymal ducts and ductus deferens. During ejaculation, a sphincter at the neck of the bladder contracts, preventing sperm from entering the bladder and preventing urine from leaving it; the seminal vesicles, prostate gland, and bulbourethral glands contract to pump their secretions into the urethra; and semen is propelled through the ducts and out the external urethral opening.

16-A. The urogenital diaphragm consists of the sphincter urethrae and deep transverse perineal muscles.

17-B. The deep dorsal vein of the penis enters the pelvis through a gap between the arcuate pubic ligament and the transverse perineal ligament.

18-C. The perineal body (central tendon of the perineum) is a fibromuscular node at the center of the perineum. It provides attachment for the bulbospongiosus, the superficial and deep transverse perineal, and the sphincter ani externus muscles.

19-D. The superficial transverse perineal muscle is located in the superficial perineal space between the inferior fascia of the urogenital diaphragm and the membranous layer of the superficial perineal fascia (Colles' fascia). The bulbourethral (Cowper's) glands and the membranous urethra are found in the deep perineal pouch.

20-B. The ducts of the prostate gland open into the prostatic sinus, which is a groove on each side of the urethral crest. The duct of the seminal vesicle and the ductus deferens form the ejaculatory duct. The ejaculatory duct opens into the prostatic urethra on the seminal colliculus. The duct of the bulbourethral gland opens into the lumen of the bulbous portion of the penile urethra.

21-A. The normal position of the uterus is anteverted (i.e., angle of 90° at the junction of the vagina and cervical canal) and anteflexed (i.e., angle of 160°–170° at the junction of the cervix and body).

22-B. The deep dorsal vein of the penis lies medial to the dorsal artery of the penis on the dorsum of the penis and superficial to Buck's fascia, drains into the prostatic plexus of veins, and is compressed against the underlying deep fascia of the penis during erection.

23-E. The pelvic splanchnic nerve contains preganglionic parasympathetic fibers, whereas the sacral splanchnic nerve contains preganglionic sympathetic fibers. Parasympathetic fibers are responsible for erection, whereas sympathetic fibers are involved with ejaculation. The right and left hypogastric nerves contain primarily sympathetic fibers and visceral sensory fibers. The dorsal nerve of the penis and the perineal nerve provide sensory nerve fibers.

24-D. The lymphatic vessels from the ovary ascend with the ovarian vessels in the suspensory ligament and terminate in the lumbar (aortic) nodes. Lymphatic vessels from the perineum, external genitalia, and lower part of the anterior abdominal wall drain into the superficial inguinal nodes.

25-D. The ischiorectal fossa contains the inferior rectal nerves and vessels and adipose tissue. The bulb of the vestibule and the great vestibular gland are located in the superficial perineal space, whereas the bulbourethral gland is found in the deep perineal space. The internal pudendal artery runs in the pudendal canal, but its branches pass through the superficial and deep perineal spaces.

26-A. The dorsal artery of the penis supplies the glans penis. The mesosalpinx is a fold of peritoneum that suspends the uterine tube, and the mesometrium is a major part of the broad ligament below the mesosalpinx and the mesovarium. The duct of the bulbourethral gland opens into the bulbous portion of the spongy urethra, whereas the greater vestibular gland opens into the vestibule between the labium minora and the hymen. The anterior lobe of the prostate is devoid of glandular substance, the middle lobe is prone to benign hypertrophy, and the posterior lobe is prone to carcinomatous transformation.

27-E. The pelvic diaphragm, particularly the levator ani, provides the most important support for the uterus, although the urogenital diaphragm as well as uterosacral and ovarian ligaments support the uterus. The arcuate pubic ligament arches across the inferior aspect of the pubic symphysis.

28-A. Extravasated urine from the penile urethra below the perineal membrane spreads into the superficial perineal space, scrotum, penis, and anterior abdominal wall. However, it does not spread into the testis, ischiorectal fossa, and thigh because Scarpa's fascia ends by firm attachment to the fascia lata of the thigh.

29-E. In addition to the uterine cervix, the uterus, uterine tubes, ovaries, and ureters can be palpated. The apex of the urinary bladder is the anterior end of the bladder, and thus it cannot be palpated. The fundus of the uterus is anterosuperior part of the uterus. The terminal part of the round ligament of the uterus emerges from the superficial inguinal ring and becomes lost in the subcutaneous tissue of the labium majus.

30-D. The uterine tubes lie in the broad ligament. The anterior surface of the ovary is attached to the posterior surface of the broad ligament of the uterus. The ureter descends retroperitoneally on the lateral pelvic wall but is crossed by the uterine artery in the base (in the inferomedial part) of the broad ligament. The terminal part of the round ligament of the uterus becomes lost in the subcutaneous tissue of the labium majus. The suspensory ligament of the ovary is a band of peritoneum that extends superiorly from the ovary to the pelvic wall.

31-A. The prostate gland may be palpated on rectal examination. The ejaculatory duct runs within the prostate gland and cannot be felt. In the male, the pelvic part of the ureter lies lateral to the ductus deferens and enters the posterosuperior angle of the bladder, where it is situated anterior to the upper end of the seminal vesicle, and thus cannot be palpated during rectal examination. However, in the female the ureter can be palpated during vaginal examination because it runs near the uterine cervix and the lateral fornix of the vagina to enter the posterosuperior angle of the bladder.

32-C. The pubococcygeus, which encircles and supports the urethra, vagina, and anal canal, may be torn during parturition. The levator ani forms the major part of the pelvic diaphragm and the medial wall of the ischiorectal fossa. It is innervated by branches of the sacral nerves (S3–S4) and perineal branches of the pudendal nerve. The iliococcygeus is the most posterolateral part of the levator ani.

33-A. The pelvic inlet (pelvic brim) is bounded by the promontory and the anterior border of the ala of the sacrum, the arcuate line of the ilium, the pectineal line, the pubic crest, and the superior margin of the pubic symphysis.

34-B. The iliohypogastric nerve innervates the skin above the pubis. The skin of the urogenital triangle is innervated by the pudendal nerve, perineal branches of the posterior femoral cutaneous nerve, anterior scrotal or labial branches of the ilioinguinal nerve, and the genital branch of the genitofemoral nerve.

35-D. The sacrospinous ligament forms a boundary of the lesser sciatic foramen. The pubic arcuate ligament, tip of the coccyx, ischial tuberosities, and sacrotuberous ligament all form part of the boundary of the perineum.

36-A. The scrotum is innervated by branches of the ilioinguinal, genitofemoral, pudendal, and posterior femoral cutaneous nerves. The scrotum receives blood from the posterior scrotal branches of the internal pudendal arteries and the anterior scrotal branches of the external pudendal arteries, but it does not receive blood from the testicular artery. Similarly, the scrotum is drained by the posterior scrotal veins into the internal pudendal vein. The lymph vessels from the scrotum drain into the superficial inguinal nodes, whereas the lymph vessels from the testis drain into the upper lumbar nodes. The dartos tunic is continuous with the membranous layer of the superficial perineal fascia (Colles' fascia).

37-A. The sphincter ani externus does not support the uterus. The pelvic and urogenital diaphragmata; the broad, ovarian, and cardinal (transverse cervical) ligaments; and the round ligament of the uterus provide the necessary support.

38-D. An obstetrician should avoid incising the levator ani and the external anal sphincter. The levator ani is the major part of the pelvic diaphragm, which forms the pelvic floor and supports all of the pelvic organs.

39-C. Of all the arteries listed, the uterine artery remains within the pelvic cavity.

40-C. The lumbosacral trunk is formed by part of the ventral ramus of the fourth lumbar nerve and the ventral ramus of the fifth lumbar nerve. This trunk contributes to the formation of the sacral plexus by joining the ventral ramus of the first sacral nerve in the pelvic cavity and does not leave the pelvic cavity.

41-D. The sphincter urethrae is found in the deep perineal space, whereas the other structures are located in the superficial perineal space.

42-D. Lymphatic vessels from the testis and epididymis ascend along the testicular vessels in the spermatic cord through the inguinal canal and continue upward in the abdomen to drain into the upper lumbar nodes. The lymph from the other structures drains into the superficial inguinal lymph nodes.

43-E. All of the listed structures do not cross the pelvic brim except the lumbosacral trunk, which arises from L4 and L5, enters the true pelvis by crossing the pelvic brim, and contributes to the formation of the sacral plexus. The deep dorsal vein of the penis enters the pelvic cavity by passing under the symphysis pubis between the arcuate and transverse perineal ligaments.

44-B. The bulbourethral glands lie on either side of the membranous urethra, embedded in the sphincter urethrae. Their ducts open into the bulbous part of the penile urethra. Semen, a thick, yellowish white, viscous, spermatozoa-containing fluid, is a mixture of the secretions of the testes, seminal vesicles, prostate, and bulbourethral glands. Sperm, or spermatozoa, are produced in the seminiferous tubules of the testis and matured in the head of the epididymis.

45-B. The sphincter urethrae is striated muscle that lies in the deep perineal space and forms the urogenital diaphragm. It is not enclosed in the pelvic fascia.

46-D. The pudendal nerve, which arises from the sacral plexus, provides sensory innervation to the scrotum or labium majus. It leaves the pelvis through the greater sciatic foramen and enters the perineum through the lesser sciatic foramen near the inferior margin of the ischial spine. Therefore, it can be blocked by injection of an anesthetic near the inferior margin of the ischial spine.

47-B. The ischiorectal fossa is bounded posteriorly by the gluteus maximus and the sacrotuberous ligament. It contains fat, the inferior rectal nerve and vessels, and perineal branches of the posterior femoral cutaneous nerve. The pudendal canal runs along its lateral wall.

48-D. The ejaculatory ducts, which open onto the seminal colliculus, may be injured. The prostate ducts open into the urethral sinus; the bulbourethral ducts open into the bulbous part of the penile urethra; and the ducts of the seminal vesicle join the ampulla of the ductus deferens to form the ejaculatory duct. The prostatic utricle is a minute pouch on the summit of the seminal colliculus.

49-D. The pectinate line is a point of demarcation between visceral and somatic portions of the anal canal. Characteristics above the pectinate line include columnar epithelium, venous drainage into the portal system, lymphatic drainage into the internal iliac nodes, visceral sensory innervation, and internal hemorrhoids.

50-C. Compared to the female pelvis, the male pelvis is characterized by larger size and greater weight, a heart-shaped as opposed to an oval-shaped inlet, a smaller outlet, a narrower and deeper cavity, a smaller subpubic angle, and a longer and narrower sacrum.

51-D. Space C is the obturator foramen. The obturator nerve passes through the obturator foramen, where it divides into anterior and posterior branches.

52-A. Space D is the lesser sciatic foramen, which transmits the pudendal nerve, internal pudendal vessels, and the obturator internus tendon.

53-C. Space A is the greater sciatic foramen, which transmits the piriformis muscle, internal pudendal vessels, superior and inferior gluteal nerves and vessels, sciatic, pudendal, and posterior femoral cutaneous nerves.

54-D. Space B deep to the inguinal ligament is separated by the iliopectineal arcus (ligament) into the lateral muscular lacunae, which transmits the iliopsoas muscle and the lateral femoral cutaneous nerve, and the medial vascular lacunae, which transmits the femoral canal and femoral nerve and vessels.

55-E. The pudendal nerve, internal pudendal vessels, and the nerve to the obturator internus muscle pass through both the greater (A) and lesser (D) sciatic foramina. The tendon of the obturator internus muscle runs only through the lesser sciatic foramen.

56-D. The vagina is the genital canal in the female, extending from the vestibule to the uterine cervix. The vagina transmits the products of menstruation and receives the penis in copulation.

57-A. In females, the urethra extends from the bladder, runs above the anterior vaginal wall, and pierces the urogenital diaphragm to reach the urethral orifice in the vestibule behind the clitoris. It is about 4 cm long. In males, the urethra is about 20 cm long.

58-E. The ischiorectal fossa lies in the anal triangle and is bound laterally by the obturator internus with its fascia and superomedially by the levator ani and external anal sphincter. It contains the inferior rectal vessels. Thus, hemorrhage occurs in the ischiorectal fossa when it is ruptured.

59-C. The mucous membrane and the circular smooth muscle layer of the rectum form three transverse folds; the middle one is called Houston's valve. The venous blood returns to the portal venous system via the superior rectal vein.

60-B. The obturator internus muscle and its fascia form the lateral wall of the ischiorectal fossa. This muscle is innervated by the nerve to the obturator internus, which passes through the greater and lesser sciatic foramen.

61-E. The greater trochanter provides an insertion site for the obturator internus muscle.

62-B. The seminal vesicle is a lobulated glandular structure and produces the alkaline constituent of the seminal fluid, which contains fructose and choline. Fructose, which is nutritive to spermatozoa, also allows forensic determination of rape, whereas choline crystals are the preferred basis for the determination of the presence of semen.

63-A. The external iliac artery becomes the femoral artery immediately after passing the inguinal ligament. Therefore, ligation of the external iliac artery reduces blood pressure in the femoral artery.

64-D. The obturator foramen transmits the obturator nerve and vessels. Therefore, the knife wound in this foramen injures the obturator nerve and vessels.

65-C. The bladder is situated in the anterior part of the pelvic cavity. Thus a stab wound superior to the pubic symphysis would injure the bladder.

7
Back

Vertebral Column

I. General Characteristics (Figures 7-1 and 7-2)

–The vertebral column consists of 33 vertebrae (7 cervical, 12 thoracic, 5 lumbar, 5 fused sacral, and 4 fused coccygeal vertebrae). It protects the spinal cord, supports the weight of the head and the trunk, and allows the movement of the rib cage for respiration by articulating with the ribs.

–The **primary curvatures** are located in the thoracic and sacral regions and developed during embryonic and fetal periods, whereas the **secondary curvatures** are located in the cervical and lumbar regions and developed after birth and during infancy.

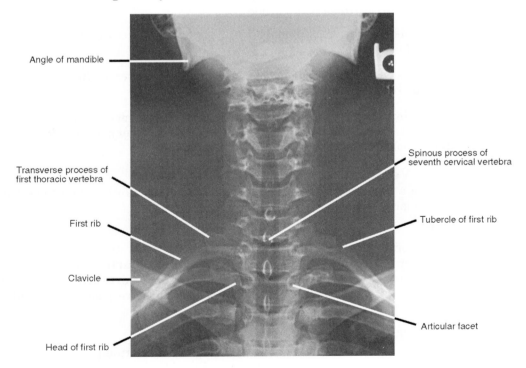

Angle of mandible

Transverse process of
first thoracic vertebra

First rib

Clavicle

Head of first rib

Spinous process of
seventh cervical vertebra

Tubercle of first rib

Articular facet

Figure 7-1. Anteroposterior radiograph of the cervical and upper thoracic vertebrae.

275

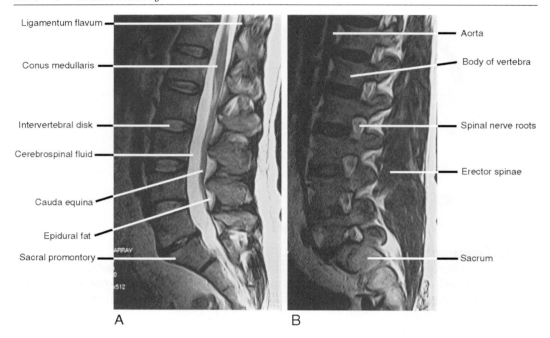

Ligamentum flavum

Conus medullaris

Intervertebral disk

Cerebrospinal fluid

Cauda equina

Epidural fat

Sacral promontory

Aorta

Body of vertebra

Spinal nerve roots

Erector spinae

Sacrum

A

B

Figure 7-2. Sagittal magnetic resonance images (MRIs) of the vertebral column.

–**Abnormal curvatures** may include the following:

A. Kyphosis (hunchback or humpback): an abnormally increased **thoracic** curvature due to osteoporosis

B. Lordosis (swayback or saddle back): an abnormally increased **lumbar** curvature due to weakened trunk musculature

C. Scoliosis: a condition of **lateral deviation** due to unequal growth of the vertebral column, pathologic erosion of vertebral bodies, or asymmetric paralysis or weakness of vertebral muscles

II. Typical Vertebra (Figure 7-3)

–consists of a **body** and a **vertebral arch** with several processes for muscular and articular attachments.

A. Body

–is a short cylinder, **supports weight,** and is separated and also bound together by the **intervertebral disks,** forming the **cartilaginous joints.**

–has **costal facets or processes of the thoracic vertebrae** anterior to the pedicles, which articulate with the heads of the corresponding and subjacent (just below) ribs.

B. Vertebral (neural) arch

–consists of paired **pedicles** laterally and paired **laminae** posteriorly.

–forms the vertebral foramen with the vertebral body and protects the spinal cord and associated structures.

–may fail to fuse, resulting in **spina bifida,** which is classified as follows:

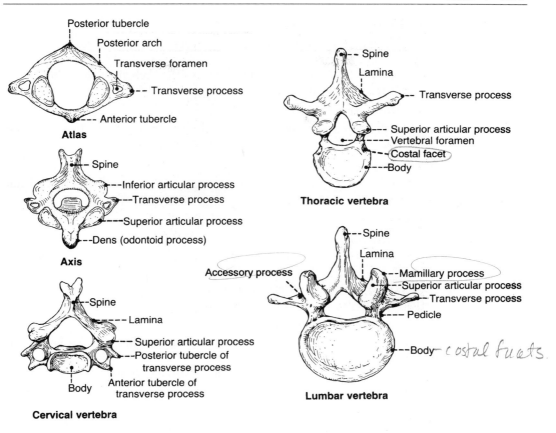

Figure 7-3. Typical cervical, thoracic, and lumbar vertebrae.

1. **Spina bifida occulta:** failure of the vertebral arch to fuse (bony defect only)

2. **Meningocele:** protrusion of the meninges through the unfused arch of the vertebra

3. **Meningomyelocele:** protrusion of the spinal cord as well as the meninges

4. **Myeloschisis (rachischisis):** a cleft spinal cord due to failure of neural folds to close

C. **Processes** associated with the vertebral arch

1. **Spinous process**

   –projects posteriorly from the junction of two laminae of the vertebral arch.
   –is bifid in the cervical region, spine-like in the thoracic region, and oblong in the lumbar region.

2. **Transverse processes**

   –project laterally on each side from the junction of the pedicle and the lamina; articulate with the tubercles of ribs 1 to 10 in the thoracic region.
   –have transverse foramina in the cervical region.

3. **Articular processes (facets)**

–are two superior and two inferior projections from the junction of the laminae and pedicles.

–articulate with other articular processes of the arch above or below, forming **plane synovial joints.**

4. **Mamillary processes**

–are tubercles on the superior articular processes of the **lumbar vertebrae.**

5. **Accessory processes**

–project backward from the base of the transverse process, lateral and inferior to the mamillary process of a lumbar vertebra.

D. **Foramina** associated with the vertebral arch

1. **Vertebral foramina**

–are formed by the vertebral bodies and vertebral arches (pedicles and laminae).

–collectively form the **vertebral canal** and transmit the **spinal cord** with its meningeal coverings, nerve roots, and associated vessels.

2. **Intervertebral foramina**

–are located between the inferior and superior surfaces of the pedicles of adjacent vertebrae.

–transmit the **spinal nerves** and accompanying vessels as they exit the vertebral canal.

3. **Transverse foramina**

–are present in **transverse processes** of the cervical vertebrae.

–transmit the **vertebral artery** (except for C7), **vertebral veins,** and **autonomic nerves.**

III. Intervertebral Disks (see Figure 7-2)

–form the secondary cartilaginous joints between the bodies of two vertebrae from the axis to the sacrum **(there is no disk between the atlas and axis).**

–consist of a central mucoid substance **(nucleus pulposus)** with a surrounding fibrocartilaginous lamina **(anulus fibrosus).**

–comprise one-fourth of the length of the vertebral column.

–allow movements between the vertebrae and serve as a **shock absorber.**

A. **Nucleus pulposus**

–is a remnant of the embryonic **notochord** and is situated in the central portion of the intervertebral disk.

–consists of reticular and collagenous fibers embedded in **mucoid material.**

–may **herniate** or protrude through the anulus fibrosus, thereby impinging on the roots of the spinal nerve.

–acts as a **shock-absorbing mechanism** by equalizing pressure.

B. **Anulus fibrosus**

–consists of concentric layers of fibrous tissue and fibrocartilage.

–**binds the vertebral column together, retains the nucleus pulposus,** and permits a limited amount of movement.

–acts as a **shock absorber.**

IV. Regional Characteristics of Vertebrae (see Figure 7-3)

A. First cervical vertebra (atlas)

–**supports the skull;** thus its name. According to Greek mythology, Atlas supported the earth on his shoulders.

–is the widest of the cervical vertebrae.

–has **no body** and **no spine** but consists of anterior and posterior arches and paired transverse processes.

–articulates superiorly with the **occipital condyles** of the skull to form the **atlanto-occipital joints** and inferiorly with the **axis** to form the **atlantoaxial joints.**

B. Second cervical vertebra (axis)

–has the **smallest transverse process.**

–is characterized by the **dens (odontoid process).** The **dens** projects superiorly from the body of the axis and articulates with the **anterior arch of the atlas,** thus forming the pivot around which the atlas rotates. It is supported by the cruciform, apical, and alar ligaments as well as the tectorial membrane.

C. Seventh cervical vertebra (C7)

–is called the **vertebra prominens** because it has a long spinous process, which is nearly horizontal, ends in a single tubercle (not bifid), and forms a visible protrusion.

–provides an attachment site for the **ligamentum nuchae, supraspinous ligaments,** and numerous back muscles.

D. Thoracic vertebra

–has costal facets. The superior costal facet on the body articulates with the head of the corresponding rib, whereas the inferior facet articulates with the subjacent rib (just below).

–has a transverse process that articulates with the tubercle of the corresponding rib.

E. Fifth lumbar vertebra (L5)

–has the **largest body** of the vertebrae. (Lumbar vertebrae are distinguished by their large bodies.)

–is characterized by a strong, massive transverse process and has **mamillary and accessory processes.**

F. Sacrum (Figure 7-4; see Figure 7-2)

–is a large, triangular, wedge-shaped bone composed of **five fused sacral vertebrae.**

–has **four pairs of foramina** for the exit of the ventral and dorsal primary rami of the first four sacral nerves.

–forms the posterior part of the pelvis and provides the strength and **stability to the pelvis.**

–is characterized by the following structures:

1. **Promontory:** the prominent anterior edge of the first sacral vertebra (S1)

2. **Ala:** the superior and lateral part of the sacrum, which is formed by the fused transverse processes and fused costal processes of the first sacral vertebra

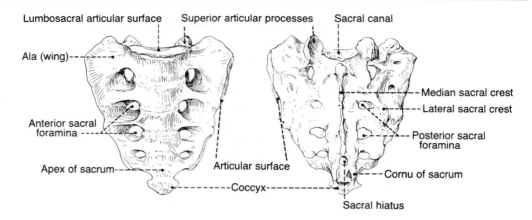

Lumbosacral articular surface   Superior articular processes   Sacral canal

Ala (wing)

Anterior sacral foramina

Apex of sacrum

Coccyx

Median sacral crest

Lateral sacral crest

Posterior sacral foramina

Articular surface

Cornu of sacrum

Sacral hiatus

Figure 7-4. Sacrum.

3. **Median sacral crest:** formed by the fused spinous processes

4. **Sacral hiatus:** formed by the failure of the **laminae** of vertebra S5 to fuse. It is used for the administration of **caudal (extradural) anesthesia.**

5. **Sacral cornu or horn:** formed by the **pedicles** of the fifth sacral verte-bra. It is an important landmark for locating the sacral hiatus.

G. Coccyx

–is a wedge-shaped bone formed by the union of the **four coccygeal ver-tebrae.**

–provides attachment for the **coccygeus and levator ani muscles.**

V. Ligaments of the Vertebral Column (Figure 7-5)

A. Anterior longitudinal ligament

–runs from the skull (occipital bone) to the sacrum on the anterior surface of the vertebral bodies and intervertebral disks.

–is narrowest at the upper end but **widens as it descends,** maintaining the stability of the joints.

–**limits extension** of the vertebral column, **supports the anulus fibrosus** anteriorly, and resists gravitational pull.

B. Posterior longitudinal ligament

–interconnects the vertebral bodies and intervertebral disks posteriorly and **narrows as it descends.**

–**supports** the posterior aspect of the **vertebral bodies** and the **anulus fibrosus,** but it runs anterior to the spinal cord within the vertebral canal.

–**limits flexion** of the vertebral column and resists gravitational pull.

C. Ligamentum flavum

–connects the **laminae** of two adjacent vertebrae and functions to **maintain the upright posture.**

–may be pierced during **lumbar (spinal) puncture.**

D. Ligamentum nuchae (back of neck)

–is a **triangular-shaped median fibrous septum** between the muscles on the two sides of the posterior aspect of the neck.

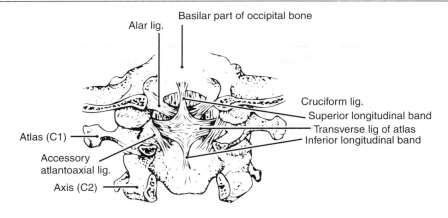

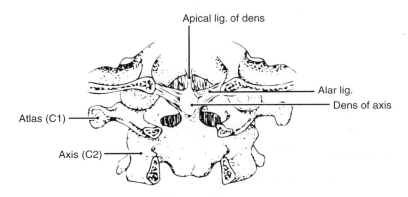

Figure 7-5. Ligaments of the atlas and the axis.

–is formed by **thickened supraspinous ligaments** that extend from vertebra C7 to the external occipital protuberance and crest.

–is also attached to the posterior tubercle of the atlas and to the spinous
processes of the other cervical vertebrae.

VI. Vertebral Venous System

–is a valveless plexiform of veins, forming interconnecting channels.

A. Internal vertebral venous plexus

–lies in the **epidural space** between the wall of the vertebral canal and the
dura mater and receives tributaries from the spinal cord and vertebrae.

–forms anterior and posterior ladder-like configurations by anastomosing longitudinal and transverse veins.

–drains into segmental veins by the **intervertebral veins** that pass through
the intervertebral and sacral foramina. The posterior veins receive the **basivertebral veins,** which lie within the vertebral bodies.

–also communicates superiorly with the cranial dural sinuses, inferiorly with
the pelvic vein, and in the thoracic and abdominal regions with both the
azygos and caval systems.

–is thought to be the **route of early metastasis of carcinoma** from the
lung, breast, and prostate gland to bones and the central nervous system
(CNS).

B. External vertebral venous plexus

–consists of the anterior part, which lies in front of the vertebral column, and the posterior part, which lies on the vertebral arch.

–communicates with the internal venous plexus by way of the **intervertebral** and **basivertebral veins.**

C. Vertebral vein

–arises from the **venous plexuses around the foramen magnum and in the suboccipital region,** passes with the vertebral artery through the transverse foramina of the upper six cervical vertebrae, and empties into the **brachiocephalic vein.**

VII. Clinical Considerations

A. Herniated (slipped) disk

–is **protrusion of the nucleus pulposus** through the anulus fibrosus of the intervertebral disk into the intervertebral foramen or into the vertebral canal, compressing the spinal nerve root.

–commonly occurs posterolaterally where the anulus fibrosus is not reinforced by the posterior longitudinal ligament and frequently affects the lumbar region.

B. Compression fracture

–is produced by **collapse of the vertebral bodies** resulting from trauma.

–may result in **kyphosis** or **scoliosis** and may cause spinal nerve compression.

C. Whiplash injury of the neck

–is produced by a force that drives the trunk forward while the head lags behind, causing **the head** (with the upper part of the neck) **to hyperextend and the lower part of the neck to hyperflex rapidly.** This may occur in a rear-end automobile collision.

–occurs frequently at the junction of vertebrae C4 and C5; thus vertebrae C1–C4 act as the lash, and vertebrae C5–C7 act as the handle of the whip.

–results in neck pain, stiff neck, and headache.

–can be treated by supporting the head and neck using a cervical collar that is higher in the back than in the front; the collar keeps the cervical vertebral column in a flexed position.

D. Hangman's fracture

–is a fracture of the vertebral arch through the pedicles of the axis (C2), which may occur as a result of judicial hanging or automobile accidents.

–may cause rupture of the anterior longitudinal ligament but may not displace the odontoid process.

Soft Tissues of the Back

I. Superficial Tissues

A. Triangles and fascia

B. Superficial muscles (Figure 7-6; Table 7-1)

Table 7–1. Superficial Muscles of the Back

Muscle	Origin	Insertion	Nerve	Action
Trapezius	External occipital protuberance, superior nuchal line, ligamentum nuchae, spines of C7–T12	Spine of scapula, acromion, and lateral third of clavicle	Spinal accessory nerve, C3–C4	Adducts, rotates, elevates, and depresses scapula
Levator scapulae	Transverse processes of C1–C4	Medial border of scapula	Nerves to levator scapulae, C3–C4; dorsal scapular nerve	Elevates scapula; rotate glenoid cavity
Rhomboid minor	Spines of C7–T1	Root of spine of scapula	Dorsal scapular nerve, C5	Adducts scapula
Rhomboid major	Spines of T2–T5	Medial border of scapula	Dorsal scapular nerve, C5	Adducts scapula
Latissimus dorsi	Spines of T7–T12, thoracodorsal fascia, iliac crest, ribs 9–12	Floor of bicipital groove of humerus	Thoracodorsal	Adducts, extends, and rotates arm medially; depresses scapula
Serratus posterior–superior	Ligamentum nuchae, supraspinal ligament, and spines of C7–T3	Upper border of ribs 2–5	Intercostal nerve, T1—T4	Elevates ribs
Serratus posterior–inferior	Supraspinous ligament and spines of T11–L3	Lower border of ribs 9–12	Intercostal nerve, T9–12	Depresses ribs

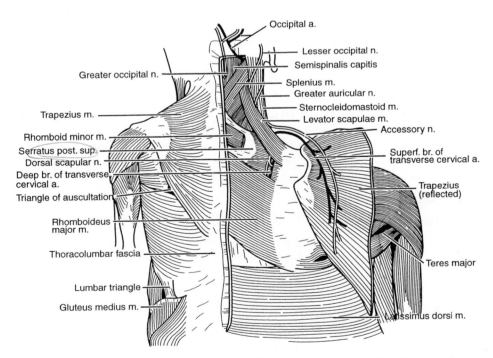

Figure 7-6. Superficial muscles of the back, with particular attention to the shoulder region.

1. **Triangle of auscultation** (see Figure 7-6)

   –is bounded by the upper border of the **latissimus dorsi,** the lateral border of the **trapezius,** and the medial border of the **scapula.**
   –has a floor formed by the **rhomboid major.**
   –is the site where **breathing sounds** can be heard most clearly.

2. **Lumbar triangle**

   –is formed by the iliac crest, latissimus dorsi, and posterior free border of the external oblique abdominis muscle.

3. **Thoracolumbar (lumbodorsal) fascia**

   –invests the deep muscles of the back.
   –has an **anterior layer** that lies anterior to the erector spinae and attaches to the vertebral **transverse process.**
   –has a **posterior layer** that lies posterior to the erector spinae and attaches to the **spinous processes.**
   –provides the origins for the latissimus dorsi and the internal oblique and transverse abdominis muscles.

C. **Blood vessels** (see Figure 7-6)

1. **Occipital artery**

   –arises from the external carotid artery, runs deep to the sternocleidomastoid muscle, and lies on the obliquus capitis superior and the semispinalis capitis.
   –pierces the trapezius, is accompanied by the **greater occipital nerve (C2),** and supplies the scalp in the occipital region.
   –gives off the **descending branch,** which divides into the **superficial branch** that anastomoses with the transverse cervical artery and the **deep branch** that anastomoses with the deep cervical artery from the costocervical trunk.

2. **Transverse cervical artery**

   –arises from the thyrocervical trunk of the subclavian artery.
   –has a **superficial branch** that accompanies the **spinal accessory nerve** on the deep surface of the trapezius.
   –has a **deep branch** that accompanies the **dorsal scapular nerve (C5)** deep to the levator scapulae and the rhomboids along the medial side of the scapula.

D. **Nerves** (see Figure 7-6)

1. **Accessory nerve**

   –consists of a cranial portion, which joins the vagus nerve, and a spinal portion, which runs deep to the sternocleidomastoid, lies on the levator scapulae, and passes deep to the trapezius.
   –supplies the sternocleidomastoid and trapezius muscles.

2. **Dorsal scapular nerve (C5)**

   –is derived from the **ventral primary ramus** of the fifth cervical spinal nerve and runs along with the deep branch of the transverse cervical artery.

3. **Greater occipital nerve (C2)**

–is derived as a medial branch of the **dorsal primary ramus,** the second cervical spinal nerve.

–crosses obliquely between the obliquus inferior and the semispinalis capitis, pierces the semispinalis capitis and the trapezius, and supplies cutaneous innervation in the occipital region.

–innervates the semispinalis capitis and communicates with the suboccipital and third occipital nerves.

4. **Third (least) occipital nerve (C3)**

–is derived from the **dorsal primary ramus** of the third cervical spinal nerve.

–ascends across the suboccipital region, pierces the trapezius, and supplies cutaneous innervation in the occipital region.

5. **Lesser occipital nerve (C2)**

–is derived from the **ventral primary ramus** of the second cervical spinal root.

–is a cutaneous branch of the cervical plexus and ascends along the posterior border of the sternocleidomastoid to the scalp behind the auricle.

II. Deep Tissues

A. Deep or intrinsic muscles

1. **Muscles of the superficial layer: spinotransverse group**

–consist of the **splenius capitis** and the **splenius cervicis.**

–originate from the spinous processes and insert into the transverse processes (splenius cervicis) and on the mastoid process and the superior nuchal line (splenius capitis).

–are innervated by the dorsal primary rami of the middle and lower cervical spinal nerves.

–**extend, rotate,** and laterally **flex** the head and neck.

2. **Muscles of the intermediate layer: sacrospinalis group**

–consist of the **erector spinae (sacrospinalis),** which is divided into three columns: iliocostalis (lateral column), longissimus (intermediate column), and spinalis (medial column).

–originate from the sacrum, ilium, ribs, and spinous processes of lumbar and lower thoracic vertebrae.

–insert on the ribs **(iliocostalis);** on the ribs, transverse processes, and mastoid process **(longissimus);** and on the spinous processes **(spinalis).**

–are innervated by the dorsal primary rami of the spinal nerves.

–**extend, rotate,** and laterally flex the vertebral column and head.

3. **Muscles of the deep layer: transversospinalis group**

–consist of the **semispinalis** (capitis, cervicis, and thoracis); the **multifidus;** and the **rotators.**

–The **semispinalis** muscles originate from the transverse processes and insert into the skull (semispinalis capitis) and the spinous processes (semispinalis cervicis and thoracis).

–The **rotators** run from the transverse processes to spinous processes two vertebrae above (longus) and one vertebra above (brevis).

–The **multifidus** originates from the sacrum, ilium, and transverse processes and inserts on the spinous processes. It is best developed in the lumbar region.

–are innervated by the dorsal primary rami of the spinal nerves.

–**extend** and **rotate** the head, neck, and trunk.

B. Segmental muscles

–are innervated by the dorsal primary rami of the spinal nerves.

–consist of the following:

1. Interspinales

–run between adjacent spinous processes and aid in extension of the vertebral column.

2. Intertransversarii

–run between adjacent transverse processes and aid in lateral flexion of the vertebral column.

3. Levatores costarum (longus and brevis)

–extend from the transverse processes to ribs and elevate ribs.

III. Suboccipital Area (Figure 7-7)

A. Suboccipital triangle

–is bound medially by the rectus capitis posterior major, laterally by the obliquus capitis superior muscle, and inferiorly by the obliquus capitis inferior muscle.

–has a roof formed by the semispinalis capitis and longissimus capitis.

–has a floor formed by the posterior arch of the atlas and posterior atlanto-occipital membrane.

–contains the vertebral artery and suboccipital nerve and vessels.

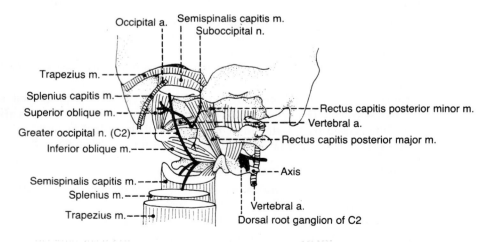

Figure 7-7. Suboccipital triangle.

B. Suboccipital muscles (Table 7-2)

Table 7-2. Suboccipital Muscles of the Back

Muscle	Origin	Insertion	Nerve	Action
Rectus capitis posterior major	Spine of axis	Lateral portion of inferior nuchal line	Suboccipital	Extends, rotates, and flexes head laterally
Rectus capitis posterior minor	Posterior tubercle of atlas	Occipital bone below inferior nuchal line	Suboccipital	Extends and flexes head laterally
Obliquus capitis superior	Transverse process of atlas	Occipital bone above inferior nuchal line	Suboccipital	Extends, rotates, and flexes head laterally
Obliquus capitis inferior	Spine of axis	Transverse process of atlas	Suboccipital	Extends and rotates head laterally

C. Suboccipital nerve

–is derived from the dorsal ramus of C1 and emerges between the vertebral artery above and the posterior arch of the atlas below.

–supplies the muscles of the suboccipital triangle and semispinalis capitis.

–contains skeletal motor fibers and no cutaneous sensory fibers but occasionally has a cutaneous branch.

D. Vertebral artery

–arises from the subclavian artery and ascends through the transverse foramina of the upper six cervical vertebrae.

–winds behind the lateral mass of the atlas, runs in a groove on the superior surface of the posterior arch of the atlas, pierces the dura mater to enter the vertebral canal, and ascends into the cranial cavity through the foramen magnum.

–gives off an anterior spinal and two posterior spinal arteries.

E. Vertebral veins

–are formed in the suboccipital triangle by union of tributaries from the venous plexus around the foramen magnum, the suboccipital venous plexus, and the intervertebral veins.

–do not emerge from the cranial cavity with the vertebral artery through the foramen magnum. Instead, they enter the transverse foramen of the atlas and descend through the next five successive foramina, emptying into the brachiocephalic vein. The small accessory vertebral veins arise from the plexus, traverse the seventh cervical transverse foramina, and end in the brachiocephalic vein.

F. Joints

1. Atlanto-occipital joint

–is an **ellipsoidal synovial joint** that occurs between the superior articular facets of the atlas and the occipital condyles.

–is involved primarily in **flexion, extension, and lateral flexion of the head.**

2. **Atlantoaxial joints**

–are **synovial joints,** consisting of two lateral **plane joints,** which are between articular facets of the atlas and axis, and one median **pivot joint** between the dens of the axis and the anterior arch of the atlas.

–are involved in **rotation of the atlas and head** as a unit on the axis.

F. **Components of the occipitoaxial ligament** (see Figure 7-5)

1. **Cruciform ligament**

a. **Transverse ligament**

–runs between the lateral masses of the atlas, arching over the dens of the axis.

b. **Longitudinal ligament**

–extends from the dens of the axis to the anterior aspect of the foramen magnum and to the body of the axis.

2. **Apical ligament**

–extends from the apex of the dens to the anterior aspect of the foramen magnum (of the occipital bone).

3. **Alar ligament**

–extends from the apex of the dens to the tubercle on the medial side of the occipital condyle.

4. **Tectorial membrane**

–is an upward extension of the posterior longitudinal ligament from the body of the axis to the basilar part of the occipital bone anterior to the foramen magnum.

–covers the posterior surface of the dens and the apical, alar, and cruciform ligaments.

Spinal Cord and Associated Structures

I. **Spinal Cord** (Figure 7-8; see Figure 7-2)

–is cylindrical, occupies about the **upper two-thirds** of the **vertebral canal,** and is enveloped by the three **meninges.**

–has cervical and lumbar enlargements for nerve supply of the upper and lower limbs, respectively.

–contains **gray matter,** which is located in the interior (in contrast to the cerebral hemispheres); the spinal cord is surrounded by **white matter.**

–has a conical end known as the **conus medullaris,** which terminates at the level of L2 vertebra or the intervertebral disk between L1 and L2 vertebrae.

–grows much more slowly than the bony vertebral column during fetal development, and thus its end gradually shifts to a higher level; ends at the level of L2 vertebra in the adult and at the level of L3 vertebra in the newborn.

–receives blood from the anterior spinal artery and two posterior spinal arteries as well as from branches of the vertebral, cervical, and posterior intercostal and lumbar arteries.

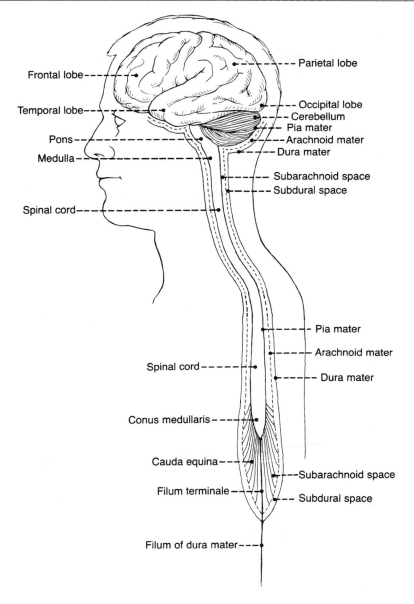

Figure 7-8. Meninges.

II. Spinal Nerves

–consist of **31 pairs** of nerves (8 cervical, 12 thoracic, 5 lumbar, 5 sacral, 1 coccygeal).

–are formed within an intervertebral foramen by union of the ventral root and the dorsal root with ganglion, which contains cell bodies of sensory neurons.

–are divided into the **dorsal primary rami,** which innervate the skin and deep muscles of the back; the **ventral primary rami,** which form the plexuses (C1–C4, cervical; C5–T1, brachial; L1–L4, lumbar; and L4–S4, sacral); and the **intercostal (T1–T11) and subcostal (T12) nerves.**

–are connected with the sympathetic chain ganglia by **rami communicantes.**

–are mixed nerves, containing all of the **general functional components** (i.e., general somatic afferent [GSA]; general somatic efferent [GSE]; general visceral afferent [GVA]; and general visceral efferent [GVE]).

–contain **sensory (GSA and GVA) fibers** with cell bodies in the dorsal root ganglion.

–contain **motor (GSE) fibers** with cell bodies in the anterior horn of the spinal cord.

–contain **preganglionic sympathetic (GVE) fibers** with cell bodies in the intermediolateral cell column in the lateral horn of the spinal cord (segments between T1 and L2).

–contain **preganglionic parasympathetic (GVE) fibers** with cell bodies in the intermediolateral cell column of the spinal cord segments between S2 and S4. These GVE fibers leave the sacral nerves via the pelvic splanchnic nerves.

III. Mepinges (see Figures 7-2 and 7-8)

A. Pia mater

–is the innermost meningeal layer; it is closely applied to the spinal cord and thus cannot be dissected from it. It also enmeshes blood vessels on the surfaces of the spinal cord.

–has lateral extensions **(denticulate ligaments)** between dorsal and ventral roots of spinal nerves and an inferior extension known as the **filum terminale.**

B. Arachnoid mater

–is a filmy, transparent, spidery layer connected to the pia mater by web-like trabeculations.

–forms the **subarachnoid space,** the space between the arachnoid layer and the pia mater that is filled with **cerebrospinal fluid (CSF)** and that extends to the second sacral vertebral level. The enlarged subarachnoid space between vertebrae L1 and S2 is called the **lumbar cistern.**

C. Dura mater

–is the tough, fibrous, outermost layer of the meninges.

–The **subdural space** is a potential space between the arachnoid and dura. It extends inferiorly to the second sacral vertebral level and contains only sufficient fluid to moisten the surfaces of two membranes.

–The **epidural space** is external to it and contains the internal vertebral venous plexus and epidural fat.

IV. Structures Associated with the Spinal Cord

A. Cauda equina ("horse's tail")

–is formed by a great lash of dorsal and ventral roots of the lumbar and sacral spinal nerves that surround the **filum terminale.**

–is located within the **subarachnoid space (lumbar cistern)** below the level of the **conus medullaris.**

–is free to float in the CSF within the lumbar cistern and therefore is not damaged during a spinal tap.

B. Denticulate ligaments

–are lateral extensions of the spinal **pia mater,** consisting of **21 pairs** of toothpick-like processes.

–extend laterally from the pia through the arachnoid to the dura mater between dorsal and ventral roots of the spinal nerves.

–help **hold the spinal cord** in position within the subarachnoid space.

C. Filum terminale (internum)

–is a prolongation of the **pia mater** from the tip (conus medullaris) of the spinal cord at the level of L2.

–lies in the midst of the cauda equina and ends at the level of S2 by attaching to the apex of the dural sac.

–blends with the dura at the apex of the dural sac, and then the dura continues downward as the **filum terminale externum** (filum of the dura mater of coccygeal ligament), which is attached to the dorsum of the coccyx.

D. Cerebrospinal fluid (CSF)

–is contained in the subarachnoid space between the arachnoid and pia mater.

–is formed by **vascular choroid plexuses** in the ventricles of the brain.

–circulates through the ventricles, enters the subarachnoid space, and eventually filters into the venous system through arachnoid villi projecting into the dural venous sinuses, particularly the superior sagittal sinus.

V. Dermatome

–is an area of skin innervated by sensory fibers derived from a particular spinal nerve or segment of the spinal cord. Knowledge of the segmental innervation is useful clinically to produce a region of anesthesia or to determine which nerve has been damaged.

VI. Clinical Considerations

A. Lumbar puncture (spinal tap)

–is the tapping of the subarachnoid space in the lumbar region, usually between the laminae of vertebrae L3 and L4 or vertebrae L4 and L5.

–allows **measurement of CSF pressure** and withdrawal of some of the fluid for **bacteriologic and chemical examinations.**

–allows introduction of **anesthesia, drugs, or radiopaque material** into the subarachnoid space.

B. Caudal (epidural) anesthesia

–is used to **block the spinal nerves in the epidural space** by injection of local anesthetic agents via the sacral hiatus located between the sacral cornua.

C. Herpes zoster (shingles)

–is an infectious disease caused by a herpes virus that remains latent in the dorsal root ganglia of spinal nerves and the sensory ganglia of cranial nerves.

–results from activation of the virus, which travels down the sensory nerve to produce severe neuralgic pain, an eruption of groups of vesicles, or a rash in the dermatome of the nerve.

D. Tethered cord syndrome

–is a congenital anomaly resulting from defective closure of the neural tube.

–is characterized by the abnormally low conus medullaris, which is tethered by a short, thickened filum terminale, leading to such conditions as progressive neurologic defects in the legs and feet and scoliosis.

E. Arnold-Chiari (or Chiari) deformity

–is a congenital cerebromedullary malformation in which the cerebellum and medulla oblongata protrude down into the vertebral canal through the foramen magnum.

–is frequently associated with spina bifida and results in such conditions as a short neck and obstructive hydrocephalus.

Review Test

Directions: Each of the numbered items or incomplete statements in this section is followed by answers or by completions of the statement. Select the **one** lettered answer or completion that is **best** in each case.

1. Lumbar punctures or spinal taps are performed to withdraw cerebrospinal fluid (CSF), which is found

(A) in the epidural space
(B) in the subdural space
(C) between the pia mater and the spinal cord
(D) in the subarachnoid space
(E) between the arachnoid layer and dura mater

2. Rupture of the internal vertebral venous plexus results in an accumulation of blood in which of the following spaces?

(A) Space deep to the pia mater
(B) Space between the arachnoid and dura maters
(C) Subdural space
(D) Epidural space
(E) Subarachnoid space

3. A patient has two masses of tumors in the intervertebral foramina between the fourth and fifth cervical vertebrae and between the fourth and fifth thoracic vertebrae. Which of the following spinal nerves may be damaged?

(A) Fourth cervical and fourth thoracic nerves
(B) Fifth cervical and fifth thoracic nerves
(C) Fourth cervical and fifth thoracic nerves
(D) Fifth cervical and fourth thoracic nerves
(E) Third cervical and fourth thoracic nerves

4. The anterior longitudinal ligament

(A) lies between the intervertebral disk and the dura
(B) extends from the coccyx to the atlas
(C) ends superiorly as the tectorial membrane
(D) limits flexion of the vertebral column
(E) is narrow at the upper end but widens as it descends

5. Which of the following structures is the primary site for absorption of cerebrospinal fluid (CSF) into the venous system?

(A) Choroid plexus
(B) Vertebral venous plexus
(C) Arachnoid villi
(D) Internal jugular vein
(E) Subarachnoid trabeculae

6. A patient is brought to the emergency department with multiple fractures of the transverse processes of the cervical and upper thoracic vertebrae. Which of the following muscles might be paralyzed?

(A) Trapezius
(B) Levator scapulae
(C) Rhomboid major
(D) Serratus posterior superior
(E) Rectus capitis posterior major

7. The body of vertebra T4 articulates with the

(A) head of the third rib
(B) neck of the fourth rib
(C) tubercle of the fourth rib
(D) head of the fifth rib
(E) tubercle of the fifth rib

8. The obliquus capitis inferior muscle in the suboccipital region

(A) originates from the posterior tubercle of the atlas
(B) inserts on the transverse process of the axis
(C) is attached to the occipital bone of the skull
(D) is innervated by the greater occipital nerve
(E) forms a boundary of the suboccipital triangle

9. A patient is brought to a hospital with multiple injuries, including lesions of the dorsal primary rami of the spinal nerves. These lesions could result in paralysis of which of the following muscles?

(A) Rhomboid major
(B) Levator scapulae
(C) Serratus posterior superior
(D) Iliocostalis
(E) Latissimus dorsi

10. A stab near the superior angle of the scapula injuring both the dorsal scapular nerve and the spinal accessory nerve would result in paralysis or weakness of which of the following muscles?

(A) Trapezius and serratus posterior superior
(B) Rhomboid major and trapezius
(C) Rhomboid minor and latissimus dorsi
(D) Splenius cervicis and sternocleidomastoid
(E) Levator scapulae and erector spinae

11. When cerebrospinal fluid (CSF) is withdrawn by lumbar puncture, which of the following structures is most likely penetrated by the needle?

(A) Pia mater
(B) Filum terminale externum
(C) Posterior longitudinal ligament
(D) Ligamentum flavum
(E) Anulus fibrosus

12. Which of the following structures would be spared if the spinal cord is crushed at the fourth lumbar spinal cord level?

(A) Dorsal horn
(B) Ventral horn
(C) Lateral horn
(D) Gray matter
(E) Pia mater

13. The internal vertebral venous plexus

(A) is formed primarily by two vertebral veins
(B) contains numerous valves
(C) has no communication with the cranial venous sinuses
(D) is located in the subdural space
(E) is the route of metastasis of carcinoma from the lung, breast, and prostate gland to the bones and the brain

14. The suboccipital nerve is injured by knife wound at the point where it emerges from between the vertebral artery and the posterior arch of the atlas. Which of the following muscles is spared from paralysis?

(A) Rectus capitis posterior major
(B) Semispinalis capitus
(C) Splenius capitis
(D) Obliquus capitis superior
(E) Obliquus capitis inferior

15. The atlantoaxial joint allows which of the following movement of the head?

(A) Extension
(B) Flexion
(C) Abduction
(D) Adduction
(E) Rotation

16. Which of the following ligaments is posterior to the spinal cord?

(A) Anterior longitudinal ligament
(B) Alar ligament
(C) Posterior longitudinal ligament
(D) Cruciform ligament
(E) Ligamentum nuchae

17. The spinal epidural space

(A) may be entered via the sacral hiatus
(B) extends from the base of the skull to the second lumbar vertebra
(C) contains an external vertebral venous plexus
(D) contains cerebrospinal fluid (CSF)
(E) is the space deep to the dura mater

18. An abnormally increased curvature of the thoracic vertebral column results in which of the following conditions?

(A) Lordosis
(B) Spina bifida occulta
(C) Meningomyelocele
(D) Meningocele
(E) Kyphosis

19. Which of the following conditions is produced by a force that drives the trunk forward while the head lags behind in a rear-end automobile collision?

(A) Scoliosis
(B) Hangman's syndrome
(C) Meningomyelocele
(D) Whiplash injury
(E) Herniated disk

20. The victim of an automobile accident is brought to the emergency department with a crushed second cervical vertebra (axis). Which of the following structures would be intact after the accident?

(A) Alar ligament
(B) Apical ligament
(C) Semispinalis cervicis muscle
(D) Rectus capitis posterior minor
(E) Obliquus capitis inferior

21. A lateral extension of the pia mater forms which of the following structures?

(A) Filum terminale internum
(B) Coccygeal ligament
(C) Denticulate ligament
(D) Choroid plexus
(E) Tectorial membrane

22. Which of the following muscles is innervated by the dorsal scapular nerve and adducts the scapula?

(A) Semispinalis capitis
(B) Rhomboid major
(C) Multifidus
(D) Rotator longus
(E) Iliocostalis

23. After an automobile accident, a back muscle, which forms the boundaries of the triangle of auscultation and the lumbar triangle, receives no blood. Which of the following muscles might be ischemic?

(A) Levator scapulae
(B) Rhomboid minor
(C) Latissimus dorsi
(D) Trapezius
(E) Splenius capitis

24. Which of the following muscles become ischemic soon after ligation of the superficial or ascending branch of the transverse cervical artery?

(A) Latissimus dorsi
(B) Multifidus
(C) Trapezius
(D) Rhomboid major
(E) Longissimus capitis

25. Which one of the following statements concerning the structure of the back is correct?

(A) Paralysis of the erector spinae may result from a lesion of the ventral primary rami of the spinal nerves
(B) Injury to the suboccipital nerve causes loss of cutaneous sensation in the occipital region
(C) The sacrum is composed of five fused sacral vertebrae and has five pairs of foramina for sacral nerves
(D) Fracture of the transverse process of the atlas may impair functions of the superior and inferior obliquus capitis muscles
(E) The posterior longitudinal ligament is penetrated by the needle during lumbar puncture

Directions: Each set of matching questions in this section consists of a list of four to twenty-six lettered options (some of which may be in figures) followed by several numbered items. For each numbered item, select the ONE lettered option that is most closely associated with it. To avoid spending too much time on matching sets with large numbers of options, it is generally advisable to begin each set by reading the list of options. Then, for each item in the set, try to generate the correct answer and locate it in the option list, rather than evaluating each option individually. Each lettered option may be selected once, more than once, or not at all.

Questions 26–30

Match each of the following descriptions with the appropriate lettered structure on the computed tomography (CT) scan of the back.

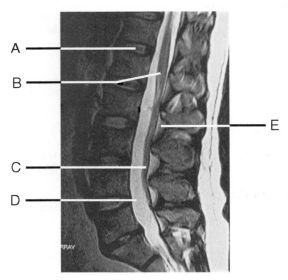

26. Indicates cerebrospinal fluid (CSF) in the subarachnoid space

27. Is formed by the dorsal and ventral roots of the lumbar and sacral nerves

28. Is a conical end of the spinal cord, which terminates at the level of the second lumbar vertebra

29. Consists of a central nucleus pulposus and the surrounding anulus fibrosus

30. Is produced by vascular choroid plexuses in the ventricles of the brain and accumulated in the subarachnoid space

Answers and Explanations

1–D. Cerebrospinal fluid (CSF) is found in the subarachnoid space, which is a wide interval between the arachnoid layer and the pia mater. The epidural space contains the internal vertebral venous plexus and epidural fat. The subdural space between the arachnoid and the dura contains a little fluid to moisten the meningeal surface. The pia mater closely covers the spinal cord and enmeshes blood vessels on the surfaces of the spinal cord. Thus, the space between the spinal cord and the pia is a potential space.

2–D. The space between the arachnoid and dura maters is the subdural space, which contains a film of fluid. The spinal cord and blood vessels lies deep to the pia mater. The space between the vertebral canal and the dura mater is the epidural space, which contains the internal vertebral venous plexus. The subarachnoid space contains cerebrospinal fluid (CSF).

3–D. All cervical spinal nerves exit through the intervertebral foramina above the corresponding vertebrae, except the eighth cervical nerves, which run inferior to the seventh cervical vertebra. All other spinal nerves exit the intervertebral foramina below the corresponding vertebrae. Therefore, the fifth cervical nerve passes between the fourth and fifth cervical vertebrae, and the fourth thoracic nerve runs between the fourth and fifth thoracic vertebrae.

4–E. The anterior longitudinal ligament extends from the base of the skull to the sacrum on the anterior surface of the vertebral bodies and intervertebral disks, and limits extension of the vertebral column. The tectorial membrane is an upward extension of the posterior longitudinal ligament from the body of the axis to the basilar part of the occipital bone.

5–C. Cerebrospinal fluid (CSF), which is produced by the choroid plexuses of the ventricles of the brain, circulates in the subarachnoid space. It is absorbed into the venous system primarily through the arachnoid villi projecting into the cranial dural venous sinuses, particularly the superior sagittal sinus.

6–B. The levator scapulae arises from the transverse processes of the upper cervical vertebrae and inserts on the medial border of the scapula. The other muscles of the back are attached to the spinous processes of the vertebrae.

7–D. The body of vertebra T4 articulates with the heads of the fourth and fifth ribs. The transverse process of vertebra T4 articulates with the tubercle of the fourth rib.

8–E. The obliquus capitis inferior originates from the spinous process of the axis, inserts on the transverse process of the atlas, does not attach to the occipital bone, is innervated by the suboccipital nerve, and forms a boundary of the suboccipital triangle. The greater occipital nerve innervates the semispinalis capitis but is mainly cutaneous, supplying the posterior part of the scalp.

9–D. The dorsal primary rami of the spinal nerves innervate the deep muscles of the back, including the iliocostalis. The superficial muscles of the back are innervated by the ventral rami of the spinal nerves.

10–B. The dorsal scapular nerve innervates the levator scapulae, and rhomboid muscles, whereas the accessory nerve innervates the trapezius and sternocleidomastoid muscles.

11–D. The cerebrospinal fluid (CSF) is located in the subarachnoid space, between the arachnoid layer and pia mater. In a lumbar puncture, the needle penetrates the skin, fascia, ligamentum flavum, epidural space, dura mater, subdural space, and arachnoid mater. The pia mater forms the internal boundary of the subarachnoid space, so it cannot be penetrated by needle. The posterior longitudinal ligament lies anterior to the spinal cord, and thus it is not penetrated by the needle. The anulus fibrosus consists of concentric layers of fibrous tissue and fibrocartilage surrounding and retaining the nucleus pulposus of the intervertebral disk, which lies anterior to the spinal cord.

12–C. The lateral horns, which contain sympathetic preganglionic neuron cell bodies, are present between the first thoracic and second lumbar spinal cord levels (T1–L2). The lateral horns of the second, third, and fourth sacral spinal cord levels (S2–S4) contain parasympathetic preganglionic neuron cell bodies. The entire spinal cord is surrounded by the pia mater and has the dorsal horn, ventral horn, and gray matter. Note that the fourth lumbar spinal cord level is not same as the fourth vertebral level.

13–E. The vertebral vein arises from the suboccipital venous plexus, runs through the transverse foramina of the cervical vertebra, forms a plexus around the vertebral artery, and opens into the brachiocephalic vein. The veins forming the plexus are valveless and lie in the epidural space. They communicate with the cranial venous sinuses and paravertebral veins in the thorax, abdomen, and pelvis. Therefore, the vertebral venous plexus provides a path for the spread of cancer cells from the lung, breast, and prostate gland to the bones and the brain.

14–C. The splenius capitis is innervated by dorsal primary rami of the middle and lower cervical nerves. The suboccipital nerve (dorsal primary ramus of C1) supplies the muscles of the suboccipital area (e.g., the rectus capitis posterior major) and the semispinalis capitis. The rectus capitis anterior is innervated by the ventral primary rami of the first and second cervical nerves.

15–E. The atlantoaxial joints are synovial joints that consist of two plane joints and one pivot joint, and are involved primarily in rotation of the head.

16–E. The ligamentum nuchae is formed of supraspinous ligaments that extend from the seventh cervical vertebra to the external occipital protuberance and crest. The anterior longitudinal ligament runs anterior to the vertebral bodies. The alar and cruciform ligaments also lie anterior to the spinal cord. Although the posterior longitudinal ligament interconnects the vertebral bodies and intervertebral disks posteriorly, it runs anterior to the spinal cord within the vertebral canal.

17–A. The spinal epidural space is external to the dura mater and contains the internal vertebral venous plexus. It extends from the base of the skull to the sacrum and can be entered through the sacral hiatus for caudal (extradural) anesthesia. The subarachnoid space contains cerebrospinal fluid (CSF).

18–E. Kyphosis is an abnormally increased thoracic curvature. Lordosis is an abnormal accentuation of the lumbar curvature. Spina bifida occulta is failure of the vertebral arch to fuse (bony defect only). Meningocele is a protrusion of the meninges through the unfused arch of the vertebra, whereas meningomyelocele is a protrusion of the spinal cord as well as the meninges.

19–D. Whiplash injury of the neck is produced by a force that drives the trunk forward while the head lags behind. Scoliosis is a lateral deviation due to unequal growth of the spinal column. Hangman's syndrome is a fracture of the neural arch through the pedicle of the axis that may occur as a result of judicial hanging or motor vehicle accidents. Meningomyelocele is a protrusion of the spinal cord and its meninges. Herniated disk compresses the spinal nerve roots when the nucleus pulposus is protruded through the anulus fibrosus.

20–D. The rectus capitis posterior minor arises from the posterior tubercle of the atlas and inserts on the occipital bone below the inferior nuchal line. The alar ligament extends from the apex of the dens to the medial side of the occipital bone. The apical ligament extends from the dens of the axis to the anterior aspect of the foramen magnum of the occipital bone. The semispinalis cervicis arises from the transverse processes and inserts on the spinous processes. The obliquus capitis inferior originates from the spine of the axis and inserts on the transverse process of the atlas.

21–C. The filum terminale (internum) is an inferior extension of the pia mater from the tip of the conus medullaris. The coccygeal ligament, which is also called the filum terminale externum or the filum of the dura, extends from the tip of the dural sac to the coccyx. The vascular choroid plexuses produce the cerebrospinal fluid (CSF) in the ventricles of the brain. The tectorial membrane is an upward extension of the posterior longitudinal ligaments from the body of the axis to the basilar part of the occipital bone.

22–B. The semispinalis capitis, multifidus, rotator longus and iliocostalis muscles are deep muscles of the back, innervated by dorsal primary rami of the spinal nerves, and have no attachment to the scapula. However, the rhomboid major is a superficial muscle of the back; is innervated by the dorsal scapular nerve, which arises from the ventral primary ramus of the fifth cervical nerve; and adducts the scapula.

23–C. The latissimus dorsi forms boundaries of the auscultation and lumbar triangles. The levator scapulae, rhomboid minor, and splenius capitis muscles do not form boundaries of these two triangles. The trapezius muscle forms a boundary of the auscultation triangle but not the lumbar triangle.

24–C. The trapezius receives blood from the superficial branch of the transverse cervical artery. The latissimus dorsi receives blood from the thoracodorsal artery. The rhomboid major receives blood from the deep or descending branch of the transverse cervical artery. The multifidus and longissimus capitis receive blood from the segmental arteries.

25–D. The obliquus capitis superior originates from the transverse process of the atlas, and the obliquus capitis inferior inserts on the same transverse process. (The transverse process of the atlas provides the origin for the obliquus capitis superior and the insertion for the obliquus capitis inferior.) The erector spinae is innervated by dorsal primary rami of the spinal nerves. The suboccipital nerve contains no cutaneous sensory fibers. The sacrum has four pairs of foramina for sacral nerves. The posterior longitudinal ligament lies anterior to the spinal cord.

26–D. The subarachnoid space is the interval between the pia and arachnoid maters, bridged by delicate trabeculae and contains cerebrospinal fluid (CSF).

27–C. The cauda equina is formed by a great lash of the dorsal and ventral roots of the lumbar and sacral nerves.

28–B. The conus medullaris is a conical end of the spinal cord and terminates at the level of the L2 vertebra or the intervertebral disk between L1 and L2 vertebrae.

29–A. The intervertebral disk lies between the bodies of two vertebrae and consists of a central mucoid substance; the nucleus pulposus, with a surrounding fibrocartilaginous lamina; and the anulus fibrosus.

30–D. The cerebrospinal fluid (CSF) is produced by vascular choroid plexuses in the ventricles of the brain, circulated in the subarachnoid space, and filtered into the venous system through the arachnoid villi and arachnoid granulations.

8

Head and Neck

Structures of the Neck

I. Major Divisions (Figure 8-1)

A. Posterior triangle

–is bounded by the posterior border of the **sternocleidomastoid** muscle, the anterior border of the **trapezius** muscle, and the superior border of the **clavicle**.

–has a roof formed by the **platysma** and the investing layer of the **deep cervical fascia.**

–has a floor formed by the splenius capitis and levator scapulae muscles, and the anterior, middle, and posterior scalene muscles.

–contains the accessory nerve, cutaneous branches of the cervical plexus, external jugular vein, transverse cervical and suprascapular vessels, subclavian vein (occasionally) and artery, posterior (inferior) belly of the omohyoid, and roots and trunks of the brachial plexus.

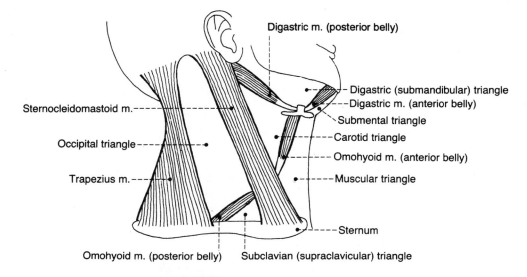

Figure 8-1. Subdivisions of the cervical triangle.

–also contains the nerve to the subclavius as well as the dorsal scapular, suprascapular, and long thoracic nerves.

–is further divided into the **occipital** and **subclavian** (supraclavicular or omoclavicular) triangles by the omohyoid posterior belly.

B. Anterior triangle

–is bounded by the anterior border of the sternocleidomastoid, the anterior midline of the neck, and the inferior border of the mandible.

–has a roof formed by the **platysma** and the **investing layer** of the deep cervical fascia.

–is further divided by the omohyoid anterior belly and the digastric anterior and posterior bellies into the **digastric** (submandibular), **submental** (suprahyoid), **carotid,** and **muscular** (inferior carotid) triangles.

II. Muscles (Figure 8-2; Table 8-1)

Table 8–1. Muscles of the Neck

Muscle	Origin	Insertion	Nerve	Action
Cervical muscles				
Platysma	Superficial fascia over upper part of deltoid and pectoralis major	Mandible; skin and muscles over mandible and angle of mouth	Facial n.	Depresses lower jaw and lip and angle of mouth; wrinkles skin of neck
Sternocleido-mastoid	Manubrium sterni and medial one-third of clavicle	Mastoid process and lateral one-half of superior nuchal line	Spinal accessory n.; C2–C3 (sensory)	Singly turns face toward opposite side; together flex head, raise thorax
Suprahyoid muscles				
Digastric	Anterior belly from digastric fossa of mandible; posterior belly from mastoid notch	Intermediate tendon attached to body of hyoid	Posterior belly by facial n.; anterior belly by mylohyoid n. of trigeminal n.	Elevates hyoid and floor of mouth; depresses mandible
Mylohyoid	Mylohyoid line of mandible	Median raphe and body of hyoid bone	Mylohyoid n. of trigeminal n.	Elevates hyoid and floor of mouth; depresses mandible
Stylohyoid	Styloid process	Body of hyoid	Facial n.	Elevates hyoid
Geniohyoid	Genial tubercle of mandible	Body of hyoid	C1 via hypo-glossal n.	Elevates hyoid and floor of mouth

(continued)

Table 8–1. Muscles of the Neck *(continued)*

Muscle	Origin	Insertion	Nerve	Action
Infrahyoid muscles				
Sternohyoid	Manubrium sterni and medial end of clavicle	Body of hyoid	Ansa cervicalis	Depresses hyoid and larynx
Sternothyroid	Manubrium sterni; first costal cartilage	Oblique line of thyroid cartilage	Ansa cervicalis	Depresses thyroid cartilage and larynx
Thyrohyoid	Oblique line of thyroid cartilage	Body and greater horn of hyoid	C1 via hypoglossal n.	Depresses and retracts hyoid and larynx
Omohyoid	Inferior belly from medial lip of suprascapular notch and suprascapular ligament; superior belly from intermediate tendon	Inferior belly to intermediate tendon; superior belly to body of hyoid	Ansa cervicalis	Depresses and retracts hyoid and larynx

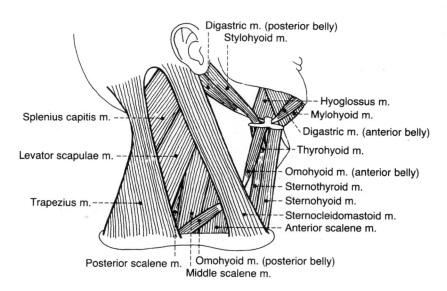

Figure 8-2. Muscles of the cervical triangle.

III. Nerves (Figures 8-3 and 8-4)

A. Accessory nerve

–is formed by the **union of cranial and spinal roots.**

–has cranial roots that arise from the medulla oblongata below the roots of the vagus.

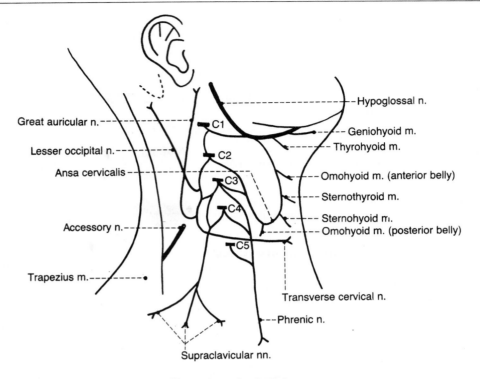

Great auricular n.

Lesser occipital n.

Ansa cervicalis

Accessory n.

Trapezius m.

C1
C2
C3
C4
C5

Hypoglossal n.

Geniohyoid m.

Thyrohyoid m.

Omohyoid m. (anterior belly)

Sternothyroid m.

Sternohyoid m.

Omohyoid m. (posterior belly)

Transverse cervical n.

Phrenic n.

Supraclavicular nn.

Figure 8-3. Cervical plexus.

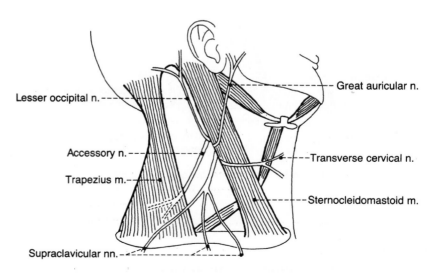

Lesser occipital n.

Accessory n.

Trapezius m.

Supraclavicular nn.

Great auricular n.

Transverse cervical n.

Sternocleidomastoid m.

Figure 8-4. Cutaneous branches of the cervical plexus.

–has spinal roots that arise from the lateral aspect of the cervical segment of the spinal cord between C1 and C3 (or C1 and C7) and unite to form a trunk that ascends between the dorsal and ventral roots of the spinal nerves in the vertebral canal and passes through the foramen magnum.

–has both spinal and cranial portions, which traverse the **jugular foramen,** where they interchange fibers. The cranial portion contains motor fibers that join the vagus nerve and innervate the soft palate, pharyngeal constrictors, and larynx. The spinal portion innervates the sternocleidomastoid and trapezius muscles.

–lies on the levator scapulae in the posterior cervical triangle and then passes deep to the trapezius.

B. Cervical plexus *anterior*

–is formed by the **ventral primary rami of C1–C4.**

1. Cutaneous branches

a. Lesser occipital nerve (C2)

–ascends along the posterior border of the sternocleidomastoid to the scalp behind the auricle.

b. Great auricular nerve (C2–C3)

–ascends on the sternocleidomastoid to innervate the skin behind the auricle and on the parotid gland.

c. Transverse cervical nerve (C2–C3)

–turns around the posterior border of the sternocleidomastoid and innervates the skin of the anterior cervical triangle.

d. Supraclavicular nerve (C3–C4)

–emerges as a common trunk from under the sternocleidomastoid and then divides into **anterior, middle, and posterior branches** to the skin over the clavicle and the shoulder.

2. Motor branches

a. Ansa cervicalis

–is a **nerve loop** formed by the union of the superior root (C1 or C1 and C2; **descendens hypoglossi**) and the inferior root (C2 and C3; **descendens cervicalis**).

–lies superficial to or within the carotid sheath in the anterior cervical triangle.

–innervates the infrahyoid (or strap) muscles such as the omohyoid, sternohyoid, and sternothyroid muscles, with the exception of the thyrohyoid muscle, which is innervated by C1 via the hypoglossal nerve.

b. Phrenic nerve (C3–C5)

–arises chiefly from the fourth cervical nerve but receives fibers from the third and fourth cervical nerves; contains motor, sensory, and sympathetic nerve fibers; and provides the motor supply to the **diaphragm** and sensation to its central part.

–descends on the anterior surface of the anterior scalene muscle under cover of the sternocleidomastoid muscle.

–passes between the subclavian artery and vein at the root of the neck and enters the thorax by crossing in front of the origin of the internal thoracic artery, where it joins the pericardiacophrenic branch of this artery.

–passes anterior to the root of the lung and between the mediastinal pleura and fibrous pericardium to supply sensory fibers to these structures.

c. Twigs from the plexus

–supply the longus capitis and cervicis or colli, sternocleidomastoid, trapezius, levator scapulae, and scalene muscles.

d. Accessory phrenic nerve (C5)

–occasionally arises as a contribution of C5 to the phrenic nerve or a branch of the nerve to the subclavius (C5), descends lateral to the phrenic nerve, enters the thorax by passing posterior to the subclavian vein, and joins the phrenic nerve below the first rib to supply the diaphragm.

C. Brachial plexus (see Figure 2-15)

–is formed by the **union of the ventral primary rami of C5–T1** and passes between the anterior scalene and middle scalene muscles.

1. Its roots give rise to the:

a. Dorsal scapular nerve (C5)

–emerges from behind the anterior scalene muscle and runs downward and backward through the middle scalene muscle and then deep to the trapezius.

–passes deep to or through the levator scapulae and descends along with the dorsal scapular artery on the deep surface of the rhomboid muscles along the medial border of the scapula, innervating the levator scapulae and rhomboid muscles.

b. Long thoracic nerve (C5–C7)

–pierces the middle scalene muscle, descends behind the brachial plexus, and enters the axilla to innervate the serratus anterior.

2. Its upper trunk gives rise to the:

a. Suprascapular nerve (C5–C6)

–passes deep to the trapezius and joins the suprascapular artery in a course toward the shoulder.

–passes through the **scapular notch** under the superior transverse scapular ligament.

–supplies the supraspinatus and infraspinatus muscles.

b. Nerve to the subclavius muscle (C5)

–descends in front of the plexus and behind the clavicle to innervate the subclavius.

–communicates with the phrenic nerve as the **accessory phrenic nerve** in many cases.

IV. Blood Vessels (Figure 8-5)

A. Subclavian artery

–is a branch of the **brachiocephalic trunk** on the right but arises directly from the **arch of the aorta** on the left.

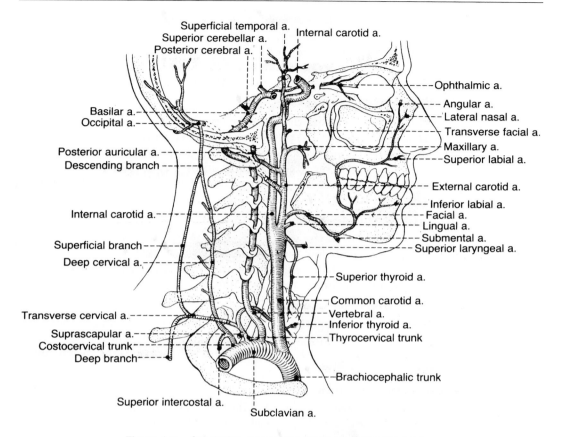

Figure 8-5. Subclavian and carotid arteries and their branches.

–is divided into three parts by the anterior scalene muscle: The first part passes from the origin of the vessel to the medial margin of the anterior scalene; the second part lies behind this muscle; and the third part passes from the lateral margin of the muscle to the outer border of the first rib.

–Its branches include the following:

1. Vertebral artery

–arises from the first part of the subclavian artery and ascends between the anterior scalene and longus colli muscles.

–ascends through the transverse foramina of vertebrae C1–C6, winds around the superior articular process of the atlas, and passes through the foramen magnum into the cranial cavity.

2. Thyrocervical trunk

–is a short trunk from the first part of the subclavian artery that divides into the following arteries:

a. Inferior thyroid artery

–ascends in front of the anterior scalene muscle, turns medially behind the carotid sheath but in front of the vertebral vessels, and then arches downward to the lower pole of the thyroid gland.

–gives rise to an **ascending cervical artery,** which ascends on the anterior scalene muscle medial to the phrenic nerve.

b. Transverse cervical artery

–runs laterally across the anterior scalene muscle, phrenic nerve, and trunks of the brachial plexus, passing deep to the trapezius.

–divides into a superficial branch and a deep branch, which takes the place of the **dorsal (descending) scapular artery.** In the absence of the deep branch, the superficial branch is known as the **superficial cervical artery.**

c. Suprascapular artery

–passes in front of the anterior scalene muscle and the brachial plexus parallel to but below the transverse cervical artery.

–passes superior to the superior transverse scapular ligament, whereas the suprascapular nerve passes inferior to this ligament.

3. Internal thoracic artery

–arises from the first part of the subclavian artery, descends through the thorax behind the upper six costal cartilages, and ends at the sixth intercostal space by dividing into the **superior epigastric and musculophrenic arteries.**

4. Costocervical trunk

–arises from the posterior aspect of the second part of the subclavian artery behind the anterior scalene muscle and divides into the following arteries:

a. Deep cervical artery

–passes between the transverse process of vertebra C7 and the neck of the first rib, ascends between the semispinalis capitis and semispinalis cervicis muscles, and anastomoses with the deep branch of the descending branch of the occipital artery.

b. Superior intercostal artery

–descends behind the cervical pleura anterior to the necks of the first two ribs and gives rise to the first two posterior intercostal arteries.

5. Dorsal (descending) scapular artery

–arises from the third part of the subclavian artery or arises as the deep (descending) branch of the transverse cervical artery.

B. Common carotid arteries

–have different origins on the right and left sides: the **right common carotid artery,** which begins at the bifurcation of the brachiocephalic artery, and the **left common carotid artery,** which arises from the aortic arch.

–ascend within the carotid sheath and divide at the level of the upper border of the thyroid cartilage into the **external and internal carotid arteries.**

1. Receptors

a. Carotid body

–lies at the bifurcation of the common carotid artery as an ovoid body.

–is a **chemoreceptor** that is stimulated by chemical changes (e.g., oxygen tension) in the circulating blood.

–is innervated by the **nerve to the carotid body,** which arises from the pharyngeal branch of the vagus nerve, and by the **carotid sinus branch** of the glossopharyngeal nerve.

b. Carotid sinus

–is a **spindle-shaped dilatation** located at the origin of the internal carotid artery, which functions as a **pressoreceptor (baroreceptor),** stimulated by changes in blood pressure.

–is innervated primarily by the **carotid sinus branch** of the glossopharyngeal nerve but also by the nerve to the carotid body.

2. Internal carotid artery

–has no branches in the neck.

–ascends within the carotid sheath in company with the vagus nerve and the internal jugular vein.

–enters the cranium through the **carotid canal** in the petrous part of the temporal bone.

–in the middle cranial fossa, gives rise to the **ophthalmic artery** and the **anterior and middle cerebral arteries.**

3. External carotid artery

–extends from the level of the upper border of the thyroid cartilage to the neck of the mandible, where it ends in the parotid gland by dividing into the maxillary and superficial temporal arteries.

–has eight named branches:

a. Superior thyroid artery

–arises below the level of the greater horn of the hyoid bone.

–descends obliquely forward in the carotid triangle and passes deep to the infrahyoid muscles to reach the superior pole of the thyroid gland.

–gives rise to an infrahyoid, sternocleidomastoid, superior laryngeal, cricothyroid, and several glandular branches.

b. Lingual artery

–arises at the level of the tip of the greater horn of the hyoid bone and passes deep to the hyoglossus to reach the tongue.

–gives rise to suprahyoid, dorsal lingual, sublingual, and deep lingual branches.

c. Facial artery

–arises just above the lingual artery and ascends forward, deep to the posterior belly of the digastric and stylohyoid muscles.

–hooks around the lower border of the mandible at the anterior margin of the masseter to enter the face.

d. Ascending pharyngeal artery

–arises from the deep surface of the external carotid artery in the carotid triangle and ascends between the internal carotid artery and the wall of the pharynx.

–gives rise to pharyngeal, palatine, inferior tympanic, and meningeal branches.

e. Occipital artery

–arises from the posterior surface of the external carotid artery, just above the level of the hyoid bone.

–passes deep to the digastric posterior belly, occupies the groove on the mastoid process, and appears on the skin above the occipital triangle.

–gives rise to the following:

(1) Sternocleidomastoid branch

–descends inferiorly and posteriorly over the hypoglossal nerve and enters the substance of the muscle.

–anastomoses with the sternocleidomastoid branch of the superior thyroid artery.

(2) Descending branch

–Its superficial branch anastomoses with the superficial branch of the transverse cervical artery.

–Its deep branch anastomoses with the deep cervical artery of the costocervical trunk.

f. Posterior auricular artery

–arises from the posterior surface of the external carotid artery just above the digastric posterior belly.

–ascends superficial to the styloid process and deep to the parotid gland and ends between the mastoid process and the external acoustic meatus.

–gives rise to stylomastoid, auricular, and occipital branches.

g. Maxillary artery

–arises behind the neck of the mandible as the larger terminal branch of the external carotid artery.

–runs deep to the neck of the mandible and enters the infratemporal fossa.

h. Superficial temporal artery

–arises behind the neck of the mandible as the smaller terminal branch of the external carotid artery.

–gives rise to the **transverse facial artery,** which runs between the zygomatic arch above and the parotid duct below.

–ascends in front of the external acoustic meatus into the scalp, accompanying the auriculotemporal nerve and the superficial temporal vein.

C. Veins (Figure 8-6)

1. Retromandibular vein

–is formed by the superficial temporal and maxillary veins.

–divides into an anterior branch, which joins the facial vein to form the common facial vein, and a posterior branch, which joins the posterior auricular vein to form the external jugular vein.

2. External jugular vein

–is formed by the union of the **posterior auricular vein** and the posterior branch of the **retromandibular vein.**

–crosses the sternomastoid obliquely, under the platysma, and ends in the subclavian (or sometimes the internal jugular) vein.

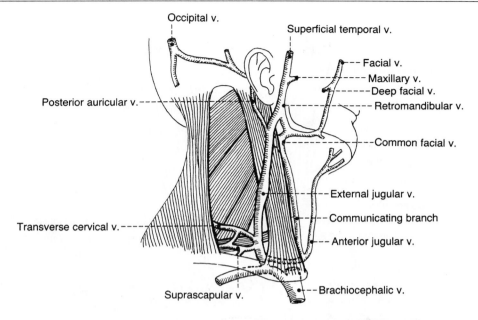

Figure 8-6. Veins of the cervical triangle.

—receives the suprascapular, transverse cervical, and anterior jugular veins.

3. **Internal jugular vein** (Figure 8-7)

—begins in the **jugular foramen** as a continuation of the sigmoid sinus, descends in the carotid sheath, and ends in the **brachiocephalic vein.**

—has the superior bulb at its beginning and the inferior bulb just above its termination.

—receives the facial, lingual, and superior and middle thyroid veins.

V. Lymphatics

A. Superficial lymph nodes of the head

—Lymph vessels from the face, scalp, and ear drain into the occipital, retroauricular, parotid, buccal (facial), submandibular, submental, and superficial cervical nodes, which in turn drain into the **deep cervical nodes** (including the jugulodigastric and jugulo-omohyoid nodes).

B. Deep lymph nodes of the head

—The middle ear drains into the retropharyngeal and upper deep cervical nodes; the nasal cavity and paranasal sinuses into the submandibular, retropharyngeal, and upper deep cervical; the tongue into the submental, submandibular, and upper and lower cervical; the larynx into the upper and lower deep cervical; the pharynx into the retropharyngeal and upper and lower deep cervical; and the thyroid gland into the lower deep cervical, prelaryngeal, pretracheal, and paratracheal.

C. Superficial cervical lymph nodes

—lie along the **external jugular vein** in the posterior triangle and along the **anterior jugular vein** in the anterior triangle.

—drain into the deep cervical nodes.

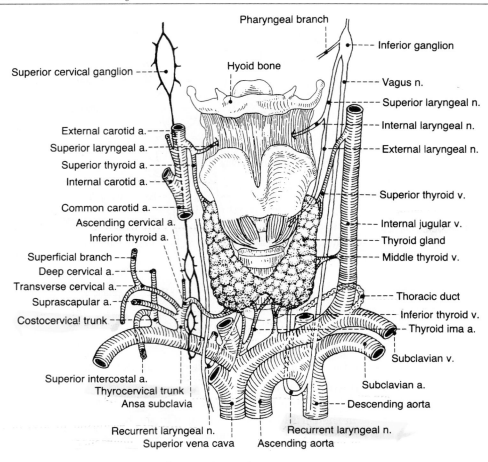

Figure 8-7. Deep structures of the neck.

D. Deep cervical lymph nodes

1. Superior deep cervical nodes

–lie along the **internal jugular vein** in the carotid triangle of the neck.
–receive afferent lymphatics from the back of the head and neck, tongue, palate, nasal cavity, larynx, pharynx, trachea, thyroid gland, and esophagus.
–has efferent vessels that join those of the inferior deep cervical nodes to form the **jugular trunk,** which empties into the thoracic duct on the left and into the junction of the internal jugular and subclavian veins on the right.

2. Inferior deep cervical nodes

–lie on the **internal jugular vein** near the subclavian vein.
–receive afferent lymphatics from the anterior jugular, transverse cervical, and apical axillary nodes.

VI. Clinical Considerations

A. Injury to the upper trunk of the brachial plexus

–may be caused by a **violent separation** of the head from the shoulder such as occurs in a fall from a motorcycle. The arm is in medial rotation owing to paralysis of the lateral rotators, resulting in **waiter's tip hand.**

–may be caused by stretching an infant's neck during a difficult delivery. This is referred to as **birth palsy** or obstetric paralysis.

B. Neurovascular compression syndrome

–produces symptoms of nerve compression of the brachial plexus and the subclavian vessels.

–is caused by abnormal insertion of the anterior and middle scalene muscles **(scalene syndrome)** and by the **cervical rib,** which is the cartilaginous accessory rib attached to vertebra C7.

–can be corrected by cutting the cervical rib or the anterior scalene muscle.

C. Torticollis (wryneck)

–is a **spasmodic contraction of the cervical muscles,** producing twisting of the neck with the chin pointing upward and to the opposite side.

–is due to injury to the sternocleidomastoid muscle or avulsion of the accessory nerve at the time of birth and unilateral fibrosis in the muscle, which cannot lengthen with the growing neck **(congenital torticollis).**

D. Lesion of the external laryngeal nerve

–may occur during **thyroidectomy** because the nerve accompanies the superior thyroid artery.

–causes **paralysis of the cricothyroid muscle,** resulting in loss of the tension of the vocal cord as well as weakness and hoarseness.

E. Lesion of the accessory nerve in the neck

–denervates the trapezius, leading to atrophy of the muscle.

–causes a downward displacement or **drooping of the shoulder.**

F. Central venous line

–is inserted into the retroclavicular portion of the **subclavian vein.** The needle should be guided medially along the long axis of the clavicle to reach the posterior surface where the vein runs over the first rib.

Deep Neck and Prevertebral Region

I. Deep Structures of the Neck (see Figure 8-7)

A. Trachea

–begins at the inferior border of the cricoid cartilage (C6).

–has **16–20 incomplete hyaline cartilaginous rings** that open posteriorly to prevent the trachea from collapsing.

B. Esophagus

–begins at the lower border of the pharynx at the level of the cricoid cartilage (C6) and descends between the trachea and the vertebral column.

–The cricopharyngeus muscle, the sphincter of the upper esophageal opening, remains closed except during deglutition (swallowing) and emesis (vomiting).

–is innervated by the recurrent laryngeal nerves and the sympathetic trunks, and receives blood from branches of the inferior thyroid arteries.

C. Thyroid gland (see Figure 8-7)

–is an endocrine gland that produces **thyroxine** and **thyrocalcitonin.**

–consists of right and left lobes connected by the **isthmus,** which crosses the second, third, and fourth tracheal rings. (The muscular band descending from the hyoid bone to the isthmus is called the **levator glandulae thyroideae.**)

–is supplied by the superior and inferior thyroid arteries and sometimes the **thyroid ima artery,** an inconsistent branch from the brachiocephalic trunk.

–drains via the superior and middle thyroid veins to the internal jugular vein and via the inferior thyroid vein to the brachiocephalic vein.

D. Parathyroid glands

–are endocrine glands that play a vital role in the regulation of calcium and phosphorus metabolism.

–usually consist of **four (can vary from two to six) small ovoid bodies** that lie against the dorsum of the thyroid under its sheath but with their own capsule.

–are supplied chiefly by the inferior thyroid artery.

E. Thyroid cartilage

–is a hyaline cartilage that forms a laryngeal prominence known as the **Adam's apple,** which is particularly apparent in males.

–has a superior horn that is joined to the tip of the greater horn of the hyoid bone by the lateral thyroid ligament and an inferior horn that articulates with the cricoid cartilage.

F. Vagus nerve

–runs through the jugular foramen and gives rise to the superior laryngeal nerve, which is divided into the external and internal laryngeal nerves.

1. External laryngeal nerve

–runs along with the superior thyroid artery.

–supplies the cricothyroid and inferior pharyngeal constrictor muscles.

2. Internal laryngeal nerve

–accompanies the superior laryngeal artery.

–supplies the sensory fibers to the larynx above the vocal cord and taste fibers to the epiglottis.

G. Sympathetic trunk

–is covered by the prevertebral fascia (the prevertebral fascia splits to enclose the sympathetic trunk).

–runs behind the carotid sheath and in front of the longus colli and longus capitis muscles.

–contains preganglionic and postganglionic sympathetic fibers, cell bodies of the postganglionic sympathetic fibers, and visceral afferent fibers with cell bodies in the upper thoracic dorsal root ganglia.

–receives gray rami communicantes but no white rami communicantes in the cervical region.

–bears the following cervical ganglia:

1. **Superior cervical ganglion**

   –lies in front of the transverse processes of vertebrae C1–C2, posterior to the internal carotid artery and anterior to the longus capitis.

   –contains cell bodies of postganglionic sympathetic fibers that pass to the visceral structures of the head and neck.

   –gives rise to the **internal carotid nerve** to form the internal carotid plexus; the **external carotid nerve** to form the external carotid plexus; the **pharyngeal branches** that join the pharyngeal branches of the glossopharyngeal and vagus nerves to form the pharyngeal plexus; and the **superior cervical cardiac nerve** to the heart.

2. **Middle cervical ganglion**

   –lies at the level of the cricoid cartilage (vertebra C6).

   –gives rise to a **middle cervical cardiac nerve,** which is the largest of the three cervical sympathetic cardiac nerves.

3. **Inferior cervical ganglion**

   –fuses with the first thoracic ganglion to become the **cervicothoracic (stellate) ganglion.**

   –lies in front of the neck of the first rib and the transverse process of vertebra C7 and behind the dome of the pleura and the vertebral artery.

   –gives rise to the **inferior cervical cardiac nerve.**

H. Ansa subclavia

   –is the cord connecting the middle and inferior cervical sympathetic ganglia, forming a loop around the first part of the subclavian artery.

II. Deep Cervical Fasciae (Figure 8-8)

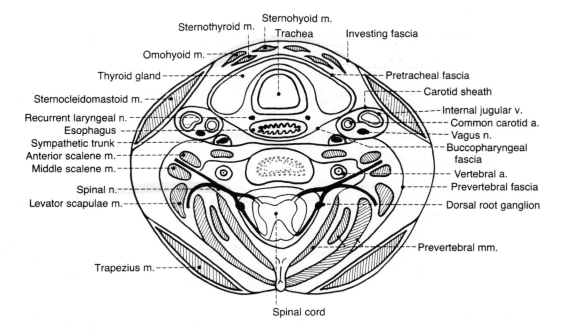

Figure 8-8. Cross-section of the neck.

A. **Superficial (investing) layer of deep cervical fascia**

–surrounds the **deeper parts of the neck.**

–splits to enclose the sternocleidomastoid and trapezius muscles.

–is attached superiorly along the mandible, mastoid process, external occipital protuberance, and superior nuchal line of the occipital bone.

–is attached inferiorly along the acromion and spine of the scapula, clavicle, and manubrium sterni.

B. **Prevertebral layer of deep cervical fascia**

–is cylindrical and encloses the **vertebral column** and its associated muscles.

–covers the scalene muscles and the deep muscles of the back.

–attaches to the external occipital protuberance and the basilar part of the occipital bone and becomes continuous with the **endothoracic fascia** and the **anterior longitudinal ligament** of the bodies of the vertebrae in the thorax.

C. **Carotid sheath**

–contains the **common and internal carotid arteries, internal jugular vein,** and **vagus nerve.**

–does not contain the sympathetic trunk, which lies posterior to the carotid sheath and anterior to the prevertebral fascia.

–blends with the prevertebral, pretracheal, and investing layers and also attaches to the base of the skull.

D. **Pretracheal layer of deep cervical fascia**

–invests the **larynx** and **trachea,** enclosing the **thyroid gland,** and contributes to the formation of the carotid sheath.

–attaches superiorly to the thyroid and cricoid cartilages and inferiorly to the pericardium.

E. **Buccopharyngeal fascia**

–covers the **buccinator muscles** and the **pharynx.**

–is attached to the pharyngeal tubercle and the pterygomandibular raphe.

F. **Pharyngobasilar fascia**

–is the **fibrous coat in the wall of the pharynx,** situated between the mucous membrane and the pharyngeal constrictor muscles.

III. Prevertebral or Deep Neck Muscles (Table 8-2)

IV. Clinical Considerations

A. **Goiter**

–is a **pathologic enlargement of the thyroid gland,** causing a swelling in the front part of the neck.

B. **Tracheotomy (tracheostomy)**

–is **opening into the trachea** by incising the third and fourth rings of the trachea, after making a vertical midline skin incision from the jugular notch of the manubrium sterni to the thyroid notch of the thyroid cartilage.

C. **Cricothyrotomy**

–is **incision through the skin and cricothyroid membrane** for relief of acute respiratory obstruction.

Table 8–2. Prevertebral or Deep Neck Muscles

Muscle	Origin	Insertion	Nerve	Action
Lateral vertebral				
Anterior scalene	Transverse processes of CV3–CV6	Scalene tubercle on first rib	Lower cervical (C5–C8)	Elevates first rib; bends neck
Middle scalene	Transverse processes of CV2–CV7	Upper surface of first rib	Lower cervical (C5–C8)	Elevates first rib; bends neck
Posterior scalene	Transverse processes of CV4–CV6	Outer surface of second rib	Lower cervical (C6–C8)	Elevates second rib; bends neck
Anterior vertebral				
Longus capitus	Transverse processes of CV3–CV6	Basilar part of occipital bone	C1–C4	Flexes and rotates head
Longus colli (L. cervicis)	Transverse processes and bodies of CV3–TV3	Anterior tubercle of atlas; bodies of CV2–CV4; transverse process of CV5–CV6	C2–C6	Flexes and rotates head
Rectus capitis anterior	Lateral mass of atlas	Basilar part of occipital bone	C1–C2	Flexes and rotates head
Rectus capitis lateralis	Transverse process of atlas	Jugular process of occipital bone	C1–C2	Flexes head laterally

–is preferable to tracheostomy for nonsurgeons in emergency respiratory obstructions.

D. Parathyroidectomy

–may occur during a total thyroidectomy and cause death if parathyroid hormone, calcium, or vitamin D is not provided.

–decreases the plasma calcium level, causing increased neuromuscular activity such as muscular spasms and nervous hyperexcitability, called **tetany.**

Face and Scalp

I. Muscles of Facial Expression (Figure 8-9; Table 8-3)

II. Nerve Supply to the Face and Scalp (Figures 8-10 and 8-11)

A. Facial nerve (Figure 8-12)

–comes through the **stylomastoid foramen** and appears posterior to the parotid gland.

Table 8–3. Muscles of Facial Expression

Muscle	Origin	Insertion	Nerve	Action
Occipitofrontalis	Superior nuchal line; upper orbital margin	Epicranial aponeurosis	Facial n.	Elevates eyebrows; wrinkles forehead (surprise)
Corrugator supercilii	Medial supraorbital margin	Skin of medial eyebrow	Facial n.	Draws eyebrows downward medially (anger, frowning)
Orbicularis oculi	Medial orbital margin; medial palpebral ligament; lacrimal bone	Skin and rim of orbit; tarsal plate; lateral palpebral raphe	Facial n.	Closes eyelids (squinting)
Procerus	Nasal bone and cartilage	Skin between eyebrows	Facial n.	Wrinkles skin over bones (sadness)
Nasalis	Maxilla lateral to incisive fossa	Ala of nose	Facial n.	Draws ala of nose toward septum
Depressor septi*	Incisive fossa of maxilla	Ala and nasal septum	Facial n.	Constricts nares
Orbicularis oris	Maxilla above incisor teeth	Skin of lip	Facial n.	Closes lips
Levator anguli oris	Canine fossa of maxilla	Angle of mouth	Facial n.	Elevates angle of mouth medially (disgust)
Levator labii superioris	Maxilla above infraorbital foramen	Skin of upper lip	Facial n.	Elevates upper lip; dilates nares (disgust)
Levator labii superioris alaeque nasi*	Frontal process of maxilla	Skin of upper lip	Facial n.	Elevates ala of nose and upper lip
Zygomaticus major	Zygomatic arch	Angle of mouth	Facial n.	Draws angle of mouth backward and upward (smile)
Zygomaticus minor	Zygomatic arch	Angle of mouth	Facial n.	Elevates upper lip
Depressor labii inferioris	Mandible below mental foramen	Orbicularis oris and skin of lower lip	Facial n.	Depresses lower lip
Depressor anguli oris	Oblique line of mandible	Angle of mouth	Facial n.	Depresses angle of mouth
Risorius	Fascia over masseter	Angle of mouth	Facial n.	Retracts angle of mouth (false smile)
Buccinator	Mandible; pterygomandibular raphe; alveolar processes	Angle of mouth	Facial n.	Presses cheek to keep it taut
Mentalis	Incisive fossa of mandible	Skin of chin	Facial n.	Elevates and protrudes lower lip
Auricularis anterior, superior, and posterior*	Temporal fascia; epicranial aponeurosis; mastoid process	Anterior, superior, and posterior sides of auricle	Facial n.	Retract and elevate ear

* Indicates less important muscles.

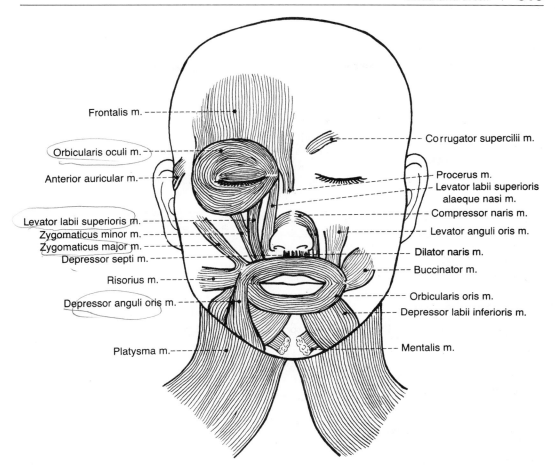

Figure 8-9. Muscles of facial expression.

–enters the parotid gland to give rise to five terminal branches—the **temporal, zygomatic, buccal, mandibular, and cervical branches**—which radiate forward in the face.

–innervates the **muscles of facial expression** and sends the **posterior auricular branch** to muscles of the auricle and the occipitalis muscle.

–also innervates the digastric posterior belly and stylohyoid muscles.

B. Trigeminal nerve

–provides sensory innervation to the **skin of the face.**

1. Ophthalmic division

–innervates the area above the upper eyelid and dorsum of the nose.

–supplies the face as the **supraorbital, supratrochlear, infratrochlear, external nasal,** and **lacrimal nerves.**

2. Maxillary division

–innervates the face below the level of the eyes and above the upper lip.

–supplies the face as the **zygomaticofacial, zygomaticotemporal,** and **infraorbital nerves.**

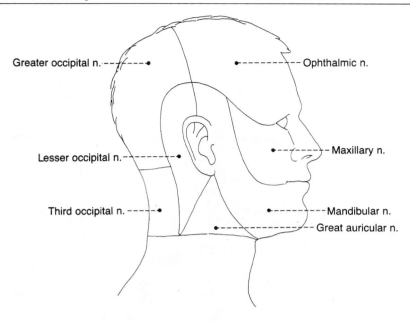

Figure 8-10. Sensory innervation of the face.

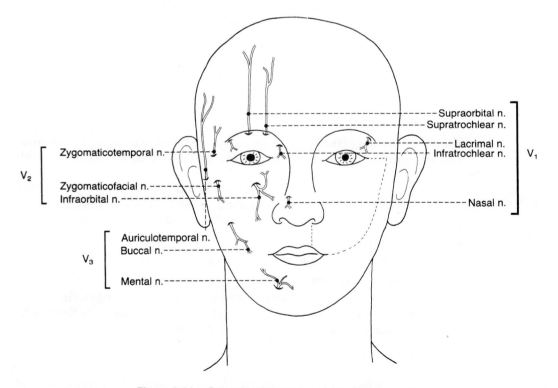

Figure 8-11. Cutaneous innervation of the face and scalp.

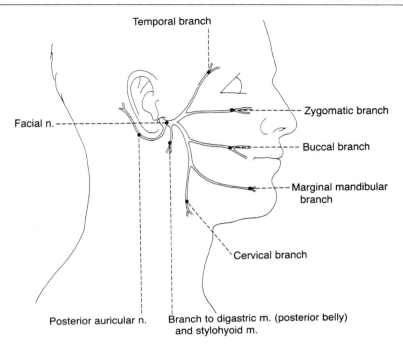

Figure 8-12. Distribution of the facial nerve.

3. Mandibular division

–innervates the face below the level of the lower lip.

–supplies the face as the **auriculotemporal, buccal, and mental nerves.**

III. Blood Vessels of the Face and Scalp (Figures 8-13 and 8-14)

A. Facial artery

–arises from the **external carotid artery** just above the upper border of the hyoid bone.

–passes deep to the mandible, winds around the lower border of the mandible, and runs upward and forward on the face.

–gives rise to the ascending palatine, tonsillar, glandular, and submental branches in the neck, as well as the inferior labial, superior labial, and lateral nasal branches in the face.

–terminates as an angular artery that anastomoses with the palpebral and dorsal nasal branches of the ophthalmic artery to establish communication between the external and internal carotid arteries.

B. Superficial temporal artery

–arises behind the neck of the mandible as the smaller terminal branch of the external carotid artery and ascends anterior to the external acoustic meatus into the scalp.

–accompanies the auriculotemporal nerve along its anterior surface.

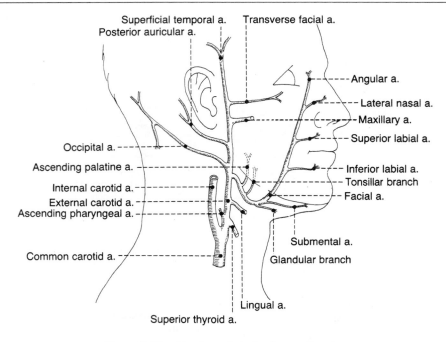

Figure 8-13. Blood supply to the face and scalp.

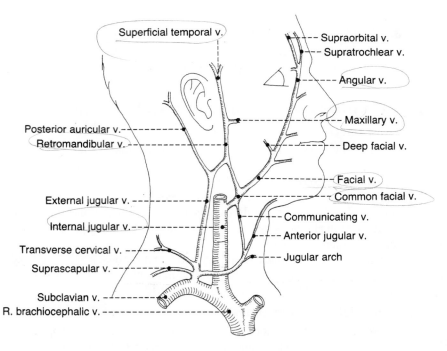

Figure 8-14. Veins of the head and neck.

–gives rise to the **transverse facial artery,** which passes forward across the masseter between the zygomatic arch above and the parotid duct below.

–also gives rise to zygomatico-orbital, middle temporal, anterior auricular, frontal, and parietal branches.

C. Facial vein

–begins as an angular vein by the confluence of the supraorbital and supratrochlear veins. The angular vein is continued at the lower margin of the orbital margin into the facial vein.

–receives tributaries corresponding to the branches of the facial artery and also receives the **infraorbital and deep facial veins.**

–drains either directly into the internal jugular vein or by joining the anterior branch of the retromandibular vein to form the **common facial vein,** which then enters the internal jugular vein.

–communicates with the superior ophthalmic vein and thus with the **cavernous sinus,** allowing a route of infection from the face to the cranial dural sinus.

D. Retromandibular vein

–is formed by the union of the superficial temporal and maxillary veins behind the mandible.

–divides into an **anterior branch,** which joins the facial vein to form the common facial vein, and a **posterior branch,** which joins the posterior auricular vein to form the external jugular vein.

IV. Scalp

A. Layers (Figure 8-15)

1. Skin

2. Connective tissue (close subcutaneous tissue)

–contains the **larger blood vessels** and nerves. Because of its toughness, the **scalp gapes** when cut and the blood vessels do not contract, which leads to severe bleeding.

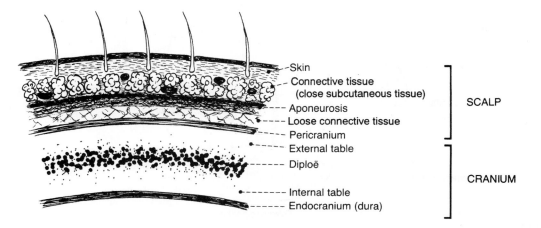

Figure 8-15. Layers of the scalp and cranium.

3. **Aponeurosis epicranialis (galea aponeurotica)**

–is a **fibrous sheet** that covers the vault of the skull and unites the occipitalis and frontalis muscles.

4. **Loose connective tissue**

–forms the **subaponeurotic space** and contains the emissary veins.

–is termed a **dangerous area** because infection (blood and pus) can spread easily in it or from the scalp to the intracranial sinuses by way of the emissary veins.

5. **Pericranium**

–is the **periosteum** over the surface of the skull.

B. **Innervation and blood supply** (Figure 8-16)

–is innervated by the supratrochlear, supraorbital, zygomaticotemporal, auriculotemporal, lesser occipital, greater occipital, and third occipital nerves.

–is supplied by the supratrochlear and supraorbital branches of the internal carotid and by the superficial temporal, posterior auricular, and occipital branches of the external carotid arteries.

V. Clinical Considerations

A. **Bell's palsy (facial paralysis)**

–is a **unilateral paralysis of the facial muscles** owing to a lesion of the facial nerve.

–is marked by characteristic **distortions of the face** such as a sagging corner of the mouth and inability to smile, whistle, or blow; drooping of the eyebrow; eversion of the lower eyelid; and inability to close or blink the eye.

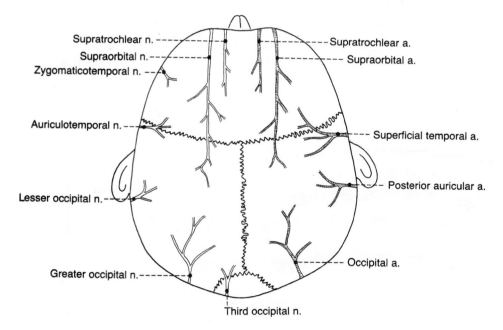

Figure 8-16. Nerves and arteries of the scalp.

–causes decreased lacrimation (as a result of a lesion of the greater petrosal nerve), loss of taste in the anterior two-thirds of the tongue (chorda tympani), painful sensitivity to sounds (nerve to the stapedius), and deviation of the lower jaw and tongue (nerve to the digastric muscle).

B. Trigeminal neuralgia (tic douloureux)

–is marked by **paroxysmal pain** along the course of the trigeminal nerve.
–may be alleviated by sectioning the sensory root of the trigeminal nerve in the trigeminal (Meckel's) cave in the middle cranial fossa.

C. Danger area of the face

–is the **area of the face drained by the facial veins.** Pustules (pimples) or other skin infections, particularly on the side of the nose and upper lip, may spread to the cavernous dural sinus through the ophthalmic veins and the pterygoid venous plexuses, which anastomose with the facial veins.

D. Corneal blink reflex

–is **closing of the eyes** caused by blowing on the cornea or touching it with a wisp of cotton wool. It is caused by bilateral contraction of the orbicularis oculi muscles.
–Its efferent limb (of the reflex arc) is the facial nerve; its afferent limb is the nasociliary nerve of the ophthalmic division of the trigeminal nerve.

Temporal and Infratemporal Fossae

I. Introduction

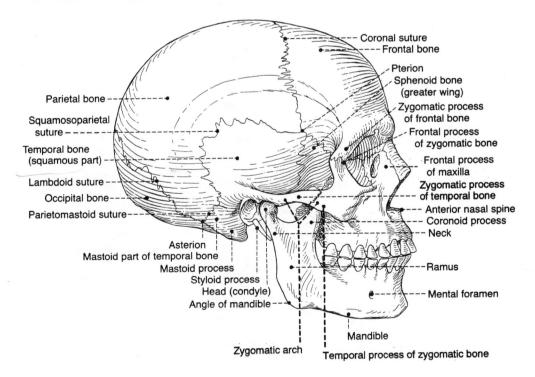

Figure 8-17. Lateral view of the skull.

A. Infratemporal fossa (Figures 8-17 and 8-18)

–contains the lower portion of the temporalis muscle, the lateral and medial pterygoid muscles, the pterygoid plexus of veins, the mandibular nerve and its branches, the maxillary artery and its branches, the chorda tympani, and the otic ganglion.

–has the following boundaries:

1. Anterior: posterior surface of the maxilla

2. Posterior: styloid process

3. Medial: lateral pterygoid plate of the sphenoid bone

4. Lateral: ramus and coronoid process of the mandible

5. Roof: infratemporal surface of the greater wing of the sphenoid bone

B. Temporal fossa (see Figures 8-17 and 8-18)

–contains the temporalis muscle, the deep temporal nerves and vessels, the auriculotemporal nerve, and the superficial temporal vessels.

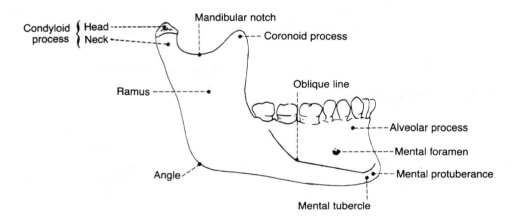

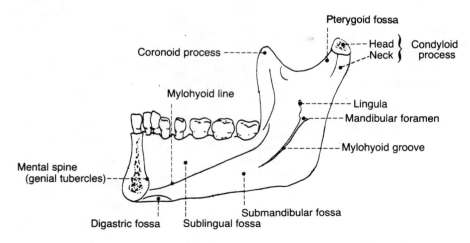

Figure 8-18. External (buccal) and internal (lingual) surfaces of the mandible.

–has the following boundaries:

1. **Anterior:** zygomatic process of the frontal bone and the frontal process of the zygomatic bone

2. **Posterior:** temporal line

3. **Superior:** temporal line

4. **Inferior:** zygomatic arch

5. **Floor:** parts of the frontal, parietal, temporal, and greater wing of the sphenoid bone

II. Muscles of Mastication (Figure 8-19; Table 8-4)

Table 8–4. Muscles of Mastication

Muscle	Origin	Insertion	Nerve	Action on mandible
Temporalis	Temporal fossa	Coronoid process and ramus of mandible	Trigeminal n.	Elevates; retracts
Masseter	Lower border and medial surface of zygomatic arch	Lateral surface of coronoid process, ramus and angle of mandible	Trigeminal n.	Elevates (superficial part); retracts (deep part)
Lateral pterygoid	Superior head from infratemporal surface of sphenoid; inferior head from lateral surface of lateral pterygoid plate of sphenoid	Neck of mandible; articular disk and capsule of temporomandibular joint	Trigeminal n.	Protracts (inferior head); depresses (superior head)
Medial pterygoid	Tuber of maxilla; medial surface of lateral pterygoid plate; pyramidal process of palatine bone	Medial surface of angle and ramus of mandible	Trigeminal n.	Protracts; elevates

The jaws are opened by the lateral pterygoid muscle and are closed by the temporalis, masseter, and medial pterygoid muscles.

III. Nerves of the Infratemporal Region (see Figure 8-19)

A. Mandibular division of the trigeminal nerve

–passes through the **foramen ovale** and innervates the tensor veli palatini and tensor tympani muscles, muscles of mastication (temporalis, masseter, and lateral and medial pterygoid), anterior belly of the digastric muscle, and the mylohyoid muscle.

–provides sensory innervation to the lower teeth and to the lower part of the face below the lower lip and the mouth.

–gives rise to the following branches:

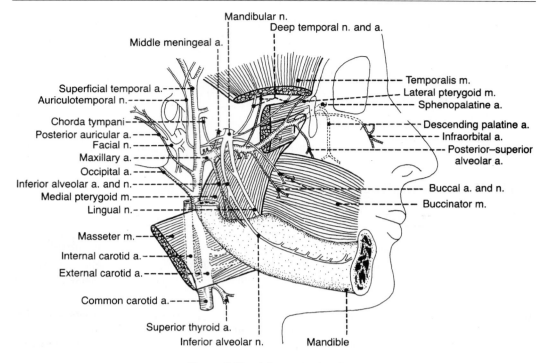

Figure 8-19. Infratemporal region.

1. **Meningeal branch**

   –accompanies the middle meningeal artery and enters the cranium through the foramen spinosum.

2. **Masseteric, deep temporal, medial pterygoid, and lateral pterygoid nerves**

   –innervate the corresponding muscles of mastication.

3. **Buccal nerve**

   –descends between the two heads of the lateral pterygoid muscle.
   –innervates skin and fascia on the buccinator muscle and penetrates this muscle to supply the mucous membrane of the cheek and gums.

4. **Auriculotemporal nerve**

   –arises from two roots that encircle the middle meningeal artery.
   –innervates sensory branches to the temporomandibular joint.
   –carries postganglionic parasympathetic and sympathetic fibers to the parotid gland in addition to general somatic afferent (GSA) fibers.
   –has terminal branches that supply the skin of the auricle and the scalp.

5. **Lingual nerve**

   –descends deep to the lateral pterygoid muscle, where it joins the **chorda tympani,** which conveys the preganglionic parasympathetic (secretomotor) fibers to the submandibular ganglion and taste fibers from the anterior two-thirds of the tongue.
   –lies anterior to the inferior alveolar nerve on the medial pterygoid muscle, deep to the ramus of the mandible.

–crosses lateral to the styloglossus and hyoglossus muscles, passes deep to the mylohyoid muscle, and descends across the submandibular duct.

–supplies general sensation for the anterior two-thirds of the tongue.

6. **Inferior alveolar nerve**

   –passes deep to the lateral pterygoid muscle and then between the spheno-mandibular ligament and the ramus of the mandible.

   –enters the mandibular canal through the mandibular foramen.

   –gives rise to the following branches:

   a. **Mylohyoid nerve,** which innervates the mylohyoid and the anterior belly of the digastric muscle

   b. **Inferior dental branch,** which innervates lower teeth

   c. **Mental nerve,** which innervates the skin over the chin

   d. **Incisive branch,** which innervates the canine and incisor teeth

B. **Otic ganglion**

   –lies in the infratemporal fossa, just below the foramen ovale between the mandibular nerve and the tensor veli palatini.

   –contains preganglionic parasympathetic fibers that run in the glossopharyngeal nerve, tympanic plexus, and lesser petrosal nerve synapse.

   –also contains postganglionic fibers that run in the **auriculotemporal nerve** to innervate the parotid gland.

IV. Blood Vessels of the Infratemporal Region (see Figure 8-19)

A. **Maxillary artery**

   –arises from the external carotid artery at the posterior border of the ramus of the mandible.

   –divides into three parts:

   1. **Mandibular part**

      –runs anteriorly between the neck of the mandible and the sphenomandibular ligament.

      –gives rise to the following branches:

      a. **Deep auricular artery**

         –supplies the external acoustic meatus.

      b. **Anterior tympanic artery**

         –supplies the tympanic cavity and tympanic membrane.

      c. **Middle meningeal artery**

         –is embraced by two roots of the auriculotemporal nerve and enters the middle cranial fossa through the foramen spinosum.

         –runs between the dura mater and the periosteum.

         –may be damaged, resulting in **epidural hematoma.**

      d. **Accessory meningeal artery**

         –passes through the foramen ovale.

      e. **Inferior alveolar artery**

         –follows the inferior alveolar nerve between the sphenomandibular ligament and the ramus of the mandible.

–enters the mandibular canal through the mandibular foramen and supplies the tissues of the chin and lower teeth.

2. Pterygoid part

–runs anteriorly deep to the temporalis and lies superficial (or deep) to the lateral pterygoid muscle.

–has branches that include the anterior and posterior deep temporal, pterygoid, masseteric, and buccal arteries, which supply chiefly the muscles of mastication.

3. Pterygopalatine part

–runs between the two heads of the lateral pterygoid muscle and then through the pterygomaxillary fissure into the pterygopalatine fossa.

–has branches that include the following arteries:

a. Posterior–superior alveolar arteries

–run downward on the posterior surface of the maxilla and supply the molar and premolar teeth and the maxillary sinus.

b. Infraorbital artery

–runs upward and forward to enter the orbit through the inferior orbital fissure.

–traverses the infraorbital groove and canal and emerges on the face through the infraorbital foramen.

–divides into branches to supply the lower eyelid, lacrimal sac, upper, lip, and cheek.

–gives rise to **anterior and middle superior alveolar branches** to the upper canine and incisor teeth and the maxillary sinus.

c. Descending palatine artery

–descends in the pterygopalatine fossa and the palatine canal.

–supplies the soft and hard palates.

–gives rise to the **greater and lesser palatine arteries,** which pass through the greater and lesser palatine foramina, respectively. The lesser palatine artery supplies the soft palate. The greater palatine artery supplies the hard palate and sends a branch to anastomose with the terminal (nasopalatine) branch of the sphenopalatine artery in the incisive canal or on the nasal septum.

d. Artery of the pterygoid canal

–passes through the pterygoid canal and supplies the upper part of the pharynx, auditory tube, and tympanic cavity.

e. Pharyngeal artery

–supplies the roof of the nose and pharynx, sphenoid sinus, and auditory tube.

f. Sphenopalatine artery

–is the terminal branch of the maxillary artery.

–enters the nasal cavity through the sphenopalatine foramen in company with the nasopalatine branch of the maxillary nerve.

–is the principal artery to the nasal cavity, supplying the conchae, meatus, and paranasal sinuses.

–may be damaged, resulting in epistaxis (nosebleed).

B. Pterygoid venous plexus (Figure 8-20)

–lies on the lateral surface of the medial pterygoid muscle.

–communicates with the cavernous sinus via emissary veins and the inferior ophthalmic vein.

–communicates with the facial vein via the deep facial vein.

C. Retromandibular vein

–is formed by the superficial temporal vein and the maxillary vein.

–divides into an anterior branch, which joins the facial vein to form the common facial vein, and a posterior branch, which joins the posterior auricular vein to form the external jugular vein.

V. Parotid Gland

–occupies the **retromandibular space** between the ramus of the mandible and the mastoid process.

–is invested with a dense fibrous capsule derived from the investing layer of the deep cervical fascia.

–is separated from the submandibular gland by the **stylomandibular ligament,** which extends from the styloid process to the angle of the mandible. (Therefore, pus does not readily exchange between these two glands.)

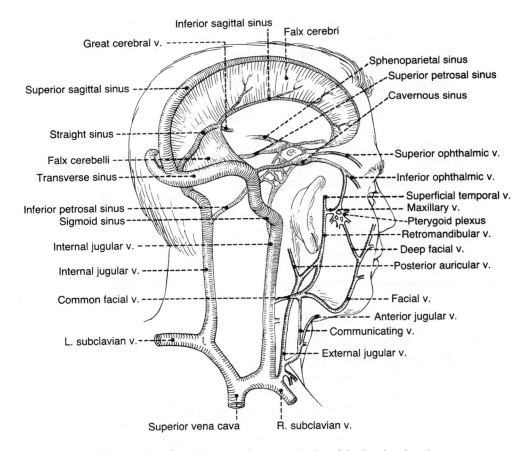

Figure 8-20. Cranial venous sinuses and veins of the head and neck.

–is innervated by parasympathetic (secretomotor) fibers of the glossopharyngeal nerve by way of the **lesser petrosal nerve, otic ganglion,** and **auriculo-temporal nerve.**

–contains Stensen's duct (the duct of the parotid), which crosses the masseter, pierces the buccinator muscle, and opens into the oral cavity opposite the second upper molar tooth.

–Complete surgical removal of the parotid may damage the facial nerve.

VI. Joints and Ligaments of the Infratemporal Region

A. Temporomandibular joint

–is a synovial joint between the **mandibular fossa** and the **articular tubercle** of the temporal bone above and the **head** of the mandible below, which has **two** (superior and inferior) **synovial cavities,** divided by an **articular disk.**

–combines an **upper gliding joint** (between the articular tubercle and mandibular fossa above and the articular disk below where **forward gliding** or protrusion and **backward gliding** or retraction takes place) and a **lower hinge joint** (between the disk and the mandibular head (condyle) where elevation (closing) and depression (opening) of the jaw takes place). During yawning, the disk and the head of the mandible glides across the articular tubercle.

–has an articular capsule that extends from the articular tubercle and the margins of the mandibular fossa to the neck of the mandible.

–is reinforced by the **lateral (temporomandibular) ligament,** which extends from the tubercle on the zygoma to the neck of the mandible, and the **sphenomandibular ligament,** which extends from the spine of the sphenoid bone to the lingula of the mandible.

–is innervated by the **auriculotemporal** and masseteric branches of the mandibular nerve.

–is supplied by the superficial temporal, maxillary (middle meningeal and anterior tympanic branches), and ascending pharyngeal arteries.

B. Pterygomandibular raphe

–is a **ligamentous band** (or a tendinous inscription) between the buccinator muscle and the superior pharyngeal constrictor.

–extends between the pterygoid hamulus superiorly and the posterior end of the mylohyoid line of the mandible inferiorly.

C. Stylomandibular ligament

–extends from the styloid process to the posterior border of the ramus of the mandible, near the angle of the mandible, separating the parotid from the submandibular gland.

VII. Clinical Considerations

A. Mumps (epidermic parotitis)

–is an acute infectious and contagious disease caused by a viral infection.

–irritates the auriculotemporal nerve, causing severe pain because of **inflammation and swelling of the parotid gland and stretching of its capsule,** and is also characterized by **inflammation of salivary glands.**

–may be accompanied by inflammation of the testes or ovaries, causing **sterility.**

B. Frey's syndrome

–produces **flushing and sweating instead of salivation in response to taste of food,** following injury of the auriculotemporal nerve, which carries parasympathetic secretomotor fibers to the parotid gland and sympathetic fibers to the sweat glands. (When the nerve is severed, the fibers can regenerate along each others pathways and innervate the wrong gland.)

–can occur after parotid surgery and may be treated by cutting the tympanic plexus in the ear.

C. Dislocation of the temporomandibular joint

–occurs anteriorly as the mandible head glides across the articular tubercle during yawning and laughing.

D. Rupture of the middle meningeal artery

–may be caused by **fracture of the squamous part of the temporal bone** as it runs through the foramen spinosum and just deep to the inner surface of the temporal bone.

–causes epidural hematoma with increased intracranial pressure.

Skull and Cranial Cavity

I. Skull (see Figure 8-17; Figures 8-21 and 8-22)

–is the skeleton of the head and may be divided into two types: 8 **cranial bones** for enclosing the brain (unpaired frontal, occipital, ethmoid, and sphenoid bones, and paired parietal and temporal bones), which **can be seen in the cranial**

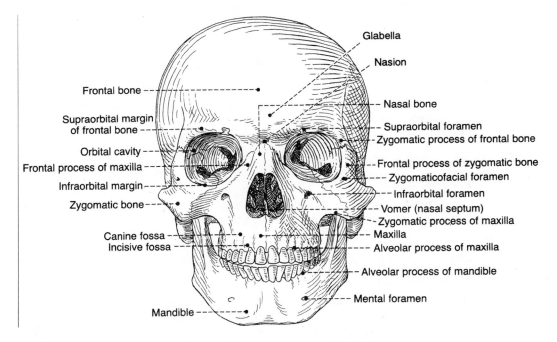

Figure 8-21. Anterior view of the skull.

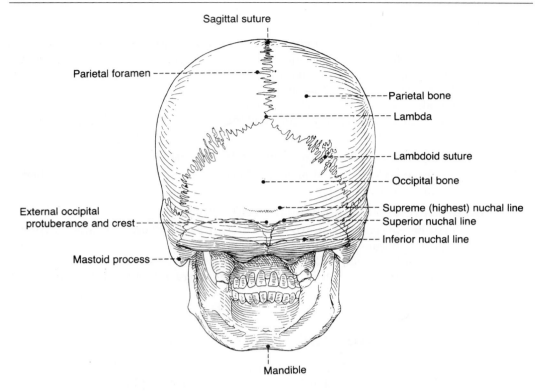

Figure 8-22. Posterior view of the skull.

cavity; and 14 **facial bones** (paired lacrimal, nasal, palatine, inferior turbinate, maxillary, and zygomatic bones, and unpaired vomer and mandible).

A. Cranium

–is sometimes restricted to the skull without the mandible.

B. Calvaria

–is the **skullcap,** which is the vault of the skull without the facial bones. It consists of the superior portions of the frontal, parietal, and occipital bones.

–Its highest point on the sagittal suture is the **vertex.**

II. Bones of the Cranium

A. Frontal bone

–underlies the forehead and the superior margin and roof of the orbit, and has a smooth median prominence called the **glabella.**

B. Parietal bone

–forms part of the superior and lateral surface of the skull.

C. Temporal bone

–consists of the **squamous part** external to the lateral surface of the temporal lobe of the brain; the **petrous part,** which encloses the internal and middle ears; the **mastoid part,** which contains mastoid air cells; and the **tympanic part,** which houses the external auditory meatus and the tympanic cavity.

D. Occipital bone

–consists of **squamous, basilar, and two lateral condylar parts.**

–encloses the foramen magnum and forms the cerebral and cerebellar fossae.

E. Sphenoid bone

–consists of the body (which houses the sphenoid sinus), the greater and lesser wings, and the **pterygoid process.**

F. Ethmoid bone

–is located between the orbits and consists of the **cribriform plate, perpendicular plate,** and two lateral masses enclosing ethmoid air cells.

III. Sutures of the Skull

–are the immovable fibrous joints between the bones of the skull.

A. Coronal suture: lies between the frontal bone and the two parietal bones

B. Sagittal suture: lies between the two parietal bones

C. Squamous (squamoparietal) suture: lies between the parietal bone and the squamous part of the temporal bone

D. Lambdoid suture: lies between the two parietal bones and the occipital bone

E. Junctions of the cranial sutures

1. **Lambda:** intersection of the lambdoid and sagittal sutures

2. **Bregma:** intersection of the sagittal and coronal sutures

3. **Pterion:** a craniometric point at the junction of the frontal, parietal, and temporal bones and the great wing of the sphenoid bone

4. **Asterion:** a craniometric point at the junction of the parietal, occipital, and temporal (mastoid part) bones

5. **Nasion:** a point on the middle of the nasofrontal suture (intersection of the frontal and two nasal bones)

6. **Inion:** most prominent point of the external occipital protuberance, which is used as a fixed point in craniometry

IV. Foramina in the Skull (Figures 8-23 and 8-24)

–include the following, which are presented here with the structures that pass through them:

A. Anterior cranial fossa

1. **Cribriform plate:** olfactory nerves

2. **Foramen cecum:** occasional small emissary vein from nasal mucosa to superior sagittal sinus

3. **Anterior and posterior ethmoidal foramina:** anterior and posterior ethmoidal nerves, arteries, and veins

B. Middle cranial fossa

1. **Optic canal:** optic nerve, ophthalmic artery, and central artery and vein of the retina

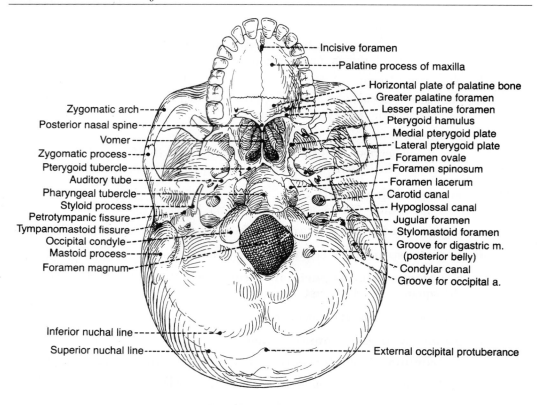

Figure 8-23. Base of the skull.

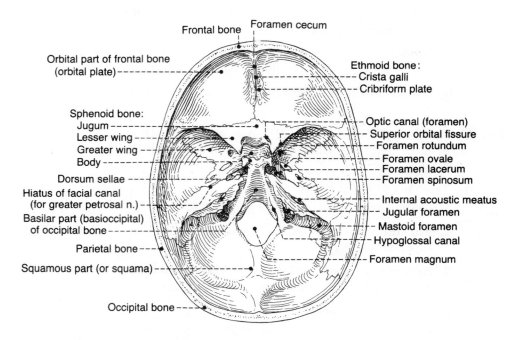

Figure 8-24. Interior of the base of the skull.

2. **Superior orbital fissure:** oculomotor, trochlear, and abducens nerves; ophthalmic division of trigeminal nerve; and ophthalmic veins

3. **Foramen rotundum:** maxillary division of trigeminal nerve

4. **Foramen ovale:** mandibular division of trigeminal nerve, accessory meningeal artery, and occasionally lesser petrosal nerve

5. **Foramen spinosum:** middle meningeal artery

6. **Foramen lacerum:** internal carotid artery and greater and deep petrosal nerves en route to the pterygoid canal

7. **Carotid canal:** internal carotid artery and sympathetic nerves (carotid plexus)

C. **Posterior cranial fossa**

1. **Internal auditory meatus:** facial and vestibulocochlear nerves and labyrinthine artery

2. **Jugular foramen:** glossopharyngeal, vagus, and spinal accessory nerves and beginning of internal jugular vein

3. **Hypoglossal canal:** hypoglossal nerve and meningeal artery

4. **Foramen magnum:** spinal cord, spinal accessory nerve, vertebral arteries, venous plexus of vertebral canal, and anterior and posterior spinal arteries

5. **Condyloid foramen:** condyloid emissary vein

6. **Mastoid foramen:** branch of occipital artery to dura mater and mastoid emissary vein

D. **Foramina in the front of the skull** (see Figure 8-21)

1. **Zygomaticofacial foramen:** zygomaticofacial nerve

2. **Supraorbital notch:** supraorbital nerve and vessels

3. **Infraorbital foramen:** infraorbital nerve and vessels

4. **Mental foramen:** mental nerve and vessels

E. **Foramina in the base of the skull** (see Figure 8-24)

1. **Petrotympanic fissure:** chorda tympani and often anterior tympanic artery

2. **Stylomastoid foramen:** facial nerve

3. **Incisive canal:** nasopalatine nerve

4. **Greater palatine foramen:** greater palatine nerve and vessels

5. **Lesser palatine foramen:** lesser palatine nerve and vessels

6. **Palatine canal:** descending palatine vessels as well as the greater and lesser palatine nerves

V. Structures in the Cranial Fossae (see Figure 8-24)

A. Foramen cecum

–is a small pit in front of the **crista galli** between the ethmoid and frontal bones.

–may transmit an emissary vein from the nasal mucosa to the superior sagittal sinus.

B. Crista galli

–is the triangular midline process of the ethmoid bone extending upward from the cribriform plate.

–provides attachment for the **falx cerebri.**

C. Cribriform plate of the ethmoid bone

–supports the olfactory bulb and transmits olfactory nerve fibers from the olfactory mucosa to the olfactory bulb.

D. Anterior clinoid processes

–are two anterior processes of the lesser wing of the sphenoid bone.

–provide attachment for the free border of the tentorium cerebelli.

E. Middle clinoid process

–is a small inconstant eminence on the body of the sphenoid, posterolateral to the tuberculum sellae.

F. Posterior clinoid processes

–are two tubercles from each side of the **dorsum sellae.**

–provide attachment for the attached border of the tentorium cerebelli.

G. Lesser wing of the sphenoid bone

–forms the anterior boundary of the middle cranial fossa.

–forms the **sphenoidal ridge** separating the anterior from the middle cranial fossa.

–forms the boundary of the **superior orbital fissure** (the space between the lesser and greater wings).

H. Greater wing of the sphenoid bone

–forms the anterior wall and the floor of the middle cranial fossa.

–presents two openings: the **foramen ovale** and **foramen spinosum.**

I. Sella turcica (Turk's saddle) of the sphenoid bone

–is bounded anteriorly by the **tuberculum sellae** and posteriorly by the **dorsum sellae**.

–has a deep central depression known as the **hypophyseal fossa,** which accommodates the pituitary gland or the hypophysis.

–lies directly above the sphenoid sinus located within the body of the sphenoid bone; its dural roof is formed by the **diaphragma sellae.**

J. Jugum sphenoidale

–forms the roof for the **sphenoidal air sinus.**

K. Clivus

–is the downward sloping surface from the dorsum sellae to the foramen magnum.

–is formed by a part of the body of the **sphenoid** and a portion of the basilar part of the **occipital** bone.

VI. Meninges of the Brain (Figure 8-25)

A. Pia mater

–is a delicate investment that is closely applied to the brain and dips into fissures and sulci.

–enmeshes blood vessels on the surfaces of the brain.

B. Arachnoid layer

–is a filmy, transparent, spidery layer that is connected to the pia mater by web-like trabeculations.

–is separated from the pia mater by the **subarachnoid space,** which is filled with cerebrospinal fluid (CSF).

–may contain blood after hemorrhage of a cerebral artery.

–projects into the venous sinuses to form **arachnoid villi,** which serve as sites where CSF diffuses into the venous blood.

1. CSF

–is formed by **vascular choroid plexuses** in the ventricles of the brain and is contained in the subarachnoid space.

–circulates through the ventricles, enters the subarachnoid space, and eventually filters into the venous system.

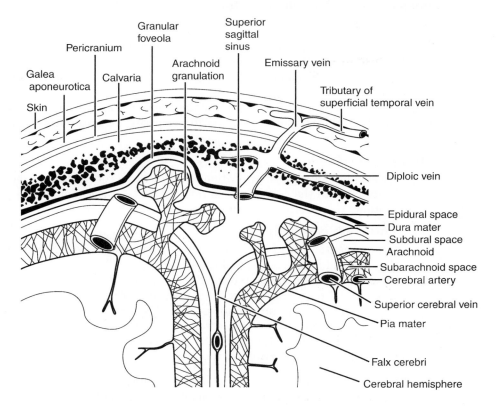

Figure 8-25. Scalp, calvaria, meninges and dural venous sinuses.

2. Arachnoid granulations

–are tuft-like collections of highly folded arachnoid (aggregations of arachnoid villi) that project into the superior sagittal sinus and the lateral lacunae, which are lateral extensions of the superior sagittal sinus.

–absorb the CSF into the dural sinuses and often produce erosion or pitting of the inner surface of the calvaria, forming the **granular pit**.

C. Dura mater

–is the tough, fibrous, outermost layer of the meninges external to the **subdural space,** the space between the arachnoid and the dura.

–lies internal to the **epidural space,** a potential space that contains the middle meningeal arteries in the cranial cavity.

–forms the **dural venous sinuses,** spaces between the periosteal and meningeal layers or between duplications of the meningeal layers.

1. Innervation of the dura mater

a. Anterior and posterior ethmoidal branches of the ophthalmic division of the trigeminal nerve in the anterior cranial fossa

b. Meningeal branches of the maxillary and mandibular divisions of the trigeminal nerve in the middle cranial fossa

c. Meningeal branches of the vagus and hypoglossal (originated from C1) nerves in the posterior cranial fossa

2. Projections of the dura mater (see Figures 8-20 and 8-25)

a. Falx cerebri

–is the sickle-shaped double layer of the dura mater, lying between the cerebral hemispheres.

–is attached anteriorly to the crista galli and posteriorly to the tentorium cerebelli.

–has a free inferior concave border that contains the **inferior sagittal sinus,** and its upper convex margin encloses the **superior sagittal sinus.**

b. Falx cerebelli

–is a small sickle-shaped projection between the cerebellar hemispheres.

–is attached to the posterior and inferior parts of the tentorium.

–contains the **occipital sinus** in its posterior border.

c. Tentorium cerebelli

–is a crescentic fold of dura mater that supports the occipital lobes of the cerebral hemispheres and covers the cerebellum.

–has a free internal concave border, that bounds the **tentorial notch,** whereas its external convex border encloses the **transverse sinus** posteriorly and the **superior petrosal sinus** anteriorly. The free border is anchored to the anterior crinoid process, whereas the attached border is attached to the posterior crinoid process.

d. Diaphragma sellae

–is a circular, horizontal fold of dura that forms the roof of the sella turcica, covering the pituitary gland or the hypophysis.

–has a central aperture for the hypophyseal stalk or infundibulum.

VII. Cranial Venous Channels (Figure 8-26; see Figure 8-20)

A. Superior sagittal sinus

–lies in the midline along the convex border of the falx cerebri.
–begins at the crista galli and receives the cerebral, diploic meningeal, and parietal emissary veins.

B. Inferior sagittal sinus

–lies in the free edge of the falx cerebri and is joined by the **great cerebral vein of Galen** to form the straight sinus.

C. Straight sinus

–runs along the line of attachment of the falx cerebri to the tentorium cerebelli.
–is formed by union of the inferior sagittal sinus and the great vein of Galen.

D. Transverse sinus

–runs laterally from the confluence of sinuses along the edge of the tentorium cerebelli.

E. Sigmoid sinus

–is a continuation of the transverse sinus; arches downward and medially in an S-shaped groove on the mastoid part of the temporal bone.
–enters the superior bulb of the internal jugular vein.

F. Cavernous sinuses

–are located on each side of the sella turcica and the body of the sphenoid bone and lie between the meningeal and periosteal layers of the dura mater.

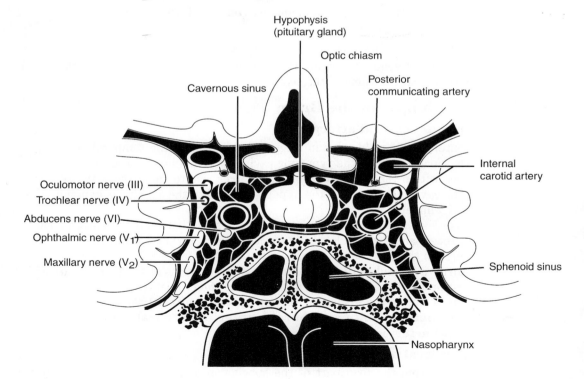

Figure 8-26. Frontal section through the cavernous sinus.

–The internal carotid artery and the abducens nerve pass through these sinuses. In addition, the oculomotor, trochlear, ophthalmic, and maxillary
nerves pass forward in the lateral wall of these sinuses.
–communicate with the pterygoid venous plexus by emissary veins and receive
the superior ophthalmic vein.

G. Superior petrosal sinus

–lies in the margin of the tentorium cerebelli, running from the posterior end
of the cavernous sinus to the transverse sinus.

H. Inferior petrosal sinus

–drains the cavernous sinus into the bulb of the internal jugular vein.
–runs in a groove between the petrous part of the temporal bone and the
basilar part of the occipital bone.

I. Sphenoparietal sinus

–lies along the posterior edge of the lesser wing of the sphenoid bone and
drains into the cavernous sinus.

J. Occipital sinus

–lies in the falx cerebelli and drains into the confluence of sinuses.

K. Basilar plexus

–consists of interconnecting venous channels on the basilar part of the occipital
bone and connects the two inferior petrosal sinuses.
–communicates with the internal vertebral venous plexus.

L. Diploic veins

–lie in the **diploë** of the skull and are connected with the cranial dura sinuses
by the emissary veins.

M. Emissary veins

–are small veins connecting the venous sinuses of the dura with the diploic
veins and the veins of the scalp.

VIII. Blood Supply of the Brain (Figure 8-27)

A. Internal carotid artery

–enters the carotid canal in the petrous portion of the temporal bone.
–is separated from the tympanic cavity by a thin bony structure.
–lies within the cavernous sinus and gives rise to small twigs to the wall of
the cavernous sinus, to the hypophysis, and to the semilunar ganglion of the
trigeminal nerve.
–pierces the dural roof of the cavernous sinus between the anterior clinoid
process and the middle clinoid process, which is a small projection posterolateral to the tuberculum sellae.
–forms a carotid **siphon** (a bent tube with two arms of unequal length), which
is the petrosal part just before it enters the cranial cavity.
–gives rise to the **superior hypophyseal, ophthalmic, posterior communicating, anterior choroid, anterior cerebral, and middle cerebral arteries.**

B. Vertebral arteries

–arise from the first part of the subclavian artery and ascend through the
transverse foramina of the vertebrae C1–C6.

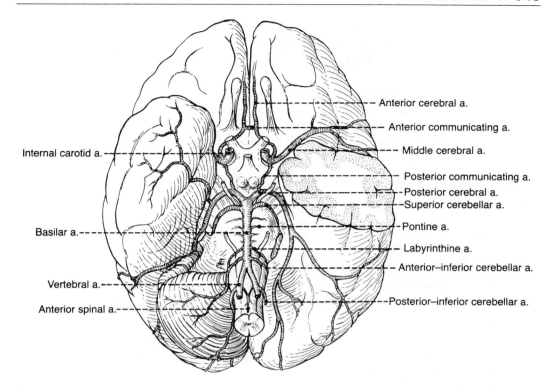

Figure 8-27. Arterial circle on the inferior surface of the brain.

–curve posteriorly behind the lateral mass of the atlas, pierce the dura mater into the vertebral canal, and then enter the cranial cavity through the foramen magnum.

–join to form the **basilar artery.**

–give rise to the following:

1. Anterior spinal artery

–arises as two roots from the vertebral arteries shortly before the junction of the vertebral arteries.

–descends in front of the medulla, and the two roots unite to form a single median trunk at the level of the foramen magnum.

2. Posterior spinal artery

–arises from the vertebral artery or the posterior–inferior cerebellar artery.

–descends on the side of the medulla, and the right and left roots unite at the lower cervical region.

3. Posterior–inferior cerebellar artery

–is the largest branch of the vertebral artery, distributes to the posterior–inferior surface of the cerebellum, and gives rise to the posterior spinal artery.

C. Basilar artery

–is formed by the union of the two vertebral arteries at the lower border of the pons.

–gives rise to the **pontine, anterior–inferior cerebellar, labyrinthine, and superior cerebellar arteries.**

–ends near the upper border of the pons by dividing into the right and left **posterior cerebral arteries.**

D. Circle of Willis (circulus arteriosus) [Figure 8-28]

–is formed by the posterior cerebral, posterior communicating, internal carotid, anterior cerebral, and anterior communicating arteries.

–forms an important means of **collateral circulation** in the event of obstruction.

IX. Clinical Considerations

A. Epidural hematoma

–is due to rupture of the middle meningeal artery.

B. Subdural hematoma

–is due to rupture of bridging cerebral veins as they pass from the brain surface into one of the venous sinuses.

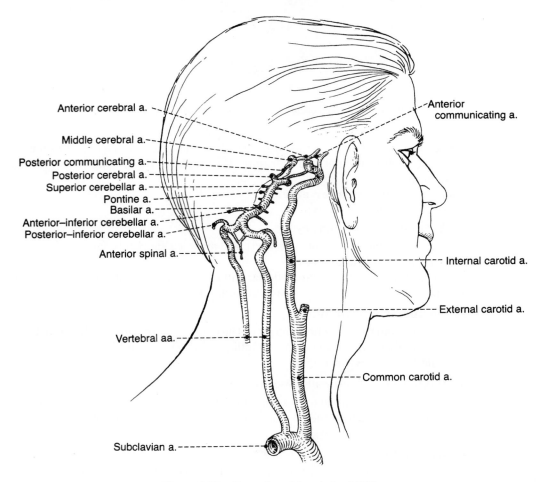

Figure 8-28. Formation of the circle of Willis.

C. Subarachnoid hemorrhage

–is due to rupture of cerebral arteries and also veins.

D. Pial hemorrhage

–is due to damage to the small vessels of the pia and brain tissue.

E. Cavernous sinus thrombophlebitis

–is an **infectious inflammation of the cavernous sinus** with secondary thrombus formation.

–is associated with significant morbidity and mortality because of the formation of **meningitis** (inflammation of the meninges).

–may produce papilledema (edema of the optic disk probably due to increased intracranial pressure), exophthalmos (protrusion of the eyeball), and ophthalmoplegia (paralysis of the eye muscles).

Nerves of the Head and Neck

I. Cranial Nerves (Figure 8-29; Table 8-5)

A. Olfactory nerves (CN I)

–consist of about 20 bundles of unmyelinated special visceral afferent (SVA) fibers that arise from olfactory neurons in the olfactory area, the upper one-third of the nasal mucosa, and mediate the sense of smell (olfaction).

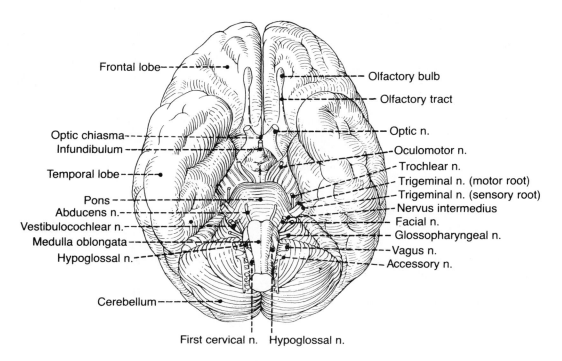

Figure 8-29. Cranial nerves on the base of the brain.

Table 8–5. Cranial Nerves

Nerve	Cranial Exit	Cell Bodies	Components	Chief Functions
I: Olfactory	Cribriform plate	Nasal mucosa	SVA	Smell
II: Optic	Optic canal	Ganglion cells of retina	SSA	Vision
III: Oculo-motor	Superior orbital fissure	Nucleus CN III (midbrain)	GSE	Eye movements (superior, inferior, and medial recti, inferior oblique, and levator palpebrae superioris mm.)
		Edinger-Westphal nucleus (midbrain)	GVE	Constriction of pupil (sphincter pupillae m.) and accommodation (ciliary m.)
IV: Trochlear	Superior orbital fissure	Nucleus CN IV (midbrain)	GSE	Eye movements (superior oblique m.)
V: Trigeminal	Superior orbital fissure; foramen rotundum and foramen ovale	Motor nucleus CN V (pons)	SVE	Muscles of mastication, mylohyoid, anterior belly of digastric, tensor veli palatini, and tensor tympani mm.
		Trigeminal ganglion	GSA	Sensation in head (skin and mucous membranes of face and head)
VI: Abducens	Superior orbital fissure	Nucleus CN VI (pons)	GSE	Eye movement (lateral rectus m.)
VII: Facial	Stylomastoid foramen	Motor nucleus CN VII (pons)	SVE	Muscle of facial expression, posterior belly of digastric, stylohyoid, and stapedius mm.
		Superior salivatory nucleus (pons)	GVE	Lacrimal and salivary secretion
		Geniculate ganglion	SVA	Taste from anterior two-thirds of tongue and palate
		Geniculate ganglion	GVA	Sensation from palate
		Geniculate ganglion	GSA	Auricle and external acoustic meatus
VIII: Vestibulocochlear	Does not leave skull	Vestibular ganglion	SSA	Equilibrium
		Spiral ganglion	SSA	Hearing

(continued)

Table 8–5. Cranial Nerves *(continued)*

Nerve	Cranial Exit	Cell Bodies	Components	Chief Functions
IX: Glosso-pharyngeal	Jugular foramen	Nucleus ambiguus (medulla)	SVE	Elevation of pharynx (stylopharyngeus m.)
		Inferior salivary nucleus (medulla)	GVE	Secretion of saliva (parotid gland)
		Inferior ganglion	GVA	Carotid sinus and body, tongue, pharynx, and middle ear
		Inferior ganglion	SVA	Taste from posterior one-third of tongue
		Inferior ganglion	GSA	External ear
X: Vagus	Jugular foramen	Nucleus ambiguus (medulla)	SVE	Muscles of pharynx, larynx, and palate
		Dorsal nucleus (medulla)	GVE	Smooth muscles and glands in thoracic and abdominal viscerae
		Inferior ganglion	GVA	Sensation in lower pharynx, larynx, trachea, and other viscerae
		Inferior ganglion	SVA	Taste on epiglottis
		Superior ganglion	GSA	Auricle and external acoustic meatus
XI: Accessory	Jugular foramen	Spinal cord (cervical)	SVE	Sternocleidomastoid and trapezius mm.
XII: Hypo-glossal	Hypoglossal canal	Nucleus CN XII (medulla)	GSE	Muscles of movements of tongue

GSA = general somatic afferent; GSE = general somatic efferent; GVA = general visceral afferent; GVE = general visceral efferent; SSA = special somatic afferent; SVA = special visceral afferent; SVE = special visceral efferent.

–pass through the foramina in the **cribriform plate** of the ethmoid bone and enter the **olfactory bulb,** where they synapse.

–Lesion (e.g., ethmoidal bone fracture) causes anosmia, or loss of olfactory sensation.

B. Optic nerve (CN II)

–is formed by the axons of **ganglion cells of the retina,** which converge at the optic disk.

–carries special somatic afferent (SSA) fibers (for vision) from the retina to the brain.

–leaves the orbit through the optic canal and forms the **optic chiasma,** where fibers from the nasal side of the retina cross over to the opposite side of the brain, but fibers from the temporal retina pass ipsilaterally through the chiasma.

–mediates the afferent limb of the pupillary light reflex, whereas parasympathetic fibers in the oculomotor nerve mediate the efferent limb.

–Lesion results in ipsilateral blindness and no direct pupillary light reflex. Lesion of the optic chiasma produces bitemporal heteronymous hemianopsia or tunnel vision, whereas lesion of the optic tract produces contralateral homonymous hemianopsia.

C. Oculomotor nerve (CN III)

–enters the orbit through the superior orbital fissure within the tendinous ring.

–supplies general somatic efferent (GSE) fibers to the extraocular muscles (i.e., medial, superior, and inferior recti; inferior oblique; and levator palpebrae superioris).

–contains preganglionic parasympathetic [general visceral efferent (GVE)] fibers with cell bodies located in the Edinger-Westphal nucleus, and postganglionic fibers derived from the ciliary ganglion that run in the **short ciliary nerves** to supply the **sphincter pupillae** (miosis) and the **ciliary muscle** (accommodation).

–contains parasympathetic fibers that mediate the efferent limb of the pupillary light reflex. Lesion causes dilation of the pupil (mydriasis) and thinning of the lens, which results in loss of accommodation to near objects. Lesion of GSE fibers causes the eye to deviate downward and laterally **(down-and-out),** and ptosis due to paralysis of levator palpebrae superioris.

D. Trochlear nerve (CN IV)

–passes through the lateral wall of the cavernous sinus during its course.

–enters the orbit by passing through the superior orbital fissure and supplies GSE fibers to the superior oblique muscle.

–is the **smallest cranial nerve** and the only cranial nerve that emerges from the dorsal aspect of the brainstem.

E. Trigeminal nerve (CN V)

–is the nerve of the first branchial arch, and supplies special visceral efferent (SVE) fibers to the muscles of mastication, the mylohyoid and the anterior belly of the digastric, and the tensor tympani and tensor veli palatini.

–provides GSA sensory fibers to the face, scalp, auricle, external auditory meatus, nose, paranasal sinuses, mouth (except the posterior one-third of the tongue), parts of the nasopharynx, auditory tube, and cranial dura mater.

–has a ganglion **(semilunar or trigeminal ganglion)** that consists of cell bodies of GSA fibers and occupies the trigeminal impression, or **Meckel's cave,** on the petrous portion of the temporal bone.

–has the following divisions:

1. Ophthalmic division (see Orbit: I B 1)

–runs in the dura of the lateral wall of the cavernous sinus and enters the orbit through the **supraorbital fissure.**

–provides sensory innervation to the eyeball, tip of the nose, and skin of the face above the eye.

–mediates the **afferent limb of the corneal reflex** by way of the nasociliary branch, whereas the facial nerve mediates the efferent limb.

2. Maxillary division (see Pterygopalatine Fossa: II A)

–passes through the lateral wall of the cavernous sinus and through the **foramen rotundum.**

–provides sensory (GSA) innervation to the midface (below the eye but above the upper lip), palate, paranasal sinuses, and maxillary teeth, with cell bodies in the trigeminal ganglion.

–mediates the **afferent limb of the sneeze reflex** (irritation of the nasal mucosa), and vagus nerve mediates the efferent limb.

3. **Mandibular division** (see Temporal and Infratemporal Fossae: III A)

–passes through the **foramen ovale** and supplies SVE fibers to the tensor veli palatini, tensor tympani, muscles of mastication (temporalis, masseter, and lateral and medial pterygoid), and the anterior belly of the digastric and mylohyoid muscles.

–provides sensory (GSA) innervation to the lower part of the face (below the lower lip and mouth), scalp, jaw, mandibular teeth, and anterior two-thirds of the tongue.

–mediates the **afferent and efferent limbs of the jaw jerk reflex.**

F. **Abducens nerve (CN VI)**

–pierces the dura on the dorsum sellae of the sphenoid bone.

–passes through the cavernous sinus, enters the orbit through the supraorbital fissure, and supplies GSE fibers to the lateral rectus.

G. **Facial nerve (CN VII)** [Figure 8-30]

–is the nerve of the second branchial arch.

–consists of a larger root, which contains SVE fibers to innervate the muscles of facial expression, and a smaller root, termed the nervus intermedius, which contains SVA (taste) fibers from the anterior two-thirds of the tongue. In addition, it contains preganglionic parasympathetic GVE fibers for the lacrimal, submandibular, sublingual, nasal, and palatine glands; GVA fibers from the palate and nasal mucosa; and GSA fibers from the external acoustic meatus and the auricle.

–enters the **internal acoustic meatus,** the **facial canal** in the temporal bone, and emerges from the **stylomastoid foramen.**

–has a sensory ganglion, the **geniculate ganglion,** which lies at the knee-shaped bend or genu (Latin for "knee") and contains cell bodies of SVA (taste), GVA, and GSA fibers.

–mediates the efferent limb of the **corneal (blink) reflex**.

–Lesion produces Bell's palsy (facial paralysis).

–gives rise to the following branches:

1. **Greater petrosal nerve**

–contains preganglionic parasympathetic GVE fibers and joins the deep **petrosal nerve** (containing postganglionic sympathetic fibers) to form the **nerve of the pterygoid canal** (vidian nerve).

–also contains SVA (taste) and GVA fibers, which pass from the palate through the pterygopalatine ganglion, the nerve of the pterygoid canal, and the greater petrosal nerve to the geniculate ganglion (where cell bodies are located).

2. **Communicating branch**

–joins the lesser petrosal nerve.

3. **Stapedial nerve**

–supplies motor (SVE) fibers to the stapedius.

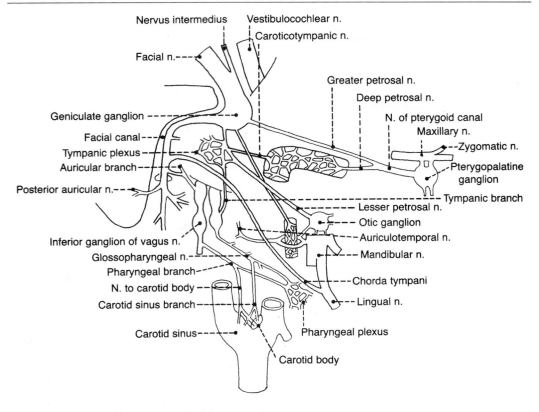

Figure 8-30. Facial nerve and its connections with other nerves.

4. Chorda tympani

–arises in the descending part of the facial canal, crosses the tympanic membrane, passing between the handle of the malleus and the long process of the incus.

–exits the skull through the **petrotympanic fissure** and joins the lingual nerve in the infratemporal fossa.

–contains preganglionic parasympathetic GVE fibers that synapse on post-ganglionic cell bodies in the **submandibular ganglion.** Their postganglionic fibers innervate the submandibular, sublingual, and lingual glands.

–also contains taste (SVA) fibers from the anterior two-thirds of the tongue and the soft palate, with cell bodies located in the geniculate ganglion.

–may communicate with the otic ganglion below the base of the skull.

5. Muscular branches

–supply motor (SVE) fibers to the stylohyoid and the posterior belly of the digastric muscle.

6. Fine communicating branch

–joins the auricular branch of the vagus nerve and the glossopharyngeal nerve to supply GSA fibers to the external ear.

7. Posterior auricular nerve

–runs behind the auricle with the posterior auricular artery.

–supplies SVE fibers to the muscles of the auricle and the occipitalis muscle.

8. Terminal branches

–arise in the parotid gland and radiate onto the face as the temporal, zygomatic, buccal, marginal mandibular, and cervical branches.

–supply motor (SVE) fibers to the muscles of facial expression.

H. Vestibulocochlear (acoustic or auditory) nerve (CN VIII)

–enters the internal acoustic meatus and remains within the temporal bone to supply SSA fibers to hair cells of the cochlea (organ of Corti), the ampullae of the semicircular ducts, and the utricle and saccule.

–is split into a **cochlear portion** (for hearing), which has bipolar neurons in the spiral (cochlear) ganglion, and a **vestibular portion** (for equilibrium), which has bipolar neurons in the vestibular ganglion.

I. Glossopharyngeal nerve (CN IX) [see Figure 8-30]

–is the nerve of the third branchial arch and contains SVE, SVA (taste), GVE, GVA, and GSA fibers.

–passes through the **jugular foramen** and gives rise to the following branches:

1. Tympanic nerve

–forms the **tympanic plexus** on the medial wall of the middle ear with sympathetic fibers from the internal carotid plexus (caroticotympanic nerves) and a branch from the geniculate ganglion of the facial nerve.

–conveys GVA fibers to the tympanic cavity, the mastoid antrum and air cells, and the auditory tube.

–continues beyond the plexus as the **lesser petrosal nerve,** which transmits preganglionic parasympathetic GVE fibers to the otic ganglion.

2. Communicating branch

–joins the auricular branch of the vagus nerve and provides GSA fibers.

3. Pharyngeal branch

–supplies GVA fibers to the pharynx and forms the **pharyngeal plexus** on the middle constrictor muscle along with the pharyngeal branch (SVE fibers) of the vagus nerve and branches from the sympathetic trunk.

–Its GVA component mediates the afferent limb of the **gag (pharyngeal) reflex.** The vagus nerve mediates the efferent limb.

4. Carotid sinus branch

–supplies GVA fibers to the **carotid sinus** and the **carotid body.**

–mediates the afferent limbs of the carotid sinus and body reflexes.

5. Tonsillar branches

–supply GVA fibers to the palatine tonsil and the soft palate.

6. Motor branch

–supplies SVE fibers to the stylopharyngeus.

7. Lingual branch

–supplies GVA and SVA (taste) fibers to the posterior one-third of the tongue and the vallate papillae.

J. Vagus nerve (CN X)

–is the nerve of the fourth and sixth branchial arches.

–passes through the jugular foramen.

–provides branchiomotor (SVE) innervation to all muscles of the larynx, pharynx (except the stylopharyngeus), and palate (except the tensor veli palatini).

–also provides motor (GVE) innervation to smooth muscle and cardiac muscle, secretory innervation to all glands, and afferent (GVA) fibers from all mucous membranes in the lower pharynx, larynx, trachea, bronchus, esophagus, and thoracic and abdominal visceral organs (except for the descending colon, sigmoid colon, rectum, and other pelvic organs).

–mediates the afferent and efferent limbs of the **cough reflex** (caused by irritation of the bronchial mucosa) as well as the efferent limbs of the **gag (pharyngeal) reflex.**

–Lesion results in deviation of the uvula toward the opposite side of the lesion on phonation.

–gives rise to the following branches:

1. **Meningeal branch**

    –arises from the superior ganglion and supplies the dura mater of the posterior cranial fossa.

2. **Auricular branch**

    –is joined by a branch from the glossopharyngeal nerve and the facial nerve and supplies GSA fibers to the external acoustic meatus.

3. **Pharyngeal branch**

    –supplies motor (SVE) fibers to all muscles of the pharynx, except the stylopharyngeus, by way of the pharyngeal plexus and all muscles of the palate except the tensor veli palatini.

    –gives rise to the **nerve to the carotid body,** which supplies GVA fibers to the carotid body and the carotid sinus.

    –Lesion causes **deviation** of the **uvula** toward the **opposite side** of the injury.

4. **Superior, middle, and inferior cardiac branches**

    –pass to the cardiac plexuses.

5. **Superior laryngeal nerve**

    –divides into internal and external branches:

    a. **Internal laryngeal nerve**

        –provides sensory (GVA) fibers to the larynx above the vocal cord, lower pharynx, and epiglottis.

        –supplies SVA (taste) fibers to the taste buds on the root of the tongue near and on the epiglottis.

    b. **External laryngeal nerve**

        –supplies motor (SVE) fibers to the cricothyroid and inferior pharyngeal constrictor muscles.

6. **Recurrent laryngeal nerve**

    –hooks around the subclavian artery on the right and around the arch of the aorta lateral to the ligamentum arteriosum on the left.

    –ascends in the groove between the trachea and the esophagus.

    –provides sensory (GVA) fibers to the larynx below the vocal cord and motor (SVE) fibers to all muscles of the larynx except the cricothyroid muscle.

–becomes the **inferior laryngeal nerve** at the lower border of the cricoid cartilage.

K. Accessory nerve (CN XI)

–passes through the jugular foramen.

–has spinal roots that originate from the anterior horn of the upper cervical segments, emerge from the lateral aspect of the spinal cord between dorsal and ventral roots of the spinal nerves, and unite to form the trunk that passes through the foramen magnum and jugular foramen.

–provides branchiomotor (SVE) fibers to the sternocleidomastoid and trapezius muscles.

–has a cranial portion that contains motor fibers that exit the medulla, pass through the jugular foramen where they join the vagus nerve, and supply muscles of the pharynx, larynx, and palate.

–When it is lesioned, the arm cannot be abducted beyond the horizontal position as a result of an inability to rotate the scapula.

L. Hypoglossal nerve (CN XII)

–passes through the **hypoglossal canal.**

–loops around the occipital artery, passes between the external carotid and internal jugular vessels, and runs deep to the digastric posterior belly and stylohyoid muscles.

–passes above the hyoid bone on the lateral surface of the hyoglossus deep to the mylohyoid muscle.

–supplies GSE fibers to all of the intrinsic and extrinsic muscles of the tongue except the palatoglossus, which is supplied by the vagus nerve.

–carries GSA fibers from C1 to supply the cranial dura mater through the meningeal branch, but the fibers are not components of the hypoglossal nerve.

–also carries GSE fibers from C1 to supply the thyrohyoid and geniohyoid muscles.

–Lesion causes **deviation of the tongue** toward the **injured side** on protrusion.

II. Parasympathetic Ganglia and Associated Autonomic Nerves (Figure 8-31; Table 8-6)

A. Ciliary ganglion

–is situated behind the eyeball, between the optic nerve and the lateral rectus muscle.

–receives preganglionic parasympathetic fibers (with cell bodies in the Edinger-Westphal nucleus of CN III in the mesencephalon), which run in the inferior division of the oculomotor nerve.

–sends its postganglionic parasympathetic fibers to the sphincter pupillae and the ciliary muscle via the **short ciliary nerves.**

–receives postganglionic sympathetic fibers (derived from the superior cervical ganglion) that reach the **dilator pupillae** by way of the sympathetic plexus on the internal carotid artery, the long ciliary nerve and/or the ciliary ganglion (without synapsing), and the short ciliary nerves.

B. Pterygopalatine ganglion

–lies in the pterygopalatine fossa just below the maxillary nerve, lateral to the sphenopalatine foramen and anterior to the pterygoid canal.

Table 8–6. Parasympathetic Ganglia and Associated Autonomic Nerves

Ganglion	Location	Parasympathetic Fibers	Sympathetic Fibers	Chief Distribution
Ciliary	Lateral to optic n.	Oculomotor n. and its inferior division	Internal carotid plexus	Ciliary muscle, and sphincter pupillae (para-sympathetic); dilator pupillae and tarsal mm. (sympathetic)
Pterygopalatine	In pterygopal-atine fossa	Facial n., greater petrosal n., and n. of pterygoid canal	Internal carotid plexus	Lacrimal gland and glands in palate and nose
Submandibular	On hyoglossus	Facial n., chorda tympani, and lingual n.	Plexus on facial a.	Submandibular and sublingual glands
Otic	Below foramen ovale	Glossopharyn-geal n., its tym-panic branch, and lesser petrosal n.	Plexus on middle meningeal a.	Parotid gland

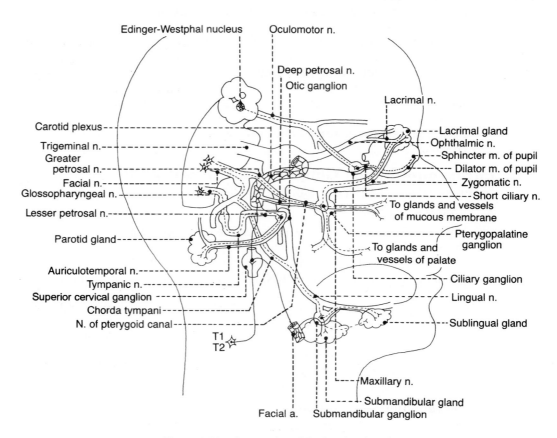

Figure 8-31. Autonomics of the head and neck.

–receives preganglionic parasympathetic fibers from the facial nerve by way of the greater petrosal nerve and the nerve of the pterygoid canal.

–sends postganglionic parasympathetic fibers to the nasal and palatine glands and to the lacrimal glands by way of the maxillary, zygomatic, and lacrimal nerves.

–also receives postganglionic sympathetic fibers (derived from the superior cervical ganglion) by way of the plexus on the internal carotid artery, the deep petrosal nerve, and the nerve of the pterygoid canal. The fibers merely pass through the ganglion and are distributed with the postganglionic parasympathetic fibers.

1. **Greater petrosal nerve**

    –arises from the **facial nerve** adjacent to the geniculate ganglion.

    –emerges at the hiatus of the canal for the greater petrosal nerve in the middle cranial fossa.

    –contains preganglionic parasympathetic fibers and joins the deep petrosal nerve (containing postganglionic sympathetic fibers) to form the **nerve of the pterygoid canal** (vidian nerve).

    –also contains taste fibers, which pass from the palate nonstop through the pterygopalatine ganglion, the nerve of the pterygoid canal, and the greater petrosal nerve to the geniculate ganglion (where cell bodies are found).

2. **Deep petrosal nerve**

    –arises from the plexus on the internal carotid artery.

    –contains postganglionic sympathetic fibers with cell bodies located in the superior cervical ganglion. These fibers run inside the nerve of the pterygoid canal, pass through the pterygopalatine ganglion without synapsing, and then join the postganglionic parasympathetic fibers in supplying the lacrimal gland and the nasal and oral mucosa.

3. **Nerve of the pterygoid canal (vidian nerve)**

    –consists of preganglionic parasympathetic fibers from the greater petrosal nerve and postganglionic sympathetic fibers from the deep petrosal nerve.

    –passes through the pterygoid canal and ends in the pterygopalatine ganglion, which is slung from the maxillary nerve. The postganglionic parasympathetic fibers have cell bodies located in the pterygopalatine ganglion, and the postganglionic sympathetic fibers are distributed to the lacrimal, nasal, and palatine glands.

    –also contains SVA (taste) and GVA fibers from the palate.

C. **Submandibular ganglion**

    –lies on the lateral surface of the hyoglossus muscle but deep to the mylohyoid muscle and is suspended from the lingual nerve.

    –receives preganglionic parasympathetic (secretomotor) fibers that run in the facial nerve, chorda tympani, and lingual nerve.

    –sends postganglionic fibers to supply the submandibular gland mostly, although some join the lingual nerve to reach the sublingual and lingual glands.

D. **Otic ganglion**

    –lies in the infratemporal fossa, just below the foramen ovale, between the mandibular nerve and the tensor veli palatini.

–receives preganglionic parasympathetic fibers that run in the glossopharyngeal nerve, tympanic plexus, and lesser petrosal nerve and synapse in the otic ganglion.

–sends postganglionic fibers that run in the auriculotemporal nerve and supply the parotid gland.

1. **Tympanic nerve**

–contains preganglionic parasympathetic (secretomotor) fibers for the parotid gland.

–arises from the inferior ganglion of the glossopharyngeal nerve.

–passes through a small canal between the jugular foramen and the carotid canal into the tympanic cavity.

–enters the tympanic plexus on the promontory of the medial wall of the tympanic cavity.

2. **Lesser petrosal nerve**

–is a continuation of the tympanic nerve beyond the tympanic plexus.

–runs just lateral to the greater petrosal nerve and leaves the middle cranial fossa through either the foramen ovale or the fissure between the petrous bone and the great wing of the sphenoid to enter the otic ganglion.

–contains preganglionic parasympathetic (secretomotor) fibers that run in the glossopharyngeal and tympanic nerves before synapsing in the otic ganglion. (The postganglionic fibers arising from the ganglion are passed to the parotid gland by the auriculotemporal nerves.)

–also transmits postganglionic sympathetic fibers to the parotid gland.

III. Clinical Considerations

A. Herpes zoster (shingles)

–is a viral disease of the spinal and certain cranial (i.e., trigeminal) ganglia.

–is characterized by an eruption of groups of vesicles due to inflammation of ganglia resulting from activation of virus that has remained latent for years.

B. Chickenpox

–is caused by the varicella-zoster virus, which later resides latent in the cranial (i.e., trigeminal) or dorsal root ganglia.

–is marked by vesicular eruption of the skin and mucous membranes.

Orbit

I. Bony Orbit (Figure 8-32)

A. Orbital margin

–is formed by the frontal, maxillary, and zygomatic bones.

B. Walls of the orbit

1. **Superior wall or roof:** orbital part of frontal bone and lesser wing of spheroid bone

2. **Lateral wall:** zygomatic bone (frontal process) and greater wing of sphenoid bone

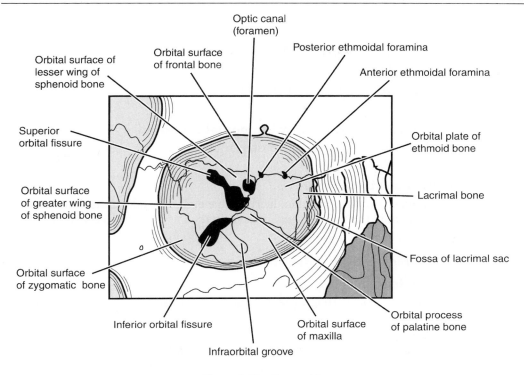

Figure 8-32. Bony orbit.

3. **Inferior wall or floor:** maxilla (orbital surface), zygomatic, and palatine bones

4. **Medial wall:** ethmoid (orbital plate), frontal, lacrimal, and sphenoid (body) bones

C. Fissures, canals, and foramina

1. Superior orbital fissure

–communicates with the middle cranial fossa and is bounded by the greater and lesser wings of the sphenoid.

–transmits the oculomotor, trochlear, abducens, and ophthalmic nerves (three branches), as well as the ophthalmic veins.

2. Inferior orbital fissure

–communicates with the infratemporal and pterygopalatine fossae.

–is bounded by the greater wing of the sphenoid (above) and the maxillary and palatine bones (below).

–transmits the maxillary (or infraorbital) nerve and its zygomatic branch and the infraorbital vessels.

–is bridged by the orbitalis (smooth) muscle.

3. Optic canal

–connects the orbit with the middle cranial fossa.

–is formed by the two roots of the lesser wing of the sphenoid and is situated in the posterior part of the roof of the orbit.

–transmits the optic nerve and ophthalmic artery.

4. Infraorbital groove and infraorbital foramen

–transmit the infraorbital nerve and vessels.

5. Supraorbital notch or foramen

–transmits the supraorbital nerve and vessels.

6. Anterior and posterior ethmoidal foramina

–transmit the anterior and posterior ethmoidal nerves and vessels, respectively.

7. Nasolacrimal canal

–is formed by the maxilla, lacrimal bone, and inferior nasal concha.
–transmits the nasolacrimal duct from the lacrimal sac to the inferior nasal meatus.

II. Nerves (Figures 8-33, 8-34, and 8-35)

A. Ophthalmic nerve

–enters the orbit through the superior orbital fissure and divides into three branches:

1. Lacrimal nerve

–enters the orbit through the superior orbital fissure.
–enters the lacrimal gland, giving rise to branches to the lacrimal gland, the conjunctiva, and the skin of the upper eyelid.

2. Frontal nerve

–enters the orbit through the superior orbital fissure.
–runs superior to the levator palpebrae superioris.
–divides into the **supraorbital nerve,** which passes through the supraorbital **notch or foramen** and supplies the scalp, forehead, frontal sinus,

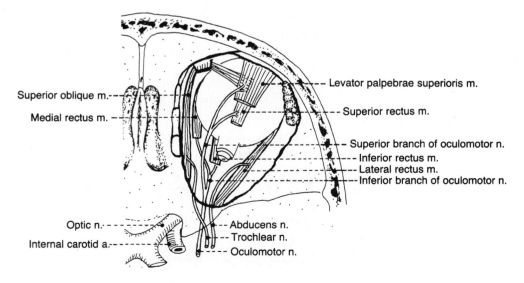

Figure 8-33. Motor nerves of the orbit.

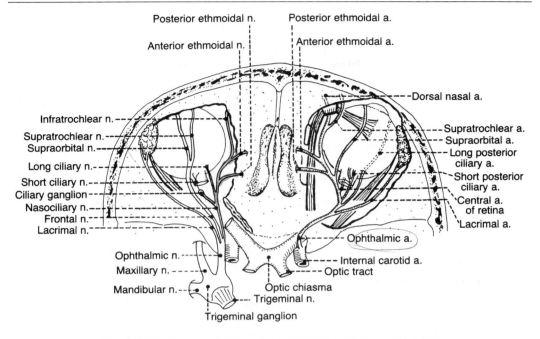

Figure 8-34. Branches of the ophthalmic nerve and ophthalmic artery.

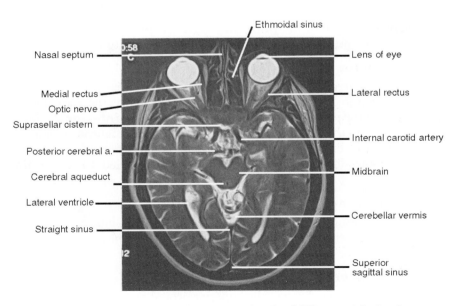

Figure 8-35. Axial magnetic resonance imaging (MRI) scan of the head.

and upper eyelid; and the **supratrochlear nerve,** which passes through the trochlea and supplies the scalp, forehead, and upper eyelid.

3. **Nasociliary nerve**

–is the sensory nerve for the eye.
–enters the orbit through the superior orbital fissure, within the common tendinous ring.
–gives rise to the following:

   a. **A communicating branch** to the ciliary ganglion

   b. **Short ciliary nerves,** which carry postganglionic parasympathetic and sympathetic fibers to the ciliary body and iris and afferent fibers from the iris and cornea.

   c. **Long ciliary nerves,** which transmit postganglionic sympathetic fibers to the dilator pupillae and afferent fibers from the iris and cornea.

   d. **The posterior ethmoidal nerve,** which passes through the posterior ethmoidal foramen to the sphenoidal and posterior ethmoidal sinuses.

   e. **The anterior ethmoidal nerve,** which passes through the anterior ethmoidal foramen to supply the anterior ethmoidal air cells. It divides into **internal nasal branches,** which supply the septum and lateral walls of the nasal cavity, and **external nasal branches,** which supply the skin of the tip of the nose.

   f. **The infratrochlear nerve,** which innervates the eyelids, conjunctiva, skin of the nose, and lacrimal sac

B. **Optic nerve**

   –consists of the axons of the ganglion cells of the retina and leaves the orbit by passing through the **optic canal.**
   –carries SSA fibers for vision from the retina to the brain and mediates the **afferent limb** of the **pupillary light reflex.**
   –joins the optic nerve from the corresponding eye to form the optic chiasma.

C. **Oculomotor nerve**

   –leaves the cranium through the superior orbital fissure.
   –divides into a **superior division,** which innervates the superior rectus and levator palpebrae superioris muscles, and an **inferior division,** which innervates the medial rectus, inferior rectus, and inferior oblique muscles.
   –Its inferior division also carries preganglionic parasympathetic fibers (with cell bodies located in the Edinger-Westphal nucleus) to the **ciliary ganglion.**

D. **Trochlear nerve**

   –passes through the lateral wall of the cavernous sinus during its course.
   –enters the orbit by passing through the superior orbital fissure and innervates the superior oblique muscle.

E. **Abducens nerve**

   –enters the orbit through the superior orbital fissure and supplies the lateral rectus muscle.

F. Ciliary ganglion

–is a parasympathetic ganglion situated behind the eyeball, between the optic nerve and the lateral rectus muscle (see Nerves of the Head and Neck: II A).

III. Blood Vessels (see Figure 8-34)

A. Ophthalmic artery

–is a branch of the internal carotid artery and enters the orbit through the **optic canal** beneath the optic nerve.

–gives rise to the **ocular and orbital vessels,** which include the following:

1. Central artery of the retina

–is the **most important branch** of the ophthalmic artery.

–travels in the optic nerve; it divides into superior and inferior branches to the optic disk, and each of those further divides into temporal and nasal branches.

–is an end artery that does not anastomose with other arteries, and thus its **occlusion results in blindness.**

2. Long posterior ciliary arteries

–pierce the sclera and supply the ciliary body and the iris.

3. Short posterior ciliary arteries

–pierce the sclera and supply the choroid.

4. Lacrimal artery

–passes along the superior border of the lateral rectus and supplies the lacrimal gland, conjunctiva, and eyelids.

–gives rise to two **lateral palpebral arteries,** which contribute to arcades in the upper and lower eyelids.

5. Medial palpebral arteries

–contribute to arcades in the upper and lower eyelids.

6. Muscular branches

–supply orbital muscles and give off the anterior ciliary arteries, which supply the iris.

7. Supraorbital artery

–passes through the supraorbital notch (or foramen) and supplies the forehead and the scalp.

8. Posterior ethmoidal artery

–passes through the posterior ethmoidal foramen to the posterior ethmoidal air cells.

9. Anterior ethmoidal artery

–passes through the anterior ethmoidal foramen to the anterior and middle ethmoidal air cells, frontal sinus, nasal cavity, and external nose.

10. Supratrochlear artery

–passes to the supraorbital margin and supplies the forehead and the scalp.

11. Dorsal nasal artery

–supplies the side of the nose and the lacrimal sac.

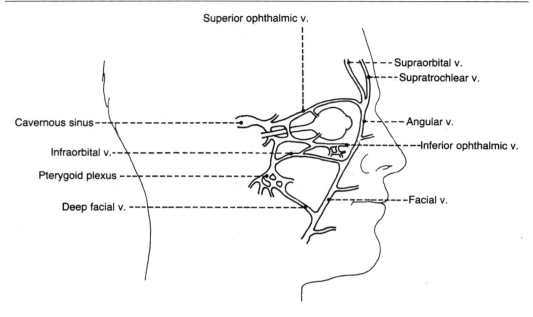

Figure 8-36. Ophthalmic veins.

B. Ophthalmic veins (Figure 8-36)

1. Superior ophthalmic vein

–is formed by the union of the supraorbital, supratrochlear, and angular veins.

–receives branches corresponding to most of those of the ophthalmic artery and, in addition, receives the inferior ophthalmic vein before draining into the cavernous sinus.

2. Inferior ophthalmic vein

–begins by the union of small veins in the floor of the orbit.

–communicates with the pterygoid venous plexus and often with the infraorbital vein and terminates directly or indirectly in the cavernous sinus.

IV. Muscles of Eye Movement (Figures 8-37 and 8-38; Table 8-7) [see Figure 8-35]

A. Innervation of muscles of the eyeball

–can be summarized as **SO$_4$**, **LR$_6$**, and **Remainder$_3$**, which means that the superior oblique muscle is innervated by the trochlear nerve, the lateral rectus by the abducens nerve, and the remainder of these muscles by the oculomotor nerve.

B. Movements of the eye

1. Intorsion

–is a **medial (inward) rotation** of the upper pole (12 o'clock position) of the cornea, caused by the superior oblique and superior rectus muscles.

2. Extorsion

–is a **lateral (outward) rotation** of the upper pole of the cornea, caused by the inferior oblique and inferior rectus muscles.

Table 8–7. Muscles of Eye Movement

Muscle	Origin	Insertion	Nerve	Actions on Eyeball
Superior rectus	Common tendinous ring	Sclera just behind cornea	Oculomotor n.	Elevates; intorts
Inferior rectus	Common tendinous ring	Sclera just behind cornea	Oculomotor n.	Depresses; extorts
Medial rectus	Common tendinous ring	Sclera just behind cornea	Oculomotor n.	Adducts
Lateral rectus	Common tendinous ring	Sclera just behind cornea	Abducens n.	Abducts
Levator palpebrae superioris	Lesser wing of sphenoid above and anterior to optic canal	Tarsal plate and skin of upper eyelid	Oculomotor n. Sympathetic n.	Elevates upper eyelid
Superior oblique	Body of sphenoid bone above optic canal	Sclera beneath superior rectus	Trochlear n.	Rotates downward and laterally; turns upper pole of cornea inward (intorsion); depresses adducted eye
Inferior oblique	Floor of orbit lateral to lacrimal groove	Sclera beneath lateral rectus	Oculomotor n.	Rotates upward and laterally; turns upper pole of cornea outward (extorsion); elevates adducted eye

(handwritten margin notes: "down + out" beside Superior oblique; "up + out" beside Inferior oblique)

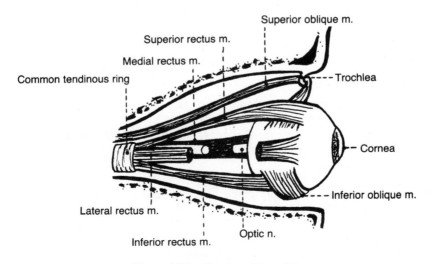

Figure 8-37. Muscles of the orbit.

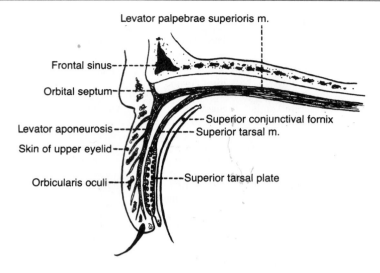

Figure 8-38. Structure of the upper eyelid.

C. Common tendinous ring (Figure 8-39)

–is a **fibrous ring** that surrounds the optic canal and the medial part of the superior orbital fissure.

–is the site of origin of the four rectus muscles of the eye and transmits the following structures:

1. **Oculomotor, nasociliary, and abducens nerves,** which enter the orbit through the superior orbital fissure and the common tendinous ring

2. **Optic nerve, ophthalmic artery, and central artery and vein of the retina,** which enter the orbit through the optic canal and the tendinous ring

3. **Superior ophthalmic vein plus the trochlear, frontal, and lacrimal nerves,** which enter the orbit through the superior orbital fissure but outside the tendinous ring

V. Lacrimal Apparatus (Figure 8-40)

A. Lacrimal gland

–lies in the upper lateral region of the orbit on the lateral rectus and the levator palpebrae superioris muscles.

–is drained by 12 **lacrimal ducts,** which open into the superior conjunctival fornix.

B. Lacrimal canaliculi

–are two curved canals, which begin as a lacrimal punctum (or pore) in the margin of the eyelid and open into the lacrimal sac.

C. Lacrimal sac

–is the upper dilated end of the **nasolacrimal duct,** which opens into the inferior meatus of the nasal cavity.

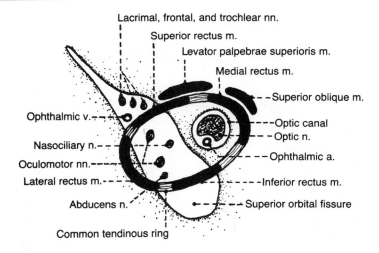

Figure 8-39. Common tendinous ring.

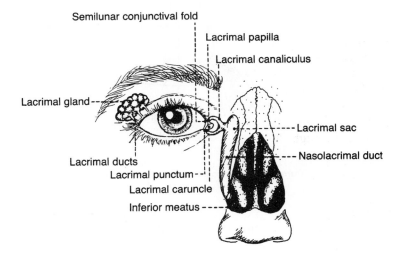

Figure 8-40. Lacrimal apparatus.

D. Tears

–are produced by the **lacrimal gland.**

–pass through excretory ductules into the superior conjunctival fornix.

–are spread evenly over the eyeball by blinking movements and accumulate in the area of the **lacrimal lake.**

–enter the lacrimal canaliculi through their lacrimal puncta (which is on the summit of the lacrimal papilla) before draining into the lacrimal sac, nasolacrimal duct, and finally the inferior nasal meatus.

VI. Eyeball (Figure 8-41; see Figure 8-35)

A. External white fibrous coat

–consists of the sclera and the cornea.

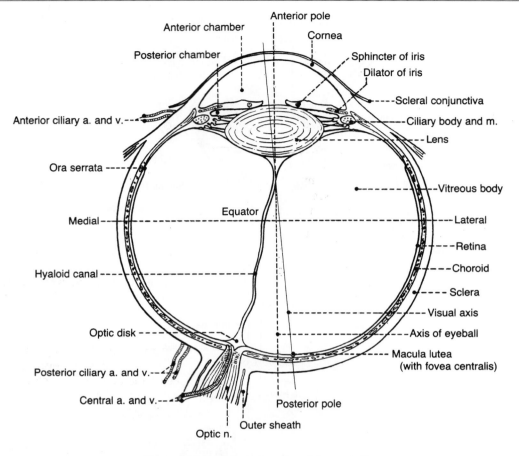

Figure 8-41. Horizontal section of the eyeball.

1. **Sclera**

   –is a tough white fibrous tunic enveloping the posterior five-sixths of the eye.

2. **Cornea**

   –is a transparent structure forming the anterior one-sixth of the external coat.

   –is responsible for the **refraction of light** entering the eye.

B. **Middle vascular pigmented coat**

   –consists of the choroid, ciliary body, and iris.

   1. **Choroid**

      –consists of an outer pigmented (dark brown) layer and an inner highly vascular layer, which invests the posterior five-sixths of the eyeball.

      –**nourishes the retina** and darkens the eye.

   2. **Ciliary body**

      –is a **thickened portion of the vascular coat** between the choroid and the iris, and consists of the ciliary ring, ciliary processes, and ciliary muscle.

a. The **ciliary processes** are radiating pigmented ridges that encircle the margin of the lens.

b. The **ciliary muscle** consists of meridional and circular fibers of smooth muscle innervated by parasympathetic fibers. It contracts to pull the **ciliary ring** and ciliary processes, relaxing the suspensory ligament of the lens and allowing it to increase its convexity.

3. Iris

–is a thin, contractile, circular, pigmented diaphragm with a central aperture, the **pupil.**

–contains circular muscle fibers **(sphincter pupillae),** which are innervated by parasympathetic fibers, and radial fibers **(dilator pupillae),** which are innervated by sympathetic fibers.

C. Internal nervous coat

–consists of the **retina,** which has an outer pigmented layer and an inner nervous layer.

–has a posterior part that is photosensitive; its anterior part, which is not photosensitive, constitutes the inner lining of the ciliary body and the posterior part of the iris.

1. Optic disk (blind spot)

–consists of **optic nerve fibers** formed by axons of the ganglion cells. These cells are connected to the rods and cones by bipolar neurons.

–is located nasal (or medial) to the fovea centralis and the posterior pole of the eye, has no receptors, and is insensitive to light.

–has a depression in its center termed the **physiological cup.**

2. Macula (yellow spot or macula lutea)

–is a yellowish area of the retina on the temporal side of the optic disk for the most distinct vision.

–contains the fovea centralis.

3. Fovea centralis

–is a **central depression** (foveola) in the macula.

–is avascular and is nourished by the choriocapillary lamina of the choroid.

–has cones only (no rods), each of which is connected with only one ganglion cell, and functions in detailed vision.

4. Rods

–are approximately 120 million in number and are most numerous about 0.5 cm from the fovea centralis.

–contain **rhodopsin,** a visual purple pigment.

–are specialized for **vision in dim light.**

5. Cones

–are 7 million in number and are most numerous in the foveal region.

–are associated with **visual acuity** and **color vision.**

D. Refractive media

–consist of the cornea, aqueous humor, lens, and vitreous body.

1. Cornea (see VI A 2)

2. Aqueous humor

–is formed by the ciliary processes and provides nutrients for the avascular cornea and lens.

–passes through the pupil from the **posterior chamber** (between the iris and the lens) into the **anterior chamber** (between the cornea and the iris) and is drained into the scleral venous plexus through the canal of Schlemm at the iridocorneal angle.

–Its impaired drainage causes an increased intraocular pressure, leading to atrophy of the retina and blindness.

3. Lens

–is a transparent **avascular biconvex structure** enclosed in an elastic capsule.

–is held in position by radially arranged **zonular fibers** (suspensory ligament of the lens), which are attached medially to the lens capsule and laterally to the ciliary processes.

–flattens to focus on distant objects by pulling the zonular fibers, and it becomes a globular shape to accommodate the eye for near objects by contracting the ciliary muscle and thus relaxing zonular fibers.

4. Vitreous body

–is a transparent gel called **vitreous humor,** which fills the eyeball posterior to the lens (vitreous chamber between the lens and the retina).

–holds the retina in place and provides support for the lens.

VII. Clinical Considerations

A. Horner's syndrome

–is caused by **injury to cervical sympathetic fibers** and characterized by:

1. **Miosis:** constriction of the pupil resulting from paralysis of the dilator muscle of the iris

2. **Ptosis:** drooping of an upper eyelid from paralysis of the smooth muscle component (superior tarsal plate) of the levator palpebrae superioris

3. **Enophthalmos:** retraction (backward displacement) of an eyeball into the orbit from paralysis of the orbitalis muscle, which is smooth muscle and bridges the inferior orbital fissure and functions in eyeball protrusion

4. **Anhidrosis:** absence of sweating

5. **Vasodilation:** increased blood flow in the facial and cervical skin

B. Crocodile tears syndrome (Bogorad's syndrome)

–is **spontaneous lacrimation during eating,** caused by a lesion of the facial nerve proximal to the geniculate ganglion.

–follows facial paralysis and is due to misdirection of regenerating parasympathetic fibers, which formerly innervated the salivary (submandibular and sublingual) glands, to the lacrimal glands.

C. Hemianopia (hemianopsia)

–is a condition characterized by loss of vision in one half of the visual field of each eye. Blindness may occur as the result of a lesion of the **optic nerve.** Types of hemianopia are:

1. **Bitemporal (heteronymous) hemianopia:** loss of vision in the temporal visual field of both eyes due to a lesion of the **optic chiasma**

2. **Right nasal hemianopia:** blindness in the nasal field of vision of the right eye as the result of a **right perichiasmal lesion** such as an aneurysm of the internal carotid artery

3. **Left homonymous hemianopia:** loss of sight in the left half of the visual field of both eyes due to a lesion of the **right optic tract** or **optic radiation**

D. Glaucoma

–is characterized by **increased intraocular pressure** due to **impaired drainage of aqueous humor** (which is produced by the ciliary processes) into the venous system through Schlemm's canal, which is a circular vascular channel at the corneoscleral junction or limbus. The increased pressure causes **impaired retinal blood flow**, producing retinal ischemia or atrophy of the retina; degeneration of the nerve fibers in the retina, particularly at the optic disk; defects in the visual field; and blindness.

–can be treated by surgical iridectomy or laser iridotomy for drainage of aqueous humor or by using drugs to inhibit the secretion of aqueous humor.

E. Cataract

–is an **opacity (milky white) of the crystalline eye lens or of its capsule,** necessitating its removal.

–results in little light to be transmitted to the retina, causing blurred images and poor vision.

F. Diplopia (double vision)

–is caused by **paralysis of one or more extraocular muscles** due to injury of the nerves supplying them.

G. Pupillary light reflex

–is constriction of the pupil in response to light stimulation.

–is mediated by parasympathetic nerve fibers in the oculomotor nerve (efferent limb). Its afferent limb is the optic nerve.

H. Accommodation

–is the adjustment or adaptation of the eye to focus on a near object.

–occurs as contraction of the ciliary muscle, causing a relaxation of the suspensory ligament (ciliary zonular fibers), an increase in thickness, convexity, and refractive power of the lens.

–is mediated by parasympathetic fibers running within the oculomotor nerve.

Oral Cavity and Palate

I. Oral Cavity (Figure 8-42)

–Its roof is formed by the **palate,** and its floor is formed by the tongue and the mucosa, supported by the geniohyoid and mylohyoid muscles.

–Its lateral and anterior walls are formed by an outer fleshy wall (cheeks and lips) and an inner bony wall (teeth and gums). (The **vestibule** is between the walls, and the **oral cavity proper** is the area inside the teeth and gums.)

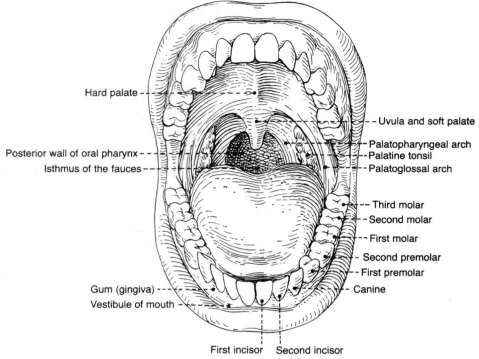

Hard palate

Uvula and soft palate

Posterior wall of oral pharynx

Isthmus of the fauces

Palatopharyngeal arch
Palatine tonsil
Palatoglossal arch

Third molar
Second molar
First molar
Second premolar
First premolar
Canine

Gum (gingiva)
Vestibule of mouth

First incisor   Second incisor

Figure 8-42.   Oral cavity.

II. Palate (Figure 8-43)

–forms the roof of the mouth and the floor of the nasal cavity.

A. Hard palate

–is the anterior four-fifths of the palate and forms a **bony framework covered with a mucous membrane** between the nasal and oral cavities.

–consists of the **palatine processes** of the maxillae and horizontal plates of the palatine bones.

–contains the incisive foramen in its median plane anteriorly and the greater and lesser palatine foramina posteriorly.

–receives sensory innervation through the greater palatine and nasopalatine nerves, and blood from the greater palatine artery.

B. Soft palate

–is a **fibromuscular fold** extending from the posterior border of the hard palate and makes up one-fifth of the palate.

–moves posteriorly against the pharyngeal wall to close the oropharyngeal (faucial) isthmus when swallowing or speaking.

–is continuous with the **palatoglossal and palatopharyngeal folds.**

–receives blood from the greater and lesser palatine arteries of the descending palatine artery of the maxillary artery, the ascending palatine artery of the facial artery, and the palatine branch of the ascending pharyngeal artery.

–receives sensory innervation through the lesser palatine nerves and skeletal motor innervation from the vagus nerve. A lesion of the vagus nerve deviates the uvula to the opposite side.

C. Muscles of the palate (Table 8-8)

Table 8–8. Muscles of the Palate

Muscle	Origin	Insertion	Nerve	Action
Tensor veli palatini	Scaphoid fossa; spine of sphenoid; cartilage of auditory tube	Tendon hooks around hamulus of medial pterygoid plate to insert into aponeurosis of soft palate	Mandibular branch of trigeminal n.	Tenses soft palate
Levator veli palatini	Petrous part of temporal bone; cartilage of auditory tube	Aponeurosis of soft palate	Vagus n. via pharyngeal plexus	Elevates soft palate
Palatoglossus	Aponeurosis of soft palate	Dorsolateral side of tongue	Vagus n. via pharyngeal plexus	Elevates tongue
Palatopharyngeus	Aponeurosis of soft palate	Thyroid cartilage and side of pharynx	Vagus n. via pharyngeal plexus	Elevates pharynx; closes nasopharynx
Musculus uvulae	Posterior nasal spine of palatine bone; palatine aponeurosis	Mucous membrane of uvula	Vagus n. via pharyngeal plexus	Elevates uvula

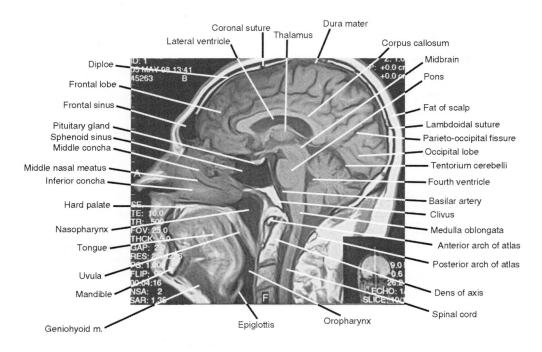

Figure 8-43. Sagittal magnetic resonance imaging (MRI) scan of the head and neck.

III. Tongue (Figure 8-44; see Figure 8-43)

–is attached by muscles to the hyoid bone, mandible, styloid process, palate, and pharynx.

–is divided by a V-shaped **sulcus terminalis** into two parts, an anterior two-thirds and a posterior one-third, which differ developmentally, structurally, and in innervation.

–The **foramen cecum** is located at the apex of the "V" and indicates the site of origin of the embryonic **thyroglossal duct.**

A. Lingual papillae

–are small, nipple-shaped projections on the anterior two-thirds of the dorsum of the tongue.

–are divided into the vallate, fungiform, filiform, and foliate papillae.

1. Vallate papillae

–are arranged in the form of a "V" in front of the sulcus terminalis.

–are studded with numerous taste buds and are innervated by the glossopharyngeal nerve.

2. Fungiform papillae

–are mushroom-shaped projections with red heads and are scattered on the sides and the apex of the tongue.

3. Filiform papillae

–are numerous, slender, conical projections that are arranged in rows parallel to the sulcus terminalis.

4. Foliate papillae

–are found in certain animals but are rudimentary in humans.

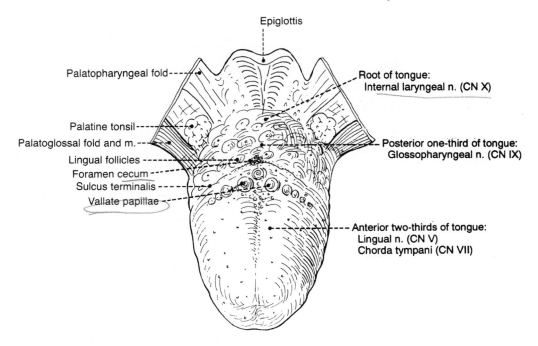

Figure 8-44. Tongue.

B. Lingual tonsil

–is the collection of **nodular masses of lymphoid follicles** on the posterior one-third of the dorsum of the tongue.

C. Lingual innervation

–The extrinsic and intrinsic muscles of the tongue are innervated by the **hypoglossal nerve** except for the palatoglossus, which is innervated by the vagus nerve. A lesion of the hypoglossal nerve deviates the tongue toward the injured side.

–The anterior two-thirds of the tongue receives general sensory innervation from the **lingual nerve** and taste sensation from the **chorda tympani.**

–The posterior one-third of the tongue and the vallate papillae receive both general and taste innervation from the **glossopharyngeal nerve.**

–The epiglottic region of the tongue and the epiglottis receive both general and taste innervation from the **internal laryngeal branch** of the vagus nerve.

D. Lingual artery

–arises from the external carotid artery at the level of the tip of the greater horn of the hyoid bone in the carotid triangle.

–passes deep to the hyoglossus and lies on the middle pharyngeal constrictor muscle.

–gives rise to the suprahyoid, dorsal lingual, and sublingual arteries and terminates as the **deep lingual artery,** which ascends between the genioglossus and inferior longitudinal muscles.

E. Muscles of the tongue (Table 8-9)

Table 8–9. Muscles of the Tongue

Muscle	Origin	Insertion	Nerve	Action
Styloglossus	Styloid process	Side and inferior aspect of tongue	Hypoglossal n.	Retracts and elevates tongue
Hyoglossus	Body and greater horn of hyoid bone	Side and inferior aspect of tongue	Hypoglossal n.	Depresses and retracts tongue
Genioglossus	Genial tubercle of mandible	Inferior aspect of tongue; body of hyoid bone	Hypoglossal n.	Protrudes and depresses tongue
Palatoglossus	Aponeurosis of soft palate	Dorsolateral side of tongue	Vagus n. via pharyngeal plexus	Elevates tongue

IV. Teeth and Gums (Gingivae)

A. Structure of the teeth

1. Enamel is the hardest substance that covers the crown.

2. Dentin is a hard substance that is nurtured through the fine dental tubules of odontoblasts lining the central pulp space.

3. Pulp fills the central cavity, which is continuous with the root canal. It contains numerous blood vessels, nerves, and lymphatics, which enter the pulp through an apical foramen at the apex of the root.

B. Parts of the teeth

1. **Crown** projects above the gingival surface and is covered by enamel.

2. **Neck** is the constricted area at the junction of the crown and root.

3. **Root,** embedded in the alveolar part of the maxilla or mandible, is covered with cement, which is connected to the bone of the alveolus by a layer of modified periosteum, the periodontal ligament. Each maxillary molar generally has three roots and each mandibular molar has two roots.

C. Basic types of teeth

1. **Incisors,** which are chisel-shaped teeth that have a single root, are used for cutting or biting.

2. **Canines,** which have a single prominent cone and a single root, are used for tearing.

3. **Premolars,** which usually have two cusps, are used for grinding. The upper first premolar tooth may be bifid and all others each have a single root.

4. **Molars,** which usually have three (sometimes three to five) cusps, are used for grinding. The upper molar teeth have three roots and the lower one two.

D. Two sets of teeth

1. **Deciduous teeth:** two incisors, one canine, and two molars in each quadrant, for a total of 20

2. **Permanent teeth:** two incisors, one canine, two premolars, and three molars in each quadrant, for a total of 32

E. Innervation of the teeth and gums (Figure 8-45)

1. **Maxillary teeth** are innervated by the anterior, middle, and posterior–superior alveolar branches of the maxillary nerve.

2. **Mandibular teeth** are innervated by the inferior alveolar branch of the mandibular nerve.

3. **Maxillary gingiva**

   a. **Outer (buccal) surface** is innervated by posterior, middle, and anterior–superior alveolar and infraorbital nerves.

   b. **Inner (lingual) surface** is innervated by greater palatine and nasopalatine nerves.

4. **Mandibular gingiva**

   a. **Outer (buccal) surface** is innervated by buccal and mental nerves.

   b. **Inner (lingual) surface** is innervated by lingual nerves.

V. Salivary Glands (see Figure 8-45)

A. Submandibular gland

–is ensheathed by the investing layer of the deep cervical fascia and lies in the **submandibular triangle.**

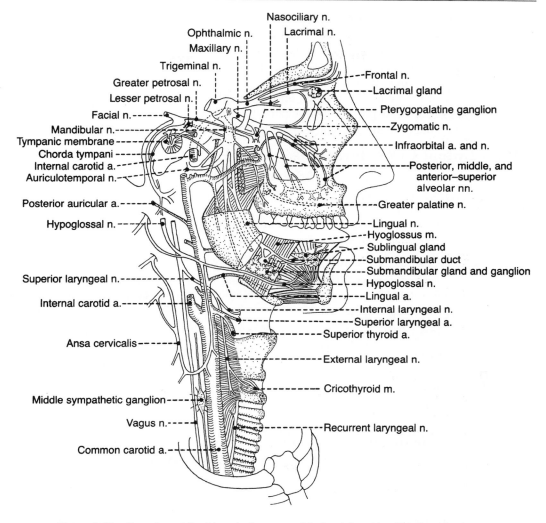

Figure 8-45. Branches of the trigeminal nerve and their relationship with other structures.

–Its superficial portion is situated superficial to the mylohyoid muscle.

–Its deep portion is located between the hyoglossus and styloglossus muscles medially and the mylohyoid muscle laterally and between the lingual nerve above and the hypoglossal nerve below.

–**Wharton's duct** arises from the deep portion and runs forward between the mylohyoid laterally and the hyoglossus medially, where it is crossed laterally by the lingual nerve. It then runs between the sublingual gland and the genioglossus and empties at the summit of the sublingual papilla (caruncle) at the side of the frenulum of the tongue.

–is innervated by parasympathetic secretomotor fibers from the facial nerve, which run in the chorda tympani and in the lingual nerve and synapse in the submandibular ganglion.

B. **Sublingual gland**

–is located in the floor of the mouth between the mucous membrane above and the mylohyoid muscle below.

–surrounds the terminal portion of the submandibular duct.

–empties mostly into the floor of the mouth along the sublingual fold by 12 short ducts, some of which enter the submandibular duct.

–is supplied by postganglionic parasympathetic (secretomotor) fibers from the submandibular ganglion either directly or through the lingual nerve.

VI. Clinical Considerations

A. Abscess or infection of the mandibular teeth

–might spread through the lower jaw to emerge on the face or in the floor of the mouth.

–irritates the **mandibular nerve,** causing pain that may be referred to the ear because this nerve also innervates a part of the ear.

B. Abscess or infection of the maxillary teeth

–irritates the **maxillary nerve,** causing upper **toothache.**

–may result in symptoms of **sinusitis** with pain referred to the distribution of the maxillary nerve.

C. Lesion of the hypoglossal nerve (hypoglossal paralysis)

–causes **deviation of the protruded tongue** toward the side of the lesion due to paralysis of the tongue muscles, especially the genioglossus muscle.

D. Lesion of the vagus nerve

–causes deviation of the uvula toward the opposite side of the lesion upon phonation.

E. Tongue-tie (ankyloglossia)

–is an **abnormal shortness of frenulum linguae,** resulting in limitation of its movement and thus a severe speech impediment.

–can be corrected surgically by cutting the frenulum.

Pharynx and Tonsils

I. Pharynx (Figure 8-46; see Figure 8-43)

–is a **funnel-shaped fibromuscular tube** that extends from the base of the skull to the inferior border of the cricoid cartilage.

–conducts food to the esophagus and air to the larynx and lungs.

II. Subdivisions of the Pharynx

A. Nasopharynx

–is situated behind the nasal cavity above the soft palate and communicates with the nasal cavities through the **nasal choanae.**

–contains the **pharyngeal tonsils** in its posterior wall.

–is connected with the tympanic cavity through the **auditory (eustachian) tube,** which equalizes air pressure on both sides of the tympanic membrane.

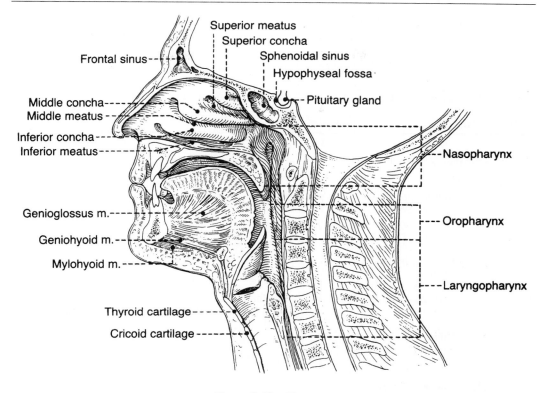

Figure 8-46. Pharynx.

B. Oropharynx

–extends between the soft palate above and the superior border of the epiglottis below and communicates with the mouth through the oropharyngeal isthmus.

–contains the **palatine tonsils,** which are lodged in the **tonsillar fossae** and are bounded by the palatoglossal and palatopharyngeal folds.

C. Laryngopharynx (hypopharynx)

–extends from the upper border of the epiglottis to the lower border of the cricoid cartilage.

–contains the **piriform recesses,** one on each side of the opening of the larynx, in which swallowed foreign bodies may be lodged.

III. Innervation and Blood Supply of the Pharynx (Figure 8-49)

A. Pharyngeal plexus

–lies on the **middle pharyngeal constrictor.**

–is formed by the **pharyngeal branches** of the glossopharyngeal and vagus nerves and the sympathetic branches from the superior cervical ganglion.

–Its **vagal branch** innervates all of the muscles of the pharynx with the exception of the stylopharyngeus, which is supplied by the glossopharyngeal nerve.

–Its **glossopharyngeal component** supplies sensory fibers to the pharyngeal mucosa.

B. Arteries of the pharynx

–are the ascending pharyngeal artery, ascending palatine branch of the facial artery, descending palatine arteries, pharyngeal branches of the maxillary artery, and branches of the superior and inferior thyroid arteries.

IV. Muscles of the Pharynx (Figures 8-47 and 8-48; Table 8-10)

Table 8–10. Muscles of the Pharynx

Muscle	Origin	Insertion	Nerve	Action
Circular muscles				
Superior constrictor	Medial pterygoid plate; pterygoid hamulus; pterygomandibular raphe; mylohyoid line of mandible; side of tongue	Median raphe and pharyngeal tubercle of skull	Vagus n. via pharyngeal plexus	Constricts upper pharynx
Middle constrictor	Greater and lesser horns of hyoid; stylohyoid ligament	Median raphe	Vagus n. via pharyngeal plexus	Constricts lower pharynx
Inferior constrictor	Arch of cricoid and oblique line of thyroid cartilages	Median raphe of pharynx	Vagus n. via pharyngeal plexus, recurrent and external laryngeal n.	Constricts lower pharynx
Longitudinal muscles				
Stylopharyngeus	Styloid process	Thyroid cartilage and muscles of pharynx	Glossopharyngeal n.	Elevates pharynx and larynx
Palatopharyngeus	Hard palate; aponeurosis of soft palate	Thyroid cartilage and muscles of pharynx	Vagus n. via pharyngeal plexus	Elevates pharynx and larynx; closes nasopharynx
Salpingopharyngeus	Cartilage of auditory tube	Muscles of pharynx	Vagus n. via pharyngeal plexus	Elevates pharynx; opens auditory tube

V. Swallowing (Deglutition)

–is described in several stages:

A. The bolus of food is pushed back by elevating the tongue by the styloglossus into the fauces, which is the passage from the mouth to the oropharynx.

B. The palatoglossus and palatopharyngeus muscles contract to squeeze the bolus backward into the oropharynx. The tensor veli palatini and levator veli palatini muscles elevate the soft palate and uvula to close the entrance into the nasopharynx.

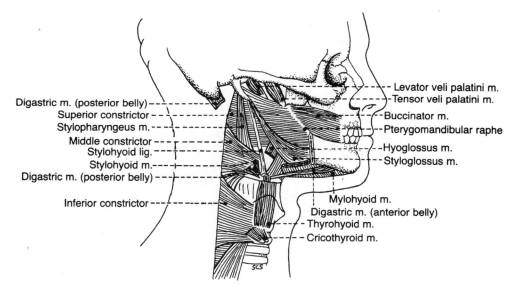

Figure 8-47. Muscles of the pharynx.

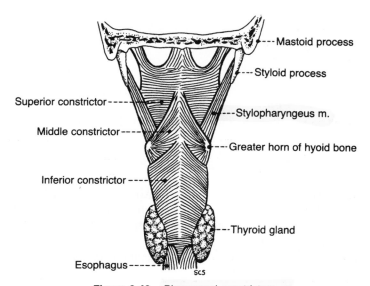

Figure 8-48. Pharyngeal constrictors.

C. The walls of the pharynx are raised by the palatopharyngeus, stylopharyngeus, and salpingopharyngeus muscles to receive the food. The suprahyoid muscles elevate the hyoid bone and the larynx to close the opening into the larynx, thus passing the bolus over the epiglottis and preventing the food from entering the respiratory passageways.

D. The serial contraction of the superior, middle, and inferior pharyngeal constrictor muscles moves the food through the oropharynx and the laryngopharynx into the esophagus, where it is propelled by peristalsis.

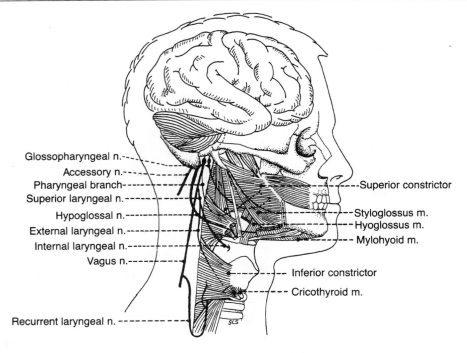

Figure 8-49. Nerve supply to the pharynx.

VI. Tonsils

A. Pharyngeal tonsil

–is found in the posterior wall and roof of the nasopharynx.

B. Palatine tonsil

–lies on each side of the oropharynx in an interval between the palatoglossal and palatopharyngeal folds.

–receives blood from the ascending palatine and tonsillar branches of the facial artery, the descending palatine branch of the maxillary artery, a palatine branch of the ascending pharyngeal artery, and the dorsal lingual branches of the lingual artery.

–is innervated by branches of the glossopharyngeal nerve and the lesser palatine branch of the maxillary nerve.

C. Tubal (eustachian) tonsil

–is the lateral prolongation of the pharyngeal tonsil and lies near the pharyngeal opening of the auditory tube.

D. Lingual tonsil

–is a collection of **lymphoid follicles** on the posterior portion of the dorsum of the tongue.

E. Waldeyer's ring

–is a **tonsillar ring** at the oropharyngeal isthmus, formed of lingual, palatine, tubal, and pharyngeal tonsils.

VII. Fascia and Space of the Pharynx (see Figure 8-8)

A. Retropharyngeal space

–is a **potential space** between the buccopharyngeal fascia and the prevertebral fascia, extending from the base of the skull to the superior mediastinum.

–permits movement of the pharynx, larynx, trachea, and esophagus during swallowing.

B. Pharyngobasilar fascia

–forms the **submucosa of the pharynx** and blends with the periosteum of the base of the skull.

–lies internal to the muscular coat of the pharynx; these muscles are covered externally by the buccopharyngeal fascia.

VIII. Clinical Considerations

A. Adenoid

–is hypertrophy or **enlargement of the pharyngeal tonsils,** obstructing passage of air from the nasal cavities through the choanae into the nasopharynx, and thus causing difficulty in nasal breathing and phonation.

–may block the pharyngeal orifices of the auditory tube, causing hearing impairment.

–The infection may spread from the nasopharynx through the auditory tube to the middle ear cavity, causing **otitis media,** which may result in deafness.

B. Tonsillectomy

–is **surgical removal of a tonsil,** carried out by dissecting the tonsil from its bed.

–may cause much bleeding because the palatine tonsils are highly vascular. Severe hemorrhage may also occur after a careless operation because the palatine tonsils are closely related to the internal carotid artery.

–could cause a loss of taste sensation in the posterior part of the tongue from injury to the lingual branches of the glossopharyngeal nerve, and also a loss of general sensation of the anterior two-thirds of the tongue from injury to the lingual nerve.

Nasal Cavity and Paranasal Sinuses

I. Nasal Cavity (Figure 8-50; see Figure 8-43)

–opens on the face through the anterior nasal apertures **(nares, or nostrils)** and communicates with the nasopharynx through a posterior opening, the **choanae.**

–has a slight dilatation inside the aperture of each nostril, the **vestibule,** which is lined largely with skin containing hair, sebaceous glands, and sweat glands.

A. Roof

–is formed by the nasal, frontal, ethmoid (cribriform plate), and sphenoid (body) bones. The **cribriform plate** transmits the olfactory nerves.

B. Floor

–is formed by the palatine process of the maxilla and the horizontal plate of the palatine bone.

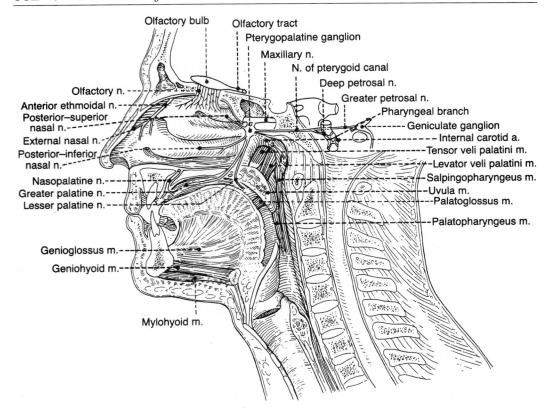

Figure 8-50. Nasal cavity.

–contains the **incisive foramen,** which transmits the nasopalatine nerve and terminal branches of the sphenopalatine artery.

C. Medial wall (nasal septum)

–is formed primarily by the perpendicular plate of the ethmoid bone, vomer, and septal cartilage.

–is also formed by processes of the palatine, maxillary, frontal, sphenoid, and nasal bones.

D. Lateral wall

–is formed by the superior and middle conchae of the ethmoid bone and the inferior concha.

–is also formed by the nasal bone, frontal process and nasal surface of the maxilla, lacrimal bone, perpendicular plate of the palatine bone, and medial pterygoid plate of the sphenoid bone.

–contains the following structures and their openings:

1. Sphenoethmoidal recess: opening of the sphenoid sinus

2. Superior meatus: opening of the posterior ethmoidal air cells

3. Middle meatus: opening of the frontal sinus into the infundibulum; openings of the middle ethmoidal air cells on the **ethmoidal bulla;** openings of the anterior ethmoidal air cells and maxillary sinus in the **hiatus semilunaris**

4. **Inferior meatus:** opening of the **nasolacrimal duct**

5. **Sphenopalatine foramen:** opening into the pterygopalatine fossa; transmits the sphenopalatine artery and nasopalatine nerve

II. Subdivisions and Mucous Membranes

A. Vestibule

–is the dilated part inside the nostril that is bound by the alar cartilages and lined by skin with hairs.

B. Respiratory region

–consists of the lower two-thirds of the nasal cavity.
–warms, moistens, and cleans incoming air with its mucous membrane.

C. Olfactory region

–consists of the superior nasal concha and the upper one-third of the nasal septum.
–is innervated by olfactory nerves, which convey the sense of smell from the olfactory cells and enter the cranial cavity through the cribriform plate of the ethmoid bone to end in the olfactory bulb.

III. Blood Supply to the Nasal Cavity

–occurs via the following routes:

A. The lateral nasal branches of the anterior and posterior ethmoidal arteries of the ophthalmic artery

B. The posterior lateral nasal and posterior septal branches of the sphenopalatine artery of the maxillary artery

C. The greater palatine branch (its terminal branch reaches the lower part of the nasal septum through the incisive canal) of the descending palatine artery of the maxillary artery

D. The septal branch of the superior labial artery of the facial artery; and the lateral nasal branch of the facial artery

IV. Nerve Supply to the Nasal Cavity

A. SVA (smell) sensation is supplied by the olfactory nerves for the olfactory area.

B. GSA sensation is supplied by the anterior ethmoidal branch of the ophthalmic nerve; the nasopalatine, posterior–superior, and posterior–inferior lateral nasal branches of the maxillary nerve via the pterygopalatine ganglion; and the anterior–superior alveolar branch of the infraorbital nerve.

V. Paranasal Sinuses (Figure 8-51; see Figures 8-35 and 8-43)

–consists of the ethmoidal, frontal, maxillary, and sphenoidal sinuses.
–is involved in a reduction of weight and resonance for voice.

A. Ethmoidal sinus

–consists of numerous **ethmoidal air cells,** which are numerous small cavities within the **ethmoidal labyrinth** between the orbit and the nasal cavity.

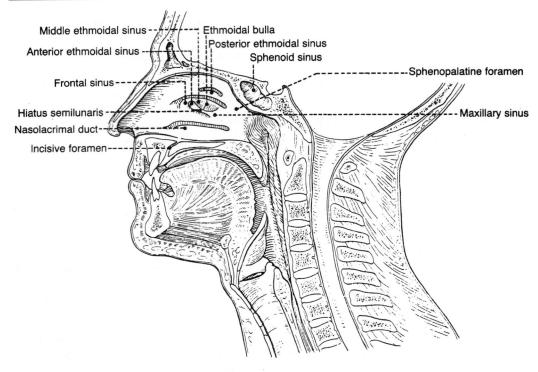

Figure 8-51. Openings of the paranasal sinuses.

—Its infection may erode through the thin orbital plate of the ethmoid bone (lamina papyracea) into the orbit.

—can be subdivided into the following groups:

1. **Posterior ethmoidal air cells,** which drain into the superior nasal meatus

2. **Middle ethmoidal air cells,** which drain into the summit of the ethmoidal bulla of the middle nasal meatus

3. **Anterior ethmoidal air cells,** which drain into the anterior aspect of the hiatus semilunaris in the middle nasal meatus

B. Frontal sinus

—lies in the **frontal bone** and opens into the hiatus semilunaris of the middle nasal meatus by way of the frontonasal duct (or infundibulum).

—is innervated by the supraorbital branch of the ophthalmic nerve.

C. Maxillary sinus

—is the largest of the paranasal air sinuses and is the only paranasal sinus that may be present at birth.

—lies in the **maxilla** on each side, lateral to the lateral wall of the nasal cavity and inferior to the floor of the orbit, and drains into the posterior aspect of the hiatus semilunaris in the middle nasal meatus.

D. Sphenoidal sinus

—is contained within the body of the **sphenoid bone.**

—opens into the **sphenoethmoidal recess** of the nasal cavity.

–is innervated by branches from the maxillary nerve and by the posterior ethmoidal branch of the nasociliary nerve.

–The pituitary gland lies above this sinus and can be reached by the **trans-sphenoidal approach,** which follows the nasal septum through the body of the sphenoid. Care must be taken not to damage the cavernous sinus and the internal carotid artery.

VI. Clinical Considerations

A. Sneeze

–is an **involuntary, sudden, violent, and audible expulsion of air** through the mouth and nose.

–The afferent limb of the reflex is carried by branches of the maxillary nerve, which convey general sensation from the nasal cavity and palate.

B. Epistaxis

–is a **nosebleed** resulting from rupture of the sphenopalatine artery. Epistaxis also occurs from nose picking, which tears the veins in the vestibule of the nose.

C. Maxillary sinusitis

–mimics the clinical signs of maxillary tooth abscess; in most cases, it is related to an infected tooth. Infection may spread from the maxillary sinus to the upper teeth and irritate the nerves to these teeth, causing toothache.

–may be confused with toothache, because only a thin layer of bone separates the roots of the maxillary teeth from the sinus cavity.

D. Nasal polyp

–is an **inflammatory polyp** developing from the mucosa of the paranasal sinus, which projects into the nasal cavity and may fill the nasopharynx.

E. Rhinoplasty

–is a type of plastic surgery that changes the shape or size of the nose.

Pterygopalatine Fossa

I. Boundaries and Openings

A. **Anterior wall:** posterior surface of the maxilla or the posterior wall of the maxillary sinus (no openings)

B. **Posterior wall:** pterygoid process and greater wing of the sphenoid. Openings and their contents include the following:

1. **Foramen rotundum to middle cranial cavity:** maxillary nerve

2. **Pterygoid canal to foramen lacerum:** nerve of the pterygoid canal

3. **Palatovaginal (pharyngeal or pterygopalatine) canal to choana:** pharyngeal branch of the maxillary artery and pharyngeal nerve from the pterygopalatine ganglion

C. **Medial wall:** perpendicular plate of the palatine. The opening is the **spheno-palatine foramen to the nasal cavity,** which transmits the sphenopalatine artery and nasopalatine nerve.

D. **Lateral wall:** open (the pterygomaxillary fissure to the infratemporal fossa)

E. **Roof:** greater wing and body of the sphenoid. The opening is the **inferior orbital fissure** to the orbit, which transmits the maxillary nerve.

F. **Floor:** fusion of the maxilla and the pterygoid process of the sphenoid. The opening is the **greater palatine foramen** to the palate, which transmits the greater palatine nerve and vessels.

II. Contents

A. **Maxillary nerve** (see Figure 8-45)

–passes through the lateral wall of the cavernous sinus and enters the pterygo-palatine fossa through the **foramen rotundum.**
–is sensory to the skin of the face below the eye but above the upper lip.
–gives rise to the following branches:

1. **Meningeal branch**

–innervates the dura mater of the middle cranial fossa.

2. **Pterygopalatine nerves (communicating branches)**

–are connected to the pterygopalatine ganglion.
–contain sensory fibers from the trigeminal ganglion.

3. **Posterior–superior alveolar nerves**

–descend through the pterygopalatine fissure and enter the posterior–superior alveolar canals.
–innervate the cheeks, gums, molar teeth, and maxillary sinus.

4. **Zygomatic nerve**

–enters the orbit through the **inferior orbital fissure,** divides into the zygomaticotemporal and zygomaticofacial branches, which supply the skin over the temporal region and over the zygomatic bone, respectively.
–joins the lacrimal nerve in the orbit and transmits postganglionic parasym-pathetic GVE fibers to the lacrimal gland.

5. **Infraorbital nerve**

–enters the orbit through the inferior orbital fissure and runs through the infraorbital groove and canal.
–emerges through the infraorbital foramen and divides in the face into the inferior palpebral, nasal, and superior labial branches.
–gives rise to the middle and anterior–superior alveolar nerves, which supply the maxillary sinus, teeth, and gums.

6. **Branches (sensory) via the pterygopalatine ganglion**

–contain GSA fibers as branches of the maxillary nerve but also carry GVA fibers from the facial nerve to the nasal mucosa and the palate.

a. **Orbital branches**

–supply the periosteum of the orbit and the mucous membrane of the posterior ethmoidal and sphenoidal sinuses.

b. Pharyngeal branch

–runs in the pharyngeal (palatovaginal) canal and supplies the roof of the pharynx and the sphenoidal sinuses.

c. Posterior–superior lateral nasal branches

–enter the nasal cavity through the sphenopalatine foramen and innervate the posterior part of the septum, the posterior ethmoidal air cells, and the superior and middle conchae.

d. Greater palatine nerve

–descends through the palatine canal and emerges through the greater palatine foramen to innervate the hard palate and the inner surface of the maxillary gingiva.

–gives rise to the posterior–inferior lateral nasal branches.

e. Lesser palatine nerve

–descends through the palatine canal and emerges through the lesser palatine foramen to innervate the soft palate and the palatine tonsil.

–contains sensory (GVA and taste) fibers that belong to the facial nerve and have their cell bodies in the geniculate ganglion.

f. Nasopalatine nerve

–runs obliquely downward and forward on the septum, supplying the septum, and passes through the incisive canal to supply the hard palate and the gum.

B. Pterygopalatine ganglion (see Figures 8-30 and 8-31)

–lies in the pterygopalatine fossa just below the maxillary nerve, lateral to the sphenopalatine foramen and anterior to the pterygoid canal.

–receives preganglionic parasympathetic fibers from the facial nerve by way of the greater petrosal nerve and the nerve of the pterygoid canal.

–sends postganglionic parasympathetic fibers to the nasal and palatine glands and to the lacrimal gland by way of the maxillary, zygomatic, and lacrimal nerves.

–also receives postganglionic sympathetic fibers (by way of the deep petrosal nerve and the nerve of the pterygoid canal), which are distributed with the postganglionic parasympathetic fibers.

C. Pterygopalatine part of the maxillary artery

–supplies blood to the maxilla and maxillary teeth, nasal cavities, and palate.

–gives rise to the posterior–superior alveolar artery, infraorbital artery (which gives rise to anterior–superior alveolar branches), descending palatine artery (which gives rise to the lesser palatine and greater palatine branches), artery of the pterygoid canal, pharyngeal artery, and sphenopalatine artery.

III. Clinical Considerations

A. Lesion of the Nerve of Pterygoid Canal

–results in vasodilation and a lack of secretion of the lacrimal, nasal, and palatine glands, and a loss of general and taste sensation of the palate.

B. Crocodile tears syndrome (see Orbit: VII B)

Larynx

I. Introduction

–is the organ of voice production and the part of the respiratory tract between the lower part of the pharynx and the trachea.

–acts as a **compound sphincter** to prevent the passage of food or drink into the airway in swallowing and to close the **rima glottidis** during the Valsalva maneuver (buildup of air pressure during coughing, sneezing, micturition, defecation, or parturition).

–regulates the flow of air to and from the lungs for vocalization (phonation).

–forms a framework of cartilage for the attachment of ligaments and muscles.

II. Cartilages (Figure 8-52)

A. Thyroid cartilage (see Deep Neck and Prevertebral Region: I E)

–is a **single hyaline cartilage** that forms a median elevation called the **laryngeal prominence (Adam's apple),** which is particularly apparent in males.

–has an **oblique line** on the lateral surface of its lamina that gives attachment for the inferior pharyngeal constrictor, sternothyroid, and thyrohyoid muscles.

B. Cricoid cartilage

–is a **single hyaline cartilage,** which is shaped like a signet ring.

–articulates with the thyroid cartilage. Its lower border marks the end of the pharynx and larynx.

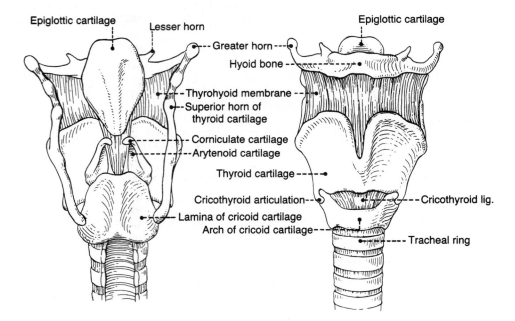

Figure 8-52. Cartilages of the larynx.

C. Epiglottis

–is a **single elastic cartilage.**

–is a spoon-shaped plate that lies behind the root of the tongue and forms the superior part of the anterior wall of the larynx.

–Its lower end is attached to the back of the thyroid cartilage.

D. Arytenoid cartilages

–are **paired elastic and hyaline cartilages.**

–are shaped liked pyramids, with bases that articulate with and rotate on the cricoid cartilage.

–have **vocal processes,** which give attachment to the vocal ligament and vocalis muscle, and **muscular processes,** which give attachment to the thyroarytenoid muscle and the lateral and posterior cricoarytenoid muscles.

E. Corniculate cartilages

–are **paired elastic cartilages** that lie on the apices of the arytenoid cartilages.

–are enclosed within the **aryepiglottic folds** of mucous membrane.

F. Cuneiform cartilages

–are **paired elastic cartilages** that lie in the aryepiglottic folds anterior to the corniculate cartilages.

III. Ligaments of the Larynx

A. Thyrohyoid membrane

–extends from the thyroid cartilage to the medial surface of the hyoid bone.

–Its middle (thicker) part is called the **middle thyrohyoid ligament,** and its lateral portion is pierced by the internal laryngeal nerve and the superior laryngeal vessels.

B. Cricothyroid ligament

–extends from the arch of the cricoid cartilage to the thyroid cartilage and the vocal processes of the arytenoid cartilages.

C. Vocal ligament

–extends from the posterior surface of the thyroid cartilage to the vocal process of the arytenoid cartilage.

–is considered the upper border of the **conus elasticus.**

D. Vestibular (ventricular) ligament

–extends from the thyroid cartilage to the anterior lateral surface of the arytenoid cartilage.

E. Conus elasticus (cricovocal ligament)

–is the paired lateral portion of the fibroelastic membrane that extends between the superior border of the entire arch of the cricoid cartilage and the vocal ligaments.

–is formed by the cricothyroid, median cricothyroid, and vocal ligaments.

IV. Cavities and Folds (Figure 8-53)

–The laryngeal cavity is divided into three portions by the vestibular and vocal folds: the vestibule, ventricle, and infraglottic cavity.

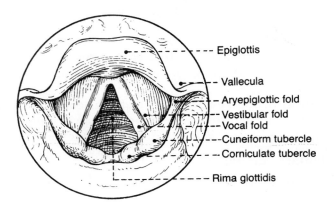

Epiglottis

Vallecula

Aryepiglottic fold

Vestibular fold

Vocal fold

Cuneiform tubercle

Corniculate tubercle

Rima glottidis

Figure 8-53.   Interior view of the larynx.

A. Vestibule

–extends from the laryngeal inlet to the **vestibular (ventricular) folds.**

B. Ventricles

–extend between the vestibular fold and the vocal fold.

C. Infraglottic cavity

–extends from the rima glottidis to the lower border of the cricoid cartilage.

D. Rima glottidis

–is the space between the vocal folds and arytenoid cartilages.
–is the narrowest part of the laryngeal cavity.

E. Vestibular folds (false vocal cords)

–extend from the thyroid cartilage above the vocal ligament to the arytenoid cartilage.

F. Vocal folds (true vocal cords)

–extend from the angle of the thyroid cartilage to the vocal processes of the arytenoid cartilages.
–contain the **vocal ligament** near their free margin and the **vocalis muscle,** which forms the bulk of the vocal fold.
–are important in **voice production** because they control the stream of air passing through the rima glottidis.
–alter the shape and size of the **rima glottidis** by movement of the arytenoids to facilitate respiration and phonation. (The rima glottidis is wide during inspiration and narrow and wedge-shaped during expiration and sound production.)

V. Muscles (Figure 8-54; Table 8-11)

Table 8–11. Muscles of the Larynx

Muscle	Origin	Insertion	Nerve	Action on Vocal Cords
Cricothyroid	Arch of cricoid cartilage	Inferior horn and lower lamina of thyroid cartilage	External laryngeal n.	Tenses; adducts; elongates
Posterior cricoarytenoid	Posterior surface of lamina of cricoid cartilage	Muscular process of arytenoid cartilage	Recurrent laryngeal n.	Abducts
Lateral cricoarytenoid	Arch of cricoid cartilage	Muscular process of arytenoid cartilage	Recurrent laryngeal n.	Adducts
Transverse arytenoid	Posterior surface of arytenoid cartilage	Opposite arytenoid cartilage	Recurrent laryngeal n.	Adducts; closes glottis
Oblique arytenoid	Muscular process of arytenoid cartilage	Apex of opposite arytenoid	Recurrent laryngeal n.	Adducts; closes glottis
Aryepiglottic	Apex of arytenoid cartilage	Side of epiglottic cartilage	Recurrent laryngeal n.	Adducts
Thyroarytenoid	Inner surface of thyroid lamina	Anterolateral surface of arytenoid cartilage	Recurrent laryngeal n.	Adducts; relaxes
Thyroepiglottic	Anteromedial surface of lamina of thyroid cartilage	Lateral margin of epiglottic cartilage	Recurrent laryngeal n.	Adducts
Vocalis	Angle between two laminae of thyroid cartilage	Vocal process of arytenoid cartilage	Recurrent laryngeal n.	Adducts; tenses (anterior part); relaxes (posterior part); controls pitch

VI. Innervation (Figure 8-55)

A. Recurrent laryngeal nerve

–innervates all of the intrinsic muscles of the larynx except the cricothyroid, which is innervated by the external laryngeal branch of the superior laryngeal branch of the vagus nerve.

–supplies sensory innervation below the vocal cord.

–has a terminal portion above the lower border of the cricoid cartilage called the **inferior laryngeal nerve.**

B. Internal laryngeal nerve

–innervates the mucous membrane above the vocal cord and taste buds on the epiglottis.

–is accompanied by the superior laryngeal artery and pierces the thyrohyoid membrane.

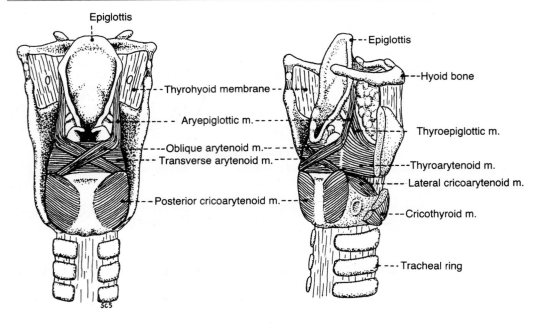

Figure 8-54. Muscles of the larynx.

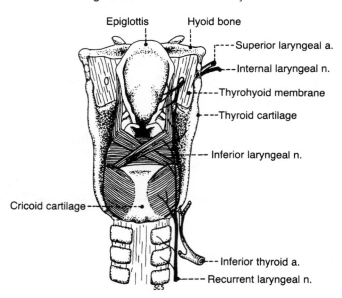

Figure 8-55. Nerve supply to the larynx.

C. External laryngeal nerve

–innervates the cricothyroid and inferior pharyngeal constrictor (cricopharyngeus part) muscles.

–is accompanied by the superior thyroid artery.

VII. Clinical Considerations

A. Laryngeal obstruction (choking)

–is caused by aspirated foods, which are usually lodged at the rima glottidis.

–can be released by compression of the abdomen to expel air from the lungs and thus dislodge the foods (e.g., the Valsalva maneuver).

B. Laryngitis

–is an **inflammation of the mucous membrane of the larynx.**

–is characterized by dryness and soreness of the throat, hoarseness, cough, and dysphagia.

C. Laryngotomy

–is an **operative opening into the larynx** through the cricothyroid membrane (cricothyrotomy), through the thyroid cartilage (thyrotomy), or through the thyrohyoid membrane (superior laryngotomy).

–is performed when severe edema or an impacted foreign body calls for rapid admission of air into the larynx and trachea.

D. Lesion of the recurrent laryngeal nerve

–could be produced during thyroidectomy or cricothyrotomy or by aortic aneurysm.

–may cause respiratory obstruction, hoarseness, and an inability to speak.

Ear

I. External Ear (Figure 8-56)

–consists of the auricle and the external acoustic meatus, and receives sound waves.

A. Auricle

–consists of cartilage connected to the skull by ligaments and muscles and is covered by skin.

–funnels sound waves into the external auditory meatus.

–receives sensory nerves from the auricular branch of the **vagus** and **facial** nerves and the **greater auricular**, auriculotemporal branch of the **trigeminal** nerve, and **lesser occipital** nerves.

–receives blood from the superficial temporal and posterior auricular arteries.

–has the following features:

1. **Helix:** the slightly curved rim of the auricle

2. **Antihelix:** a broader curved eminence internal to the helix, which divides the auricle into an outer scaphoid fossa and the deeper concha

3. **Concha:** the deep cavity in front of the antihelix

4. **Tragus:** a small projection from the anterior portion of the external ear anterior to the concha

5. **Lobule:** a structure made up of areolar tissue and fat but no cartilage

B. External acoustic (auditory) meatus

–is about 2.5 cm long, extending from the concha to the tympanic membrane.

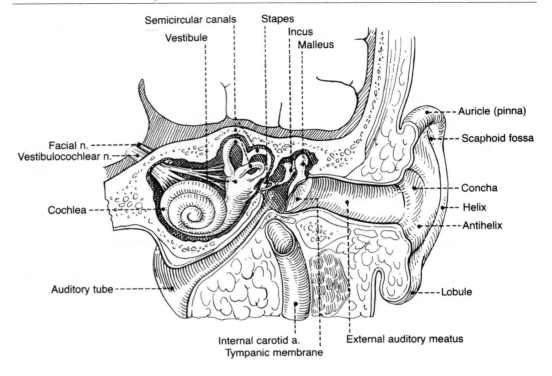

Figure 8-56. External, middle, and inner ear.

—Its external one-third is formed by cartilage, and its internal two-thirds is formed by bone. The cartilaginous portion is wider than the bony portion and has numerous **ceruminous glands** that produce earwax.

—is innervated by the auriculotemporal branch of the **trigeminal** nerve and the auricular branch of the **vagus** nerve, which is joined by a branch of the **facial** nerve and the **glossopharyngeal** nerve.

—receives blood from the superficial temporal, posterior auricular, and maxillary arteries (a deep auricular branch).

C. Tympanic membrane (eardrum)

—lies obliquely across the end of the meatus sloping medially from posterosuperiorly to anteroinferiorly; thus, the anterior–inferior wall is longer than the posterior–superior wall.

—consists of **three layers:** an outer (cutaneous), an intermediate (fibrous), and an inner (mucous) layer.

—has a thickened fibrocartilaginous ring at the greater part of its circumference, which is fixed in the tympanic sulcus at the inner end of the meatus.

—has a small triangular portion between the anterior and posterior malleolar folds called the **pars flaccida** (deficient ring and lack of fibrous layer). The remainder of the membrane is called the **pars tensa.**

—contains the **cone of light,** which is a triangular reflection of light seen in the anterior–inferior quadrant.

—contains the most depressed center point of the concavity, called the **umbo** (Latin for "knob").

—conducts sound waves to the middle ear.

–Its external (lateral) concave surface is covered by skin and is innervated by the auriculotemporal branch of the **trigeminal** nerve and the auricular branch of the **vagus** nerve. The auricular branch is joined by branches of the **glossopharyngeal** and **facial** nerves. This surface is supplied by the deep auricular artery of the maxillary artery.

–Its internal (medial) surface is covered by mucous membrane, is innervated by the tympanic branch of the **glossopharyngeal** nerve, and serves as an attachment for the handle of the **malleus.** This surface receives blood from the auricular branch of the occipital artery and the anterior tympanic artery.

II. Middle Ear (Figures 8-57 and 8-58)

–consists of the tympanic cavity with its **ossicles.**

–transmits the sound waves from air to auditory ossicles and then to the inner ear.

A. Tympanic (middle ear) cavity

–includes the **tympanic cavity proper,** the space internal to the tympanic membrane; and the **epitympanic recess,** the space superior to the tympanic membrane that contains the head of the malleus and the body of the incus.

–communicates anteriorly with the nasopharynx via the **auditory (eustachian) tube** and posteriorly with the **mastoid air cells** and the **mastoid antrum** through the **aditus ad antrum.**

–is traversed by the chorda tympani and lesser petrosal nerve.

1. Boundaries of the tympanic cavity

a. Roof: tegmen tympani

b. Floor: jugular fossa

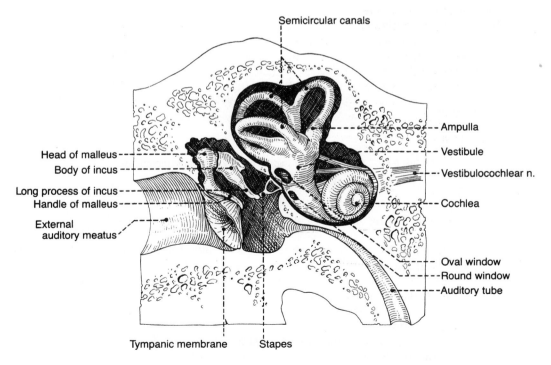

Figure 8-57. Middle and inner ear.

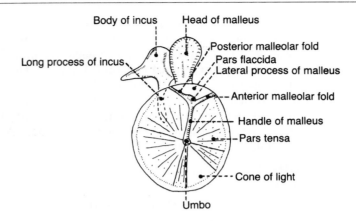

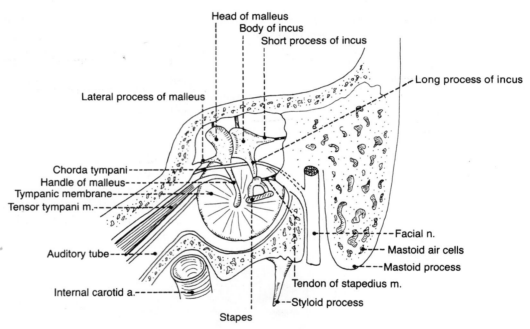

Figure 8-58. Ossicles of the middle ear and tympanic membrane.

c. **Anterior:** carotid canal

d. **Posterior:** mastoid air cells and mastoid antrum through the aditus ad antrum

e. **Lateral:** tympanic membrane

f. **Medial:** lateral wall of the inner ear, presenting the **promontory** formed by the basal turn of the cochlea; the fenestra vestibuli **(oval window);** the fenestra cochlea **(round window);** and the prominence of the facial canal

2. **Oval window (fenestra vestibuli)**

–is pushed back and forth by the footplate of the stapes and **transmits the sonic vibrations** of the ossicles into the perilymph of the scala vestibuli in the inner ear.

3. **Round window (fenestra cochlea or tympani)**

–is closed by the secondary tympanic (mucous) membrane of the middle ear and accommodates the pressure waves transmitted to the perilymph of the scala tympani.

B. **Muscles**

1. **Stapedius muscle**

–is the **smallest of the skeletal muscles** in the human body.
–arises from the pyramidal eminence, and its tendon emerges from the eminence.
–inserts on the neck of the stapes.
–is innervated by a branch of the facial nerve.
–pulls the head of the stapes posteriorly, thereby tilting the base of the stapes.
–prevents (or reduces) excessive oscillation of the stapes and thus protects the inner ear from injury from a loud noise.
–Its paralysis results in **hyperacusis**.

2. **Tensor tympani muscle**

–arises from the cartilaginous portion of the auditory tube.
–inserts on the handle (manubrium) of the malleus.
–is innervated by the mandibular branch of the trigeminal nerve.
–draws the tympanic membrane medially and tightens it (in response to loud noises), thereby increasing the tension and reducing the vibration of the tympanic membrane.

C. **Auditory ossicles**

–consist of the malleus, incus, and stapes.
–form a bridge by synovial joints in the middle ear cavity, transmit sonic vibrations from the tympanic membrane to the inner ear, and amplify the force.

1. **Malleus (hammer)**

–consists of a head, neck, handle (manubrium), and anterior and lateral processes.
–Its rounded head articulates with the incus in the epitympanic recess.
–Its handle is fused to the medial surface of the tympanic membrane and serves as an attachment for the **tensor tympani muscle.**

2. **Incus (anvil)**

–consists of a body and two processes (crura).
–Its long process descends vertically, parallel to the handle of the malleus, and articulates with the stapes.
–Its short process extends horizontally backward to the fossa of the incus and provides the attachment for the posterior ligament of the incus.

3. **Stapes (stirrup)**

–consists of a head and neck, two processes (crura), and a base (footplate).

–Its neck provides insertion of the **stapedius muscle.**

–has a hole through which the stapedial artery is transmitted in the embryo; this hole is obturated by a thin membrane in the adult.

–Its base (footplate) is attached by the annular ligament to the margin of the oval window (fenestra vestibuli). Abnormal ossification between the footplate and the oval window **(otosclerosis)** limits the movement of the stapes, causing deafness.

D. Auditory (eustachian) tube

–connects the middle ear to the nasopharynx.

–allows air to enter or leave the middle ear cavity and thus balances the pressure in the middle ear with atmospheric pressure, allowing free movement of the tympanic membrane.

–Its cartilaginous portion remains closed except during swallowing or yawning.

–is opened by the simultaneous contraction of the tensor veli palatini and salpingopharyngeus muscles.

E. Sensory nerve and blood supply to the middle ear

–is innervated by the **tympanic** branch of the **glossopharyngeal** nerve, which forms the **tympanic plexus** with **caroticotympanic** nerves from the internal carotid plexus of sympathetic fibers. The tympanic nerve continues beyond the plexus as the **lesser petrosal** nerve, which transmits preganglionic parasympathetic fibers to the otic ganglion.

–receives blood from the stylomastoid branch of the posterior auricular artery and the anterior tympanic branch of the maxillary artery.

III. Inner Ear (see Figure 8-57)

–consists of the **acoustic apparatus,** the cochlea housing the cochlear duct for auditory sense, and the **vestibular apparatus,** the vestibule housing the utricle and saccule, and the semicircular canals housing the semicircular ducts for the sense of equilibrium.

–is the place where vibrations are transduced to specific nerve impulses that are transmitted through the acoustic nerve to the central nervous system (CNS).

–is composed of the bony labyrinth and the membranous labyrinth.

A. Bony labyrinth

–consists of three parts: the vestibule, the three semicircular canals, and the cochlea, all of which contain the **perilymph,** in which the membranous labyrinth is suspended.

–The **vestibule** is a cavity of the bony labyrinth communicating with the cochlea anteriorly and the semicircular canals posteriorly.

–The **bony cochlea** consists of two adjacent ducts, the upper **scala vestibuli,** which begins in the vestibule and receives the vibrations transmitted to the perilymph at the oval window, and the lower **scala tympani,** which communicates with the scala vestibuli through the helicotrema at the apex of the cochlea and ends at the round window, where the sound pressure waves are dissipated.

B. Membranous labyrinth

–is suspended in perilymph within the bony labyrinth, is filled with **endolymph,** and contains the sensory organs.

–has comparable parts and arrangement as the bony labyrinth.

–Its **utricle** and **saccule** are dilated membranous sacs in the vestibule and contain sense organs called maculae.

–Its **semicircular ducts** consist of anterior (superior), lateral, and posterior, and their dilated ends are called ampullae.

–Its **cochlear duct (scala media)** is wedged between the scala vestibuli and scala tympani and contains the spiral organ of Corti.

IV. Clinical Considerations

A. Hyperacusis (hyperacusia)

–is **excessive acuteness of hearing,** due to paralysis of the stapedius muscle (causing uninhibited movements of the stapes), resulting from a lesion of the facial nerve.

B. Otosclerosis

–is a condition of **abnormal bone formation** around the stapes and the oval window, limiting the movement of the stapes and thus resulting in **progressive conduction deafness.**

C. Conductive deafness

–is hearing impairment caused by **defect of the sound-conducting apparatus** such as the auditory meatus, eardrum, or ossicles.

D. Neural or sensorineural deafness

–is hearing impairment due to a lesion of the auditory nerve or the central afferent neural pathway.

E. Otitis media

–is a condition of **middle ear infection** that may be spread from the nasopharynx through the auditory tube, causing temporary or permanent deafness.

F. Meniere's disease (endolymphatic or labyrinthine hydrops)

–is characterized by a **loss of balance** (vertigo), ringing or buzzing in the ears, and **progressive deafness** due to edema of the labyrinth or inflammation of the vestibular division of the vestibulocochlear nerve.

Review Test

Directions: Each of the numbered items or incomplete statements in this section is followed by answers or by completions of the statement. Select the **one** lettered answer or completion that is **best** in each case.

1. Damage to the external laryngeal nerve during thyroid surgery could result in the inability to

(A) relax the vocal cords
(B) rotate the arytenoid cartilages
(C) tense the vocal cords
(D) widen the rima glottidis
(E) abduct the vocal cords

2. On ligation of the superior laryngeal artery, care must be taken to avoid injury to which of the following nerves?

(A) External laryngeal nerve
(B) Internal laryngeal nerve
(C) Superior laryngeal nerve
(D) Hypoglossal nerve
(E) Vagus nerve

3. In a patient who demonstrates a lack of general sensation in the nasopharynx, a lesion of which of the following nerves would be expected?

(A) Maxillary nerve
(B) Superior cervical ganglion
(C) External laryngeal nerve
(D) Glossopharyngeal nerve
(E) Vagus nerve

4. During surgery, a surgeon notices profuse bleeding from the deep cervical artery. Which of the following arteries must be ligated immediately?

(A) Inferior thyroid artery
(B) Transverse cervical artery
(C) Thyrocervical trunk
(D) Costocervical trunk
(E) Ascending cervical artery

5. The phrenic nerve passes by which of the following structures in the neck?

(A) Anterior to the subclavian vein
(B) Posterior to the subclavian artery
(C) Deep to the anterior scalene muscle
(D) Medial to the common carotid artery
(E) Superficial to the anterior scalene muscle

6. Which of the following muscles is a landmark for locating the glossopharyngeal nerve in the neck?

(A) Inferior pharyngeal constrictor muscle
(B) Stylopharyngeus muscle
(C) Posterior belly of the digastric muscle
(D) Longus colli muscle
(E) Rectus capitis anterior muscle

7. A lesion of the external laryngeal branch of the superior laryngeal nerve may cause weakness of which of the following muscles?

(A) Inferior pharyngeal constrictor muscle
(B) Middle pharyngeal constrictor muscle
(C) Superior pharyngeal constrictor muscle
(D) Thyroarytenoid muscle
(E) Thyrohyoid muscle

8. A patient with crocodile tears syndrome has spontaneous lacrimation during eating due to misdirection of regenerating autonomic nerve fibers. Which of the following nerves has been injured?

(A) Facial nerve proximal to the geniculate ganglion
(B) Auriculotemporal nerve
(C) Chorda tympani in the infratemporal fossa
(D) Facial nerve at the stylomastoid foramen
(E) Lacrimal nerve

9. A 13-year-old girl complains of dryness of the nose and the palate, indicating a lesion of which of the following ganglia?

(A) Nodose ganglion
(B) Otic ganglion
(C) Pterygopalatine ganglion
(D) Submandibular ganglion
(E) Ciliary ganglion

400

10. Bell's palsy can involve corneal inflammation and subsequent corneal ulceration, which results from

(A) sensory loss of the cornea and conjunctiva
(B) lack of secretion of the salivary glands
(C) absence of the corneal blink reflex due to paralysis of the muscles that close the eyelid
(D) absence of the corneal blink reflex due to paralysis of the muscles that open the eyelid
(E) constriction of the pupil due to paralysis of the dilator pupillae

11. Which of the following sinuses lies in the margin of the tentorium cerebelli, running from the posterior end of the cavernous sinus to the transverse sinus?

(A) Straight sinuses
(B) Inferior sagittal sinus
(C) Sphenoparietal sinus
(D) Superior petrosal sinuses
(E) Cavernous sinus

12. Which of the following conditions results from severance of the abducens nerve proximal to its entrance into the orbit?

(A) Ptosis of the upper eyelid
(B) Loss of the ability to dilate the pupil
(C) External strabismus (lateral deviation)
(D) Loss of visual accommodation
(E) Internal strabismus (medial deviation)

13. Death may result from bilateral severance of which of the following nerves?

(A) Trigeminal nerve
(B) Facial nerve
(C) Vagus nerve
(D) Spinal accessory nerve
(E) Hypoglossal nerve

14. When the middle meningeal artery is ruptured but the meninges remain intact, blood enters which of the following spaces?

(A) Subarachnoid space
(B) Subdural space
(C) Epidural space
(D) Subpial space
(E) Cranial dural sinuses

15. Which of the following structures contains cell bodies of preganglionic parasympathetic neurons?

(A) Cervical and sacral spinal cord
(B) Cervical and thoracic spinal cord
(C) Brainstem and cervical spinal cord
(D) Thoracic and lumbar spinal cord
(E) Brainstem and sacral spinal cord

16. Following radical resection of a primary tongue tumor, a patient has lost general sensation on the anterior two-thirds of the tongue. This is probably due to injuries to branches of which of the following nerves?

(A) Trigeminal nerve
(B) Facial nerve
(C) Glossopharyngeal nerve
(D) Vagus nerve
(E) Hypoglossal nerve

17. The pituitary gland lies in the sella turcica, immediately posterior and superior to which of the following structures?

(A) Frontal sinus
(B) Maxillary sinus
(C) Ethmoid air cells
(D) Mastoid air cells
(E) Sphenoid sinus

18. After tonsillectomy, a 7-year-old boy is unable to distinguish the sensation of taste on the posterior one-third of his tongue. Which of the following nerves most likely has been injured?

(A) Internal laryngeal nerve
(B) Lingual nerve
(C) Lingual branch of the glossopharyngeal nerve
(D) Greater palatine nerve
(E) Chorda tympani

19. Damage to the sella turcica is probably due to fracture of which of the following bones?

(A) Frontal bone
(B) Ethmoid bone
(C) Temporal bone
(D) Basioccipital bone
(E) Sphenoid bone

20. The scalenus anterior muscle

(A) inserts on the second rib
(B) is innervated by the phrenic nerve
(C) passes anterior to the subclavian vein
(D) descends posterior to the subclavian artery
(E) runs anterior to the roots of the brachial plexus

21. A patient has an infectious inflammation of the dural venous sinus nearest to the pituitary gland, with secondary thrombus formation. Which of the following is the most likely site of infection?

(A) Straight sinus
(B) Cavernous sinus
(C) Superior petrosal sinus
(D) Sigmoid sinus
(E) Confluence of sinuses

22. A patient with a pituitary tumor would exhibit which of the following disorders?

(A) Blindness
(B) Bitemporal (heteronymous) hemianopia
(C) Right nasal hemianopia
(D) Left homonymous hemianopia
(E) Binasal hemianopia

23. If a patient is unable to abduct the vocal cords during quiet breathing, which of the following muscles is paralyzed?

(A) Vocalis muscle
(B) Cricothyroid muscle
(C) Oblique arytenoid muscle
(D) Posterior cricoarytenoid muscle
(E) Thyroarytenoid muscle

24. Which of the following pairs of muscles is most instrumental in preventing food from entering the larynx and trachea during swallowing?

(A) Sternohyoid and sternothyroid muscles
(B) Oblique arytenoid and aryepiglottic muscles
(C) Inferior pharyngeal constrictor and thyrohyoid muscles
(D) Levator veli palatini and tensor veli palatini muscles
(E) Musculus uvulae and geniohyoid muscles

25. The veins of the brain are direct tributaries of the

(A) emissary veins
(B) pterygoid venous plexus
(C) diploic veins
(D) dural venous sinuses
(E) internal jugular vein

26. Which of the following conditions or actions results from stimulation of the parasympathetic fibers to the eyeball?

(A) Enhanced vision for distant objects
(B) Dilation of the pupil
(C) Contraction of capillaries in the iris
(D) Contraction of the ciliary muscle
(E) Flattening of the lens

27. The tympanic nerve

(A) is a branch of the facial nerve
(B) contains postganglionic parasympathetic fibers
(C) synapses with fibers in the lesser petrosal nerve
(D) is a branch of the glossopharyngeal nerve
(E) forms the tympanic plexus in the external auditory meatus

28. Which of the following cavities are separated from the middle cranial fossa by a thin layer of bone?

(A) Auditory tube and bony orbit
(B) Middle ear cavity and sphenoid sinus
(C) Sigmoid sinus and frontal sinus
(D) Sphenoid sinus and ethmoid sinus
(E) Maxillary sinus and middle ear cavity

29. Loss of general sensation in the dura of the middle cranial fossa indicates a lesion of the

(A) vagus nerve
(B) facial nerve
(C) hypoglossal nerve
(D) trigeminal nerve
(E) glossopharyngeal nerve

30. The carotid sinus

(A) is located at the origin of the external carotid artery
(B) is innervated by the facial nerve
(C) functions as a chemoreceptor
(D) is stimulated by changes in blood pressure
(E) communicates freely with the cavernous sinus

31. During a game, a 26-year-old baseball player receives a severe blow to the head that fractures the optic canal. Which of the following pairs of structures is most likely to be damaged?

(A) Optic nerve and ophthalmic vein
(B) Ophthalmic vein and ophthalmic nerve
(C) Ophthalmic artery and optic nerve
(D) Ophthalmic nerve and optic nerve
(E) Ophthalmic artery and ophthalmic vein

32. Paralysis of the posterior belly of the digastric muscle would result from a lesion of which of the following nerves?

(A) Accessory nerve
(B) Trigeminal nerve
(C) Ansa cervicalis
(D) Facial nerve
(E) Glossopharyngeal nerve

33. Contraction of the tensor tympani and the stapedius prevents damage to the eardrum and middle ear ossicles. These muscles are most likely controlled by which of the following nerves?

(A) Chorda tympani and tympanic nerve
(B) Trigeminal and facial nerves
(C) Auditory and vagus nerves
(D) Facial and auditory nerves
(E) Trigeminal and accessory nerves

34. If a patient's pupil remains small when room lighting is subdued, which of the following nerves would be injured?

(A) Trochlear nerve
(B) Superior cervical ganglion
(C) Oculomotor nerve
(D) Ophthalmic nerve
(E) Abducens nerve

35. Which of the following statements concerning the frontal sinus is correct?

(A) It extends into the parietal bone
(B) It communicates with the superior nasal meatus
(C) It receives sensory innervation from the maxillary nerve
(D) It is supplied with blood by branches of the ophthalmic artery
(E) It is a cranial dural venous sinus that receives the ophthalmic vein

36. A patient can move his eyeball normally and see distant objects clearly but cannot focus on near objects. This condition may indicate damage to the

(A) ciliary ganglion and oculomotor nerve
(B) oculomotor nerve and long ciliary nerve
(C) short ciliary nerves and ciliary ganglion
(D) superior cervical ganglion and long ciliary nerve
(E) oculomotor, trochlear, and abducens nerves

37. Which of the following structures enters the orbit through the superior orbital fissure and the common tendinous ring?

(A) Frontal nerve
(B) Lacrimal nerve
(C) Trochlear nerve
(D) Abducens nerve
(E) Ophthalmic vein

38. Which of the following groups of cranial nerves is damaged if the muscles attached to the styloid process are paralyzed?

(A) Facial, glossopharyngeal, and hypoglossal nerves
(B) Hypoglossal, vagus, and facial nerves
(C) Glossopharyngeal, trigeminal, and vagus nerves
(D) Vagus, spinal accessory, and hypoglossal nerves
(E) Facial, glossopharyngeal, and vagus nerves

39. A 32-year-old woman has hoarseness in her voice, and her uvula is deviated to the left upon phonation. Which of the following nerves is damaged?

(A) Right trigeminal nerve
(B) Left trigeminal nerve
(C) Right vagus nerve
(D) Left vagus nerve
(E) Left glossopharyngeal nerve

40. When a low tracheotomy is performed below the isthmus of the thyroid, which of the following vessels may be encountered?

(A) Inferior thyroid artery
(B) Inferior thyroid vein
(C) Costocervical trunk
(D) Superior thyroid artery
(E) Right brachiocephalic vein

41. If a patient has no cutaneous sensation on the anterior cervical triangle, it is likely that damage has occurred to which of the following nerves?

(A) Phrenic nerve
(B) Greater auricular nerve
(C) Transverse cervical nerve
(D) Supraclavicular nerve
(E) Lesser occipital nerve

42. In a patient with swelling of the mucous membranes of the superior nasal meatus, which of the openings of the paranasal sinuses are plugged?

(A) Middle ethmoidal sinus
(B) Maxillary sinus
(C) Posterior ethmoidal sinus
(D) Anterior ethmoidal sinus
(E) Frontal sinus

43. The tongue of a 45-year-old patient deviates to the left on protrusion. Which of the following nerves is injured?

(A) Right lingual nerve
(B) Left lingual nerve
(C) Right hypoglossal nerve
(D) Left hypoglossal nerve
(E) Left glossopharyngeal nerve

44. Which condition would most likely result in a patient's inability to move his right eye laterally?

(A) A tumor of the pituitary gland
(B) Occlusion of the right posterior cerebral artery
(C) An infection in the right maxillary sinus
(D) An infection in the right cavernous sinus
(E) A tumor in the right anterior cranial fossa

45. If the lingual nerve is damaged as it enters the oral cavity, which of the following structures contain cell bodies of injured nerve fibers?

(A) Geniculate and otic ganglia
(B) Trigeminal and submandibular ganglia
(C) Trigeminal and dorsal root ganglia
(D) Geniculate and trigeminal ganglia
(E) Geniculate and pterygopalatine ganglia

46. A tumor located in the optic canal would most likely damage which of the following structures?

(A) Ophthalmic vein
(B) Ophthalmic nerve
(C) Oculomotor nerve
(D) Trochlear nerve
(E) Ophthalmic artery

47. A horizontal cut through the cricothyroid ligament in the neck would sever which of the following structures?

(A) Inferior laryngeal nerves
(B) External carotid arteries
(C) Inferior thyroid veins
(D) Thyrocervical trunks
(E) Internal laryngeal nerves

48. Severance of the oculomotor nerve can cause which of the following conditions?

(A) Complete ptosis
(B) Abduction of the eyeball
(C) A constricted pupil
(D) Impaired lacrimal secretion
(E) Paralysis of the ciliary muscle

49. Which of the following nerves supply striated muscles and are of branchiomeric origin?

(A) Oculomotor nerves
(B) Trochlear nerves
(C) Trigeminal nerves
(D) Abducens nerves
(E) Hypoglossal nerves

50. During surgery for malignant parotid tumors, the main trunk of the facial nerve is lacerated, resulting in paralysis of which of the following muscles?

(A) Masseter muscle
(B) Stylopharyngeus muscle
(C) Anterior belly of the digastric muscle
(D) Buccinator muscle
(E) Tensor tympani

51. During gang fighting, the nasal septum of a 17-year-old boy injured by a fist. Which of the following structures would be damaged?

(A) Septal cartilage and nasal bone
(B) Inferior concha and vomer
(C) Vomer and perpendicular plate of ethmoid
(D) Septal cartilage and middle concha
(E) Cribriform plate and incisive foramen

52. The tensor tympani

(A) inserts on the long process of the incus
(B) is innervated by a branch of the facial nerve
(C) runs parallel to the external acoustic meatus
(D) arises chiefly from the tympanic membrane
(E) functions to tighten the tympanic membrane

53. Infection within the carotid sheath may damage which of the following structures?

(A) Vagus nerve and middle cervical ganglion
(B) Common carotid artery and recurrent laryngeal nerve
(C) Internal jugular vein and vagus nerve
(D) Sympathetic trunk and common carotid artery
(E) External carotid artery and ansa cervicalis

54. An occlusion of the costocervical trunk could produce a marked decrease in the blood flow in which of the following arteries?

(A) Superior thoracic artery
(B) Transverse cervical artery
(C) Ascending cervical artery
(D) Deep cervical artery
(E) Inferior thyroid artery

55. The internal laryngeal nerve

(A) is a branch of the superior laryngeal nerve
(B) may contain taste fibers from the palate
(C) provides sensory innervation to the laryngeal mucosa below the vocal cord
(D) provides motor innervation to the cricothyroid muscle
(E) is accompanied by the superior thyroid artery

56. Which of the following nerves would be spared from infection in the cavernous sinus?

(A) Oculomotor nerves
(B) Abducens nerves
(C) Trochlear nerves
(D) Mandibular nerves
(E) Ophthalmic nerves

57. Which of the following tonsils is called the adenoid when enlarged?

(A) Palatine tonsil
(B) Pharyngeal tonsil
(C) Tubal tonsil
(D) Lingual tonsil
(E) Eustachian tonsil

58. An eroded lesion in the jugular foramen may damage which of the following pairs of structures?

(A) Vagus nerve and internal carotid artery
(B) Accessory nerve and external jugular vein
(C) Internal jugular vein and hypoglossal nerve
(D) Glossopharyngeal and vagus nerves
(E) Hypoglossal and spinal accessory nerves

59. A 12-year-old girl is unable to close her lips. Which of the following muscles is paralyzed?

(A) Levator labii superioris
(B) Zygomaticus minor
(C) Orbicularis oris
(D) Lateral pterygoid
(E) Depressor labii inferioris

60. Severance of the greater petrosal nerve would produce which of the following conditions?

(A) Increased lacrimal gland secretion
(B) Loss of taste sensation in the epiglottis
(C) Dryness in the nose and palate
(D) Decreased parotid gland secretion
(E) Loss of general visceral sensation in the pharynx

61. A benign tumor in the pterygoid canal could injure which of the following nerve fibers?

(A) Postganglionic parasympathetic fibers
(B) Taste fibers from the epiglottis
(C) General somatic afferent (GSA) fibers
(D) Preganglionic sympathetic fibers
(E) General visceral afferent (GVA) fibers

62. The pupillary light reflex can be eliminated by cutting which of the following nerves?

(A) Short ciliary, ophthalmic, and oculomotor nerves
(B) Long ciliary, optic, and short ciliary nerves
(C) Oculomotor, short ciliary, and optic nerves
(D) Optic and long ciliary nerves; ciliary ganglion
(E) Ophthalmic and optic nerves; ciliary ganglion

63. A 22-year-old patient has a dry corneal surface due to a lack of moistening fluid. Which of the following nerves is damaged?

(A) Proximal portion of the lacrimal nerve
(B) Zygomatic branch of the facial nerve
(C) Lesser petrosal nerve
(D) Greater petrosal nerve
(E) Deep petrosal nerve

64. Which of the following statements concerning the tongue is correct?

(A) The palatoglossus muscles are innervated by the hypoglossal nerves
(B) Taste buds in the vallate papillae are innervated by the chorda tympani of the facial nerve
(C) Its anterior two-thirds receives general sensory innervation from the facial nerve
(D) It receives taste fibers from the facial and glossopharyngeal nerves
(E) It is retracted by the genioglossus

65. A patient has a functional impediment and cannot perform the act of swallowing. Which of the following nerves is functioning normally?

(A) Hypoglossal nerve
(B) Spinal accessory nerve
(C) Vagus nerve
(D) Facial nerve
(E) Trigeminal nerve

66. Which of the following muscles would most likely open the jaw?

(A) Masseter muscle
(B) Medial pterygoid muscle
(C) Lateral pterygoid muscle
(D) Buccinator muscle
(E) Temporalis muscle

67. Which of the following muscles would most likely open the eye?

(A) Orbicularis oculi
(B) Orbicularis oris
(C) Frontalis
(D) Levator palpebrae superioris
(E) Superior rectus

68. Fracture of the foramen rotundum would cause a lesion of which of the following nerves?

(A) Ophthalmic nerve
(B) Optic nerve
(C) Maxillary nerve
(D) Mandibular nerve
(E) Trochlear nerve

69. A lack of salivary secretion from the submandibular gland may indicate a lesion of which of the following nervous structures?

(A) Lingual nerve at its origin
(B) Chorda tympani in the middle ear cavity
(C) Superior cervical ganglion
(D) Lesser petrosal nerve
(E) Auriculotemporal nerve

70. Lack of accommodation results from paralysis of which of the following muscles?

(A) Tarsal muscle
(B) Sphincter pupillae
(C) Dilator pupillae
(D) Ciliary muscles
(E) Orbitalis muscles

Directions: Each set of matching questions in this section consists of a list of four to twenty-six lettered options (some of which may be in figures) followed by several numbered items. For each numbered item, select the ONE lettered option that is most closely associated with it. To avoid spending too much time on matching sets with large numbers of options, it is generally advisable to begin each set by reading the list of options. Then, for each item in the set, try to generate the correct answer and locate it in the option list, rather than evaluating each option individually. Each lettered option may be selected once, more than once, or not at all.

Questions 71–75

Match the following descriptions with the appropriate lettered structure in this radiograph—a lateral view of the head.

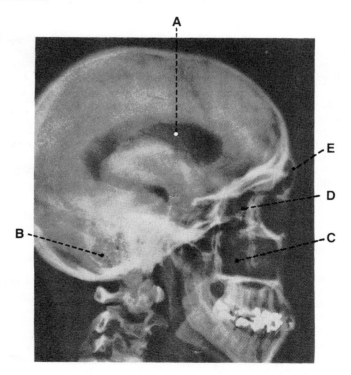

71. Structure that lies lateral to the lateral wall of the nasal cavity and inferior to the floor of the orbit

72. Structure into which a middle ear infection may spread

73. Structure that has numerous small cavities and lies between the orbit and the nasal cavity

74. Structure from which infection would spread into the anterior part of the middle nasal meatus through the frontonasal duct

75. Structure in which cerebrospinal fluid (CSF) is formed by vascular choroid plexus

Questions 76–80

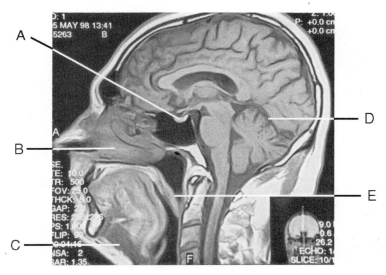

Match the following descriptive statements with the appropriate lettered structure in this magnetic resonance image (MRI)—a sagittal section through the head and neck.

76. A lesion of the right nerve that innervates this structure would deviate this structure to the left side.

77. A lesion of the first cervical spinal nerve would cause impairment of function of this structure.

78. Tears may drain below this structure through the nasolacrimal duct.

79. The straight sinus runs long the line of attachment of the falx cerebri to this structure.

80. A tumor of this structure can be removed through the transsphenoidal approach following the septum of the nose through the body of the sphenoid.

Questions 81–85

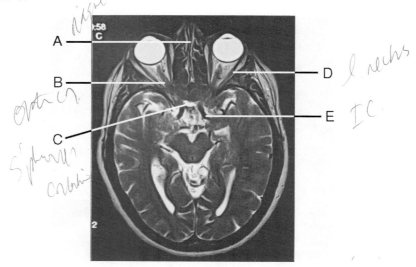

Match the following descriptions with the appropriate lettered structure in this magnetic resonance image (MRI)—a transaxial section through the head.

81. Structure that mediates the afferent limb of the pupillary light reflex

82. Structure that is formed by the perpendicular plate of the ethmoid bone, vomer, and septal cartilage

83. Structure that may be paralyzed as a result of infection of the cavernous sinus

84. Structure that pierces the dural roof of the cavernous sinus between the anterior and middle clinoid processes

85. Structure that may be obliterated by the pituitary tumor

Questions 86–90

Match the following descriptions with the most appropriate sinus.

(A) Cavernous sinus
(B) Sigmoid sinus
(C) Superior sagittal sinus
(D) Transverse sinus
(E) Straight sinus

86. Lies at the junction of the falx cerebri and the tentorium cerebelli

87. Curves laterally and forward in the convex outer border of the tentorium cerebelli

88. Lies in the superior convex border of the falx cerebri

89. Communicates directly with the ophthalmic veins

90. Becomes continuous with the internal jugular vein at the jugular foramen

Questions 91–95

Match the following descriptive statements with the most appropriate opening of the skull.

(A) Foramen ovale
(B) Foramen magnum
(C) Petrotympanic fissure
(D) Cribriform plate
(E) Foramen rotundum
(F) Pterygoid canal
(G) Superior orbital fissure
(H) Sphenopalatine foramen
(I) Internal auditory meatus
(J) Jugular foramen

91. Injury to the nerve passing through this structure causes a loss of general sensation of the maxillary teeth

92. Injury to the nerve passing through this structure causes a loss of sensation of the temporomandibular joints

93. This structure is traversed by sensory fibers from the posterior one-third of the tongue

94. This structure is traversed by sensory fibers from the mucosa of the nasal septum, posterior lateral nasal wall, and anterior portion of the hard palate

95. This structure is traversed by preganglionic parasympathetic fibers to the lacrimal gland

Questions 96–100

For each clinical condition described, select the lesion or other insult most closely related to it.

(A) Lesion of the glossopharyngeal nerve
(B) Destruction of the supraorbital notch
(C) Lesion of the facial nerve
(D) Rupture of cerebral arteries
(E) Lesion of the vagus nerve
(F) Lesion of the trigeminal nerve
(G) Rupture of cerebral veins
(H) Lesion of the oculomotor nerve
(I) Lesion of the trochlear nerve
(J) Laceration of the middle meningeal artery
(K) Lesion of the deep petrosal nerve
(L) Lesion of the greater petrosal nerve

96. A radiograph of a patient's skull reveals a fracture of the squamous part of the temporal bone and a fracture line through the foramen spinosum

97. After an automobile accident, a 21-year-old woman is unable to close her lips

98. A patient presents with a complaint of ptosis—drooping of an upper eyelid

99. A baseball pitcher who receives a blow on the head is found to have subdural hematoma

100. A patient develops a vasodilation in the lacrimal gland

Answers and Explanations

1-C. The external laryngeal nerve innervates the cricothyroid muscle, which tenses the vocal cord. This muscle cannot rotate the arytenoid cartilage. The rima glottidis is widened by the posterior cricoarytenoid muscle. Other laryngeal muscles adduct the vocal cords.

2-B. The internal laryngeal nerve accompanies the superior laryngeal artery, whereas the external laryngeal nerve accompanies the superior thyroid artery.

3-D. The glossopharyngeal nerve supplies sensory innervation to the mucosa of the upper pharynx, whereas the vagus nerve supplies sensory innervation to the lower pharynx and larynx. The maxillary nerve supplies sensory innervation to the face below the level of the eye and above the level of the upper lip.

4-D. The surgeon should ligate the costocervical trunk because it divides into the deep cervical and superior intercostal arteries. The thyrocervical trunk gives off the suprascapular, transverse cervical, and inferior thyroid artery. The ascending cervical artery is a branch of the inferior thyroid artery.

5-E. The phrenic nerve descends on the superficial surface of the anterior scalene muscle and passes into the thorax posterior to the subclavian vein, anterior to the subclavian artery, and lateral to the common carotid artery.

6-B. The glossopharyngeal nerve innervates the stylopharyngeus. This muscle is a landmark for locating the glossopharyngeal nerve because, as the nerve enters the pharyngeal wall, it curves posteriorly around the lateral margin of the stylopharyngeus.

7-A. The external laryngeal branch of the superior laryngeal nerve supplies the cricothyroid and inferior pharyngeal constrictor muscles. The superior, middle, and inferior pharyngeal constrictors are innervated by the vagus nerve through the pharyngeal plexus. The recurrent (or inferior) laryngeal nerve supplies the thyroarytenoid muscle, and the C1 via the hypoglossal nerve supplies the thyrohyoid muscle.

8-A. Crocodile tears syndrome (Bogorad's syndrome) is caused by a lesion of the facial nerve proximal to the geniculate ganglion, due to misdirection of regenerating parasympathetic fibers, which formerly innervated the salivary glands, to the lacrimal glands.

9-C. Postganglionic parasympathetic fibers originating in the pterygopalatine ganglion innervate glands in the palate and nasal mucosa. The postganglionic parasympathetic fibers from the otic ganglion supply the parotid gland, those from the submandibular ganglion supply the submandibular and sublingual glands, and those from the ciliary ganglion supply the ciliary muscle and sphincter pupillae. The nodose (inferior) ganglion of the vagus nerve is a sensory ganglion.

10-C. Bell's palsy (facial paralysis) can involve inflammation of the cornea leading to corneal ulceration, which probably is attributable to an absence of the corneal blink reflex due to paralysis of the orbicularis oculi, which closes the eyelid.

11-D. The straight sinus runs along the line of attachment of the falx cerebri to the tentorium cerebelli, the inferior sagittal sinus lies in the free edge of the falx cerebri, the sphenoparietal sinus lies along the posterior edge of the lesser wing of the sphenoid bone, and the cavernous sinus lies on each side of the sella turcica and the body of the sphenoid bone. The superior petrosal sinus runs from the cavernous sinus to the transverse sinus along the attached margin of the tentorium cerebelli.

12-E. The abducens nerve (CN VI) innervates the lateral rectus muscle, which abducts the eyeball. A lesion of the abducens nerve results in medial strabismus and diplopia (double vision). Ptosis of the upper eyelid is caused by lesions of the oculomotor nerve or sympathetic nerve to the levator palpebrae superioris. Inability to dilate the pupil is caused by a lesion of the sympathetic nerve to

410

the dilator pupillae. Loss of visual accommodation is due to a lesion of parasympathetic nerve fibers to the ciliary muscle. The external strabismus (lateral deviation) is caused by paralysis of the medial rectus muscle, which is innervated by the oculomotor nerve.

13-C. Bilateral severance of the vagus nerve (CN X) causes a loss of reflex control of circulation due to an increase in heart rate and blood pressure; poor digestion results due to decreased gastrointestinal (GI) motility and secretion; and difficulty in swallowing, speaking, and breathing occurs due to paralysis of laryngeal and pharyngeal muscles. All of these effects may result in death.

14-C. Rupture of the middle meningeal artery in the cranial cavity causes an epidural hemorrhage.

15-E. Preganglionic neurons of the parasympathetic nervous system are located in the brainstem (cranial outflow) and sacral spinal cord segments S2–S4 (sacral outflow).

16-A. The anterior two-thirds of the tongue are innervated by the lingual nerve, a branch of the mandibular division of the trigeminal nerve (CN V). The posterior one-third of the tongue is innervated by the glossopharyngeal nerve (CN IX).

17-E. The pituitary gland lies in the hypophyseal fossa of the sella turcica of the sphenoid bone, which lies immediately posterior and superior to the sphenoid sinus and medial to the cavernous sinus.

18-C. The posterior one-third of the tongue receives both general and taste innervation from the lingual branch of the glossopharyngeal nerve.

19-E. The sella turcica is part of the sphenoid bone and lies superior to the sphenoid sinus.

20-E. The scalenus anterior inserts on the first rib, is innervated by the cervical nerves, and passes anterior to the root of the brachial plexus and the subclavian artery but posterior to the subclavian vein.

21-B. The dural venous sinus nearest the pituitary gland is the cavernous sinus. Cavernous sinus thrombophlebitis is an infectious inflammation of the sinus that may produce meningitis, papilledema, exophthalmos, and ophthalmoplegia.

22-B. Lesion of the optic chiasma by the pituitary tumor results in bitemporal hemianopia due to loss in the nasal field of vision of both eyes. Lesion of the optic nerve causes blindness. The right perichiasmal lesion by an aneurysm of the internal carotid artery leads to right nasal hemianopia as a result of loss of vision in the nasal field of the right eye. Lesion of the right optic tract or optic radiation causes left homonymous hemianopia due to loss of the left half of the visual fields of both eyes. Aneurysms of the both internal carotid arteries cause the right and left perichiasmal lesions, leading to loss of vision in the nasal fields of both eyes.

23-D. The posterior cricoarytenoid muscle is the only muscle that abducts the vocal cords during quiet breathing. All other laryngeal muscles adduct the vocal cords.

24-B. The oblique arytenoid and aryepiglottic muscles tilt the arytenoid cartilages and approximate them, assisting in closing off the larynx and preventing food from entering the larynx and trachea during the process of swallowing. The cricopharyngeus fibers of the inferior pharyngeal constrictors act as a sphincter that prevents air from entering the esophagus. Other muscles are not involved in closing or opening the airway.

25-D. The veins of the brain are direct tributaries of the dural venous sinuses. The emissary veins connect the dural venous sinuses with the veins of the scalp; the pterygoid venous plexus communicates with the cavernous sinus through an emissary vein; and the diploic veins lie in channels in the diploë of the skull and communicate with the dural sinuses, the veins of the scalp, and the meningeal veins.

26-D. When the parasympathetic fibers to the eyeball are stimulated, the pupil constricts and the ciliary muscle contracts, resulting in a thicker lens and enhanced vision for near objects (accommodation). Contraction of capillaries in the iris and enhanced ability to see distant objects (flattening of the lens) result from stimulation of sympathetic nerves.

27-D. The tympanic nerve or Jacobson's nerve is a branch of the glossopharyngeal nerve, contains preganglionic parasympathetic fibers, and forms a tympanic plexus on the medial wall of the middle ear with sympathetic fibers. The tympanic nerve continues beyond the plexus as the lesser petrosal nerve, which transmits preganglionic parasympathetic fibers to the otic ganglion for synapse.

28-B. The middle ear cavity is separated from the middle cranial fossa by the tegmen tympani, a thin plate of the petrous part of the temporal bone. A part of the roof of the sphenoid bone forms the floor of the hypophyseal fossa.

29-D. The cranial dura is innervated by the ophthalmic division of the trigeminal nerve in the anterior cranial fossa, the maxillary and mandibular divisions of the trigeminal nerve in the middle cranial fossa, and the vagus and hypoglossal nerves in the posterior cranial fossa.

30-D. The carotid sinus, a spindle-shaped dilatation of the origin of the internal carotid artery, is a pressoreceptor that is stimulated by changes in blood pressure. The carotid sinus is innervated by the carotid sinus branch of the glossopharyngeal nerve and by a branch of the vagus nerve.

31-C. The optic canal transmits the optic nerve, ophthalmic artery, and the central vein of the retina. The superior orbital fissure transmits the ophthalmic nerve and ophthalmic vein.

32-D. The digastric anterior belly is innervated by the trigeminal nerve, whereas the digastric posterior belly is innervated by the facial nerve.

33-B. The tensor tympani is innervated by the trigeminal nerve, and the stapedius is innervated by the facial nerve.

34-B. When the pupil remains small in a dimly lit room, it is an indication that postganglionic sympathetic fibers that originate from the superior cervical ganglion and innervate the dilator pupillae (radial muscles of the iris) are damaged.

35-D. The frontal sinus, a paranasal air sinus, receives blood from branches of the ophthalmic artery. It lies in the frontal bone, communicates with the middle nasal sinus, and is innervated by the supraorbital branch of the ophthalmic nerve.

36-C. Damage to the parasympathetic fibers in the ciliary ganglion or in the short ciliary nerves impairs the ability to focus on close objects (accommodation). The patient is able to see distant objects clearly because the long ciliary nerve also carries sympathetic fibers to the dilator pupillae. The ability to move the eyeball normally indicates that the oculomotor, trochlear, and abducens nerves are intact.

37-D. The abducens, oculomotor, and nasociliary nerves enter the orbit through the superior orbital fissure and the common tendinous ring. The trochlear, lacrimal, and frontal nerves and the ophthalmic vein enter the orbit through the superior orbital fissure outside the common tendinous ring.

38-A. The stylohyoid muscle is innervated by the facial nerve, the styloglossus muscle by the hypoglossal nerve, and the stylopharyngeus muscle by the glossopharyngeal nerve. No other muscles are attached to the styloid process.

39-C. A lesion of the vagus nerve causes deviation of the uvula toward the opposite side of the injury. Hoarseness is caused by a paralysis of the laryngeal muscles due to damages of skeletal motor fibers in the recurrent laryngeal branch of the vagus nerve.

40-B. A low tracheotomy is a surgical incision of the trachea through the neck, below the isthmus of the thyroid gland. The inferior thyroid veins drain the thyroid gland, descend in front of the trachea, and enter the brachiocephalic veins. Consequently, these veins are closely associated with the isthmus of the thyroid gland.

41-C. The transverse cervical nerve turns around the posterior border of the sternocleidomastoid and innervates the skin of the anterior cervical triangle. The phrenic nerve, a branch of the cervical plexus, contains motor and sensory fibers but no cutaneous nerve fibers.

42-C. The posterior ethmoidal sinus opens into the superior nasal meatus. The maxillary, frontal, and anterior and middle ethmoidal sinuses drain into the middle nasal meatuses.

43-D. A lesion of the hypoglossal nerve causes deviation of the tongue toward the injured side on protrusion. The lingual and glossopharyngeal nerves do not supply tongue muscles.

44-D. The abducens nerve, which innervates the lateral rectus muscle, runs through the middle of the cavernous sinus. Other conditions do not injure the abducens nerve. The tumor in the pituitary gland may injure the optic chiasma.

45-D. The lingual nerve is joined by the chorda tympani in the infratemporal fossa. Therefore, the lingual nerve contains general somatic afferent (GSA) fibers whose cell bodies are located in the trigeminal ganglion and special somatic afferent (SSA) [taste] fibers that have cell bodies located in the geniculate ganglion. In addition, the lingual nerve carries parasympathetic preganglionic general visceral efferent (GVE) fibers that originated from the chorda tympani; the cell bodies are located in the superior salivatory nucleus in the pons.

46-E. The optic canal transmits the ophthalmic artery and optic nerve. The ophthalmic nerve, ophthalmic vein, and oculomotor and trochlear nerves enter the orbit through the superior orbital fissure.

47-A. A horizontal cut through the cricothyroid ligament severs the inferior laryngeal nerves, which are the terminal portion of the recurrent laryngeal nerves above the lower border of the cricoid cartilage. The external carotid arteries and the internal laryngeal nerves lie above the cricothyroid ligament, and the inferior thyroid veins and the thyrocervical trunks lie below the ligament.

48-E. The oculomotor nerve carries parasympathetic fibers to the constrictor pupillae and ciliary muscles. The levator palpebrae superioris inserts on the tarsal plate in the upper eyelid, which is innervated by sympathetic fibers. Thus a lesion of the oculomotor nerve does not cause complete ptosis. The abducens nerve supplies the lateral rectus, which is an abductor of the eye. The secretomotor fibers for lacrimal secretion come through the pterygopalatine ganglion. Thus severance of the oculomotor nerve has no effect on lacrimal secretion.

49-C. Special visceral efferent (SVE) nerve fibers originate from the first branchial arch (trigeminal), the second arch (facial), the third arch (glossopharyngeal), and the fourth and sixth arches (vagus). Nerves that supply the muscles of the eyeball and tongue are not of branchiomeric origin.

50-D. The buccinator muscle is innervated by the facial nerve. The masseter, tensor tympani, and anterior belly of the digastric muscles are innervated by the mandibular division of the trigeminal nerve. The stylopharyngeus muscle is innervated by the glossopharyngeal nerve.

51-C. The nasal septum is formed primarily by the vomer, the perpendicular plate of ethmoid bone, and the septal cartilage. The superior, middle and inferior conchae form the lateral wall of the nasal cavity. The ethmoid (cribriform plate), nasal, frontal and sphenoid (body) bones form the roof. The floor is formed by the palatine process of the maxilla and the horizontal plate of the palatine bone.

52-E. The tensor tympani inserts on the handle of the malleus, is innervated by the mandibular branch of the trigeminal nerve, runs parallel to the auditory tube, arises chiefly from the cartilaginous portion of the auditory tube, and functions to tighten the tympanic membrane by drawing it medially.

53-C. The carotid sheath contains the vagus nerve, the common and internal carotid arteries, and the internal jugular vein. The ansa cervicalis lies superficial to or within the carotid sheath.

54-D. The costocervical trunk gives rise to the superior intercostal and deep cervical arteries. The thyrocervical trunk gives rise to the suprascapular, transverse cervical, and inferior thyroid arteries. The ascending cervical artery arises from the inferior thyroid artery. The superior thoracic artery arises from the axillary artery.

55-A. The internal laryngeal nerve is a branch of the superior laryngeal nerve, provides sensory innervation to the mucosa of the larynx above the vocal cord, and contains taste fibers from the epiglottis and the root of the tongue adjacent to it. The external laryngeal nerve innervates the cricothyroid and inferior pharyngeal constrictor muscles.

56-D. The mandibular division of the trigeminal nerve does not lie in the wall of the cavernous sinus, whereas the oculomotor, abducens, trochlear, and ophthalmic nerves do lie in the wall of the cavernous sinus.

57-B. The enlarged pharyngeal tonsil is called the adenoid. The tubal tonsil is also called the eustachian tonsil.

58-D. The jugular foramen transmits the glossopharyngeal, spinal accessory, and vagus nerves, as well as the internal jugular vein.

59-C. The lips are closed by the orbicularis oris muscles. The lips are opened by the levator labii superioris, zygomaticus minor and depressor labii inferioris muscles. The lateral pterygoid muscle can open the mouth by depressing the lower jaw.

60-C. The greater petrosal nerve carries parasympathetic (preganglionic) fibers, which are secretomotor fibers to the lacrimal glands and mucous glands in the nasal cavity and palate; taste fibers from the palate; and general visceral afferent (GVA) fibers from the nasal cavity, palate, and roof of the oral cavity, but not from the pharynx and larynx. A lesion of the lesser petrosal nerve causes decreased parotid gland secretion. Taste sensation in the epiglottis is carried by the internal laryngeal branch of the superior laryngeal nerve. General visceral sensation in the pharynx is carried by the glossopharyngeal nerve.

61-E. The nerve of the pterygoid canal (vidian nerve) contains taste fibers from the palate, general visceral afferent (GVA) fibers, postganglionic sympathetic fibers, and preganglionic parasympathetic fibers.

62-C. The efferent limbs of the reflex are involved in the pupillary light reflex (i.e., constriction of the pupil in response to illumination of the retina) are composed of parasympathetic preganglionic fibers in the oculomotor nerve, parasympathetic fibers and ganglionic cells in the ciliary ganglion, and parasympathetic postganglionic fibers in the short ciliary nerves. The afferent limbs of this reflex are optic nerve fibers. The long ciliary nerves contain postganglionic sympathetic fibers. The ophthalmic nerve contains general somatic afferent (GSA) fibers.

63-D. The secretomotor fibers to the lacrimal gland are parasympathetic fibers that run in the facial, greater petrosal, vidian (nerve of the pterygoid canal), maxillary, zygomatic, zygomaticotemporal, and lacrimal (terminal portion) nerves. The lesser petrosal nerve carries secretomotor (preganglionic parasympathetic) fibers to the parotid gland. The deep petrosal nerve contains postganglionic sympathetic fibers.

64-D. The chorda tympani of the facial nerve supplies the taste fibers to the anterior two-thirds of the tongue, and the glossopharyngeal nerve supplies taste fibers to the posterior one-third of the tongue. The palatoglossus is innervated by the vagus nerve. The vallate papillae are located in the anterior two-thirds of the tongue, but their taste buds are innervated by the glossopharyngeal nerve, which supplies both general and taste sensations to the posterior one-third of the tongue. The anterior two-thirds of the tongue receive general sensory innervation from the trigeminal nerve. The genioglossus can retract or extend the tongue.

65-B. The spinal accessory nerve supplies the sternocleidomastoid and trapezius muscles, which are not involved in the act of swallowing. Swallowing involves movements of the tongue to push the food into the oropharynx, elevation of the soft palate to close the entrance of the nasopharynx, elevation of the hyoid bone and the larynx to close the opening into the larynx, and contraction of the pharyngeal constrictors to move the food through the pharynx. The hypoglossal nerve supplies all of the tongue muscles except the palatoglossus, which is innervated by the vagus nerve. The vagus nerve innervates the muscles of the palate, the larynx, and the pharynx. The mandibular division of the trigeminal nerve supplies the suprahyoid muscles (e.g., the anterior belly of the digastric and the mylohyoid muscles).

66-C. The lateral pterygoid muscle opens the mouth by depressing the jaw. The masseter, medial pterygoid, and temporalis muscles close the jaw. The buccinator muscle is a muscle of facial expression.

67-D. The levator palpebrae superioris muscle opens the eye by elevating the upper eyelid. The orbicularis oculi closes the eye, the orbicularis oris closes the lips, the frontalis elevates the eyebrow, and the superior rectus elevates the eyeball.

68-C. The ophthalmic nerve runs through the supraorbital fissure, the optic nerve runs through the optic foramen, the maxillary nerve runs through the foramen rotundum, the mandibular nerve passes through the foramen ovale, and the trochlear nerve passes through the superior orbital fissure.

69-B. The superior cervical ganglion provides sympathetic fibers, which supply blood vessels in the submandibular gland. The lingual nerve at its origin is not yet joined by the chorda tympani; the chorda tympani nerve contains preganglionic parasympathetic fibers responsible for secretion of the submandibular gland; the lesser petrosal nerve contains preganglionic parasympathetic fibers; and the auriculotemporal nerve contains postganglionic parasympathetic fibers, both of which are responsible for secretion of the parotid gland.

70-D. Accommodation occurs with contraction of the ciliary muscles and is mediated by parasympathetic fibers running within the oculomotor nerve. The levator palpebrae superioris inserts on the tarsal smooth muscle plate in the upper eyelid and opens the eye. The sphincter pupillae and dilator pupillae constrict and dilate the pupil, respectively. The orbitalis muscle is smooth muscle that bridges the inferior orbital fissure and protrudes the eye.

71-C. The maxillary sinus lies lateral to the lateral wall of the nasal cavity and inferior to the floor of the orbit.

72-B. Mastoid air cells communicates with the middle ear cavity through the antrum and aditus.

73-D. The ethmoidal sinus has numerous small cavities and lies between the orbit and the nasal cavity.

74-E. The frontal sinus drains into the anterior part of the middle nasal meatus via frontonasal duct or infundibulum.

75-A. Cerebrospinal fluid (CSF) is formed by vascular choroid plexus in the ventricles in the brain; the letter "A" indicates the lateral ventricle.

76-E. The musculus uvulae is innervated by the vagus nerve. A lesion of the right vagus nerve causes deviation of the uvula to the left side.

77-C. The geniohyoid muscle is innervated by the first cervical nerve through the hypoglossal nerve.

78-B. The inferior nasal meatus below the inferior concha receives the nasolacrimal duct.

79-D. The straight sinus runs along the line of the attachment of the falx cerebri to the tentorium cerebelli, which supports the occipital lobe of the cerebrum and covers the cerebellum.

80-A. The pituitary gland can be reached through the transsphenoidal approach following the septum of the nose through the body of the sphenoid.

81-B. The optic nerve mediates the afferent limb of the pupillary light reflex, whereas the efferent limb is mediated by the facial nerve.

82-A. The nasal septum is formed primarily by the perpendicular plate of the ethmoid bone, vomer, and septal cartilage.

83-D. The lateral rectus is innervated by the abducens nerve, which runs through the cavernous sinus.

84-E. The internal carotid artery pierces the dural roof of the cavernous sinus between the anterior and middle clinoid processes.

85-C. The suprasellar cistern can be obliterated by the pituitary tumor.

86-E. The straight sinus runs along the line where the falx cerebri attaches to the tentorium cerebelli.

87-D. The transverse sinus runs laterally and forward in the convex outer border of the tentorium cerebelli.

88-C. The superior sagittal sinus lies in the superior convex border of the falx cerebri.

89-A. The cavernous sinus communicates directly with the ophthalmic veins.

90-B. The sigmoid sinus becomes continuous with the internal jugular vein at the jugular foramen.

91-E. The foramen rotundum transmits the maxillary division of the trigeminal nerve. Injury to this nerve causes a loss of general sensation of the maxillary teeth.

92-A. The foramen ovale transmits the mandibular division of the trigeminal nerve. Injury to this nerve causes a loss of sensation of the temporomandibular joint.

93-J. The jugular foramen transmits the glossopharyngeal nerve, which carries sensory fibers from the posterior one-third of the tongue.

94-H. The sphenopalatine foramen transmits the nasopalatine nerve, which carries sensory fibers from the mucosa of the nasal septum, the posterior lateral nasal wall, and the anterior portion of the hard palate.

95-F. The pterygoid canal transmits the nerve of the pterygoid canal, which contains preganglionic parasympathetic fibers to the lacrimal gland.

96-J. A fracture of the foramen spinosum would result in a laceration of the middle meningeal artery, which it transmits.

97-C. The lips are closed by the orbicularis oris muscles, which are innervated by the facial nerve. However, the mouth or jaws are closed by the temporalis, masseter, and medial pterygoid muscles, which are innervated by the trigeminal nerve.

98-H. The eyes are opened by the levator palpebrae superioris muscles, which are innervated by the oculomotor nerve.

99-G. Subdural hematoma is caused by rupture of cerebral veins as they pass from the brain surface into one of the venous sinuses.

100-K. Sympathetic postganglionic fibers running in the deep petrosal nerve supply blood vessels in the lacrimal glands.

Comprehensive Examination

Directions: Each of the numbered items or incomplete statements in this section is followed by answers or by completions of the statement. Select the **one** lettered answer or completion that is **best** in each case.

1. If a stab wound lacerates the posterior humeral circumflex artery passing through the quadrangular space on the shoulder region, which of the following nerves might be injured?

(A) Radial nerve
(B) Axillary nerve
(C) Thoracodorsal nerve
(D) Suprascapular nerve
(E) Accessory nerve

2. A victim of an automobile accident has lost the function of all abductors of the arm. This indicates damage to which of the following parts of the brachial plexus?

(A) Middle trunk and posterior cord
(B) Middle trunk and lateral cord
(C) Lower trunk and lateral cord
(D) Upper trunk and posterior cord
(E) Lower trunk and medial cord

3. Which of the following muscles flexes the elbow and is innervated by the radial nerves?

(A) Flexor digitorum longus
(B) Brachioradialis
(C) Brachialis
(D) Extensor digitorum longus
(E) Biceps brachii

4. A lesion of the radial nerve in the spiral groove of the humerus would cause which of the following conditions?

(A) Numbness over the medial side of the forearm
(B) Inability to oppose the thumb
(C) Weakness in pronating the forearm
(D) Weakness in abducting the arm
(E) Inability to extend the hand

5. A patient with a fracture of the medial epicondyle of the humerus might have which of the following conditions?

(A) Impaired abduction of the hand
(B) Carpal tunnel syndrome
(C) Wrist drop
(D) Thenar atrophy
(E) Inability to sweat on the medial part of the hand

6. A 24-year-old man is unable to abduct his fingers. Which of the following nerves is injured?

(A) Ulnar nerve
(B) Median nerve
(C) Radial nerve
(D) Musculocutaneous nerve
(E) Axillary nerve

7. When the hand is in a resting supine position, the radius is in articulation at the radiocarpal joint with which of the following bones?

(A) Triquetrum and trapezium
(B) Lunate and trapezium
(C) Lunate and scaphoid
(D) Scaphoid and hamate
(E) Capitate and scaphoid

8. An injury to the thoracodorsal nerve would probably affect the strength of which of the following movements?

(A) Abduction of the arm
(B) Lateral rotation of the arm
(C) Adduction of the scapula
(D) Extension of the arm
(E) Elevation of the scapula

9. The cell bodies of nerve fibers in the lateral antebrachial cutaneous nerve are located in the

(A) collateral ganglia and dorsal root ganglia
(B) sympathetic trunk and anterior horn of spinal cord
(C) dorsal root ganglia and sympathetic trunk
(D) lateral horn of spinal cord and sympathetic trunk
(E) dorsal root ganglia and anterior horn of spinal cord

10. A patient cannot extend the proximal interphalangeal joint of the ring finger. Which of the following pairs of nerves is damaged?

(A) Radial and median nerves
(B) Radial and axillary nerves
(C) Radial and ulnar nerves
(D) Ulnar and median nerves
(E) Ulnar and axillary nerves

11. Which of the following pairs of nerves innervates the muscle that moves the metacarpophalangeal joint of the fourth digit (ring finger)?

(A) Median and ulnar nerves
(B) Radial and median nerves
(C) Musculocutaneous and ulnar nerves
(D) Ulnar and radial nerves
(E) Radial and axillary nerves

12. A 21-year-old man receives a knife wound that severs the roots of C5 and C6 of the brachial plexus. Which of the following muscles is likely to be paralyzed?

(A) Infraspinatus
(B) Flexor carpi ulnaris
(C) Palmar interossei
(D) Adductor pollicis
(E) Palmaris brevis

13. In a patient with carpal tunnel syndrome, compression could occur in which of the following structures?

(A) Ulnar artery
(B) Ulnar nerve
(C) Median nerve
(D) Flexor carpi radialis tendon
(E) Palmaris longus tendon

14. The anterior cruciate ligament of the knee joint

(A) becomes taut during flexion of the leg
(B) resists posterior displacement of the femur on the tibia
(C) inserts into the medial femoral condyle
(D) helps prevent hyperflexion of the knee joint
(E) is lax when the knee is extended

15. Which of the following actions is most seriously affected by paralysis of the deep peroneal nerve?

(A) Plantar flexion of the foot
(B) Dorsiflexion of the foot
(C) Abduction of the toes
(D) Eversion of the foot
(E) Adduction of the toes

16. The first vascular channel likely to be obstructed or occluded by an embolus from the deep veins of a lower limb is the

(A) tributaries of the renal veins
(B) branches of the coronary arteries
(C) sinusoids of the liver
(D) tributaries of the pulmonary veins
(E) branches of the pulmonary arteries

17. A patient presents with the condition known as flat foot. The foot is displaced laterally and everted, and the head of the talus is no longer supported. Which of the following ligaments probably is stretched?

(A) Plantar calcaneonavicular (spring)
(B) Calcaneofibular
(C) Anterior talofibular
(D) Plantar calcaneocuboid (short plantar)
(E) Anterior tibiotalar

18. Which of the following ligaments is important in preventing forward displacement of the femur on the tibia when the weight-bearing knee is flexed?

(A) Medial meniscus
(B) Fibular collateral ligament
(C) tibial collateral ligament
(D) Posterior cruciate ligament
(E) Anterior cruciate ligament

19. Which of the following bones is associated with the lateral longitudinal arch of the foot?

(A) Talus
(B) Medial three metatarsals
(C) Navicular
(D) Cuneiform
(E) Cuboid

20. A 72-year-old woman fell down in the bathtub and suffered a dislocation of the hip joint that may result in a vascular necrosis of the femoral head and neck due to injuries to the arteries. Which of the following arteries might remain intact?

(A) Lateral femoral circumflex artery
(B) Obturator artery
(C) Medial femoral circumflex artery
(D) Inferior gluteal artery
(E) Deep iliac circumflex artery

21. The lateral meniscus of the knee joint

(A) is C-shaped or forms a semicircle
(B) is attached to the fibular collateral ligament
(C) is larger than the medial meniscus
(D) lies outside the synovial cavity
(E) is more frequently torn in injuries than the medial meniscus

22. Cell bodies of nerve fibers in the ventral root of a thoracic spinal nerve are located in the

(A) dorsal root ganglia and sympathetic trunk
(B) lateral horn of spinal cord and dorsal root ganglia
(C) anterior horn and lateral horn of spinal cord
(D) sympathetic trunk and lateral horn of spinal cord
(E) anterior horn of spinal cord and sympathetic trunk

23. Which of the following veins drains directly into the superior vena cava?

(A) Internal thoracic vein
(B) Azygos vein
(C) Hemiazygos vein
(D) Right superior intercostal vein
(E) Left superior intercostal vein

24. Inadequate blood flow in the artery that runs aside the great cardiac vein in the anterior interventricular sulcus of the heart results from occlusion of the

(A) circumflex branch of the left coronary artery
(B) marginal branch of the right coronary artery
(C) left coronary artery
(D) right coronary artery
(E) posterior interventricular artery

25. Severely diminished blood flow in the coronary arteries most likely results from embolization of an atherosclerotic plaque at the origin of which of the following vascular structures?

(A) Pulmonary trunk
(B) Ascending aorta
(C) Coronary sinus
(D) Descending aorta
(E) Aortic arch

26. A 21-year-old woman comes to the emergency department with chylothorax due to rupture of the thoracic duct. Lymphatic drainage remains normal in which of the following areas?

(A) Left thorax
(B) Right thorax
(C) Left abdomen
(D) Right pelvis
(E) Left lower limb

27. The manubrium of the sternum is free from articulation with which of the following structures?

(A) Body of the sternum
(B) First rib
(C) Second rib
(D) Third rib
(E) Clavicle

28. A lesion of gray rami communicantes injures which of the following nerve fibers?

(A) General somatic afferent (GSA) fibers
(B) Postganglionic parasympathetic fibers
(C) Preganglionic sympathetic fibers
(D) Postganglionic sympathetic fibers
(E) General visceral afferent (GVA) fibers

29. General somatic afferent (GSA) fibers are contained in which of the following structures?

(A) Sympathetic trunk
(B) Dorsal root
(C) Greater splanchnic nerve
(D) Gray rami communicantes
(E) White rami communicantes

30. Even if thrombosis is present in the coronary sinus, which of the following cardiac veins might remain normal in diameter?

(A) Great cardiac vein
(B) Middle cardiac vein
(C) Anterior cardiac vein
(D) Small cardiac vein
(E) Oblique cardiac vein

31. A 35-year-old man is suffering from an infected mediastinum after neck and chest injuries resulting from a head-on automobile collision. Which of the following structures is free from infection?

(A) Thymus gland
(B) Esophagus
(C) Trachea
(D) Lungs
(E) Heart

32. Which of the following statements concerning the lung and bronchi is correct?

(A) The right lung has a lingula
(B) The lobar bronchi contain C-shaped cartilaginous rings
(C) The left lung has a larger volume than the right lung
(D) The right main bronchus is shorter and wider than the left bronchus
(E) The right lung usually receives three bronchial arteries

33. Which of the following structures carries or comes in contact with oxygenated blood?

(A) Pulmonary artery
(B) Crista terminalis
(C) Septomarginal trabecula
(D) Pulmonary vein
(E) Pectinate muscle

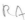

34. Aponeurosis of the internal abdominal oblique muscle forms which of the following structures?

(A) Floor of the inguinal canal
(B) Posterior wall of the inguinal canal
(C) Falx inguinalis (conjoint tendon)
(D) Posterior layer of the rectus sheath below the arcuate line
(E) Internal spermatic fascia

35. Which of the following structures forms part of the anterior wall of the inguinal canal?

(A) Transversalis fascia
(B) Aponeurosis of the transverse abdominal muscle
(C) Aponeurosis of the external abdominal oblique muscle
(D) Falx inguinalis
(E) Lacunar ligament

36. An indirect inguinal hernia occurs

(A) lateral to the inferior epigastric artery
(B) between the inferior epigastric and obliterated umbilical arteries
(C) medial to the obliterated umbilical artery
(D) between the median and medial umbilical folds
(E) between the linea alba and linea semilunaris

37. A lesion of parasympathetic fibers in the vagus nerve interferes with glandular secretory or smooth muscle functions in which of the following organs?

(A) Bladder
(B) Transverse colon
(C) Sigmoid colon
(D) Prostate gland
(E) Rectum

38. A slowly growing tumor in the head of the pancreas could compress which of the following structures?

(A) Duodenojejunal junction
(B) Gastroduodenal artery
(C) Bile duct
(D) Inferior mesenteric artery
(E) Common hepatic duct

39. Which of the following organs may be spared from ischemia in the presence of an occlusive lesion in the celiac trunk?

(A) Liver
(B) Spleen
(C) Pancreas
(D) Gallbladder
(E) Stomach

40. The portal venous system includes which of the following veins?

(A) Left suprarenal vein
(B) Inferior epigastric vein
(C) Superior rectal vein
(D) Azygos vein
(E) Hepatic vein

41. The sigmoid colon

(A) is a retroperitoneal organ
(B) receives parasympathetic fibers from the vagus nerve
(C) receives blood mainly from the superior mesenteric artery
(D) is the site of digestion and absorption of foods
(E) drains its venous blood into the portal venous system

42. The deep perineal space

(A) is formed superiorly by the perineal membrane
(B) contains the superficial transverse perineal muscles
(C) contains a segment of the dorsal nerve of the penis
(D) is formed inferiorly by Colles' fascia
(E) contains the greater vestibular glands

43. If the urethra in males is torn distal to the urogenital diaphragm, urine might accumulate in the

(A) retropubic space
(B) medial aspect of the thigh
(C) ischiorectal fossa
(D) superficial perineal space
(E) paravesical fossa

44. The inferior hypogastric (pelvic) plexus contains parasympathetic nerve fibers from the

(A) lumbar splanchnic nerves
(B) pelvic splanchnic nerves
(C) sacral sympathetic ganglia
(D) vagus nerve
(E) sacral splanchnic nerves

45. Parasympathetic fibers that supply the urinary bladder are derived from which of following nerves?

(A) Vagus nerve
(B) Pelvic splanchnic nerve
(C) Sacral splanchnic nerve
(D) Lesser splanchnic nerve
(E) Greater splanchnic nerve

46. Carcinoma of the uterus can spread directly to the labia majus through lymphatics that follow the

(A) ovarian ligament
(B) suspensory ligament of the ovary
(C) round ligament of the uterus
(D) uterosacral ligaments
(E) pubocervical ligaments

47. A man complains of having no tactile or pain sensation in his scrotum after a race car accident. Which of the following nerves carries undamaged sensory nerve fibers?

(A) Ilioinguinal nerve
(B) Genitofemoral nerve
(C) Iliohypogastric nerve
(D) Perineal branch of the pudendal nerve
(E) Perineal branch of the posterior femoral cutaneous nerve

48. A patient has a damaged pelvic outlet as the result of an automobile accident. Which of the following structures is intact?

(A) Sacrotuberous ligament
(B) Inferior pubic ramus
(C) Pubic crest
(D) Ischial tuberosity
(E) Coccyx

49. Which of the following statements contrasting male and female pelvic structures is correct?

(A) The pelvic inlet is oval in females and heart-shaped in males
(B) The pelvic outlet is smaller in females than in males
(C) The pubic angle is lesser in females than in males
(D) The sacrum is narrower and longer in females than in males
(E) The pelvic cavity is narrower and deeper in females than in males

50. A 26-year-old woman experiences severe back pain from an automobile accident. A computed tomography (CT) scan shows that the L5 vertebral foramen is completely obliterated by the collapsed L5 laminae and pedicles. In this injury, which of the following structures is crushed?

(A) Vertebral artery
(B) Spinal cord
(C) Filum terminale externus (filum of the dura)
(D) Denticulate ligament
(E) Cauda equina

51. A lesion of the suboccipital nerve results in paralysis of which of the following muscles?

(A) Splenius capitis
(B) Trapezius
(C) Rectus capitis posterior major
(D) Levator scapulae
(E) Iliocostalis

52. When withdrawing cerebrospinal fluid (CSF) by lumbar puncture, the needle might penetrate which of the following pairs of structures?

(A) Dura mater and denticulate ligament
(B) Arachnoid mater and pia mater
(C) Dura mater and arachnoid mater
(D) Anulus fibrosus and pia mater
(E) Arachnoid mater and nucleus pulposus

53. A patient has been in an automobile accident; as a result of the accident, the transverse processes of the cervical and thoracic regions are crushed. Which of the following muscles might be paralyzed?

(A) Trapezius
(B) Latissimus dorsi
(C) Rhomboid major
(D) Levator scapulae
(E) Serratus posterior superior

54. Numbness of the skin over the anterior triangle of the neck may be due to injury to which of the following nerves?

(A) Great auricular nerve
(B) Transverse cervical nerve
(C) Superior ramus of the ansa cervicalis
(D) Inferior ramus of the ansa cervicalis
(E) Superior laryngeal nerve

55. If a benign tumor is found where the common carotid artery usually bifurcates, it would be located at the level of the

(A) thyroid isthmus
(B) cricoid cartilage
(C) angle of the mandible
(D) superior border of the thyroid cartilage
(E) jugular notch

56. Damage to the articular disk and capsule of the temporomandibular joint results in paralysis of which of the following muscles?

(A) Masseter
(B) Temporalis
(C) Medial pterygoid
(D) Lateral pterygoid
(E) Buccinator

57. A patient exhibits ptosis (drooping of the upper eyelid). Which of the following nerves is probably damaged?

(A) Trochlear nerve
(B) Abducens nerve
(C) Oculomotor nerve
(D) Ophthalmic nerve
(E) Facial nerve

58. The superior petrosal sinus lies in the margin of the

(A) tentorium cerebelli
(B) falx cerebri
(C) falx cerebelli
(D) diaphragma sellae
(E) straight sinus

59. The arachnoid granulations

(A) allow cerebrospinal fluid (CSF) to pass from the subarachnoid space into the venous sinuses of the dura mater
(B) are storage areas for CSF
(C) increase the surface area available for the production of CSF
(D) provide a shunt that allows CSF to return to the ventricles of the brain
(E) receive blood from the diploë of the skull

60. The great cerebral vein of Galen drains directly into the

(A) superior sagittal sinus
(B) inferior sagittal sinus
(C) cavernous sinus
(D) transverse sinus
(E) straight sinus

61. While making a local excision for a tumor in the palate, a surgical intern accidentally cuts a tendon that loops around the pterygoid hamulus. Which of the following muscles would most likely be paralyzed?

(A) Tensor tympani
(B) Tensor veli palatini
(C) Levator veli palatini
(D) Superior pharyngeal constrictor
(E) Stylohyoid

62. If a vertical stab wound lacerates the pterygomandibular raphe, which of the following muscles would be paralyzed?

(A) Superior and middle pharyngeal constrictors
(B) Middle and inferior pharyngeal constrictors
(C) Superior pharyngeal constrictor and buccinator muscles
(D) Medial and lateral pterygoid muscles
(E) Tensor veli palatini and levator veli palatini

63. In which of the following muscle–nerve pairs is the muscle paired with the nerve that innervates it?

(A) Tensor veli palatini–vagus nerve
(B) Palatoglossus muscle–hypoglossal nerve
(C) Cricothyroid muscle–recurrent laryngeal nerve
(D) Tensor tympani–trigeminal nerve
(E) Geniohyoid muscle–facial nerve

64. Which of the following muscles indents the submandibular gland and divides it into superficial and deep parts?

(A) Hyoglossus
(B) Genioglossus
(C) Styloglossus
(D) Superior constrictor muscle
(E) Mylohyoid muscle

65. An abscess in the auditory tube may block a communication between the nasopharynx and which of the following structures?

(A) Vestibule of the inner ear
(B) Middle ear
(C) Semicircular canals
(D) External ear
(E) Inner ear

66. A man is unable to open his jaw because of paralysis of which of the following muscles?

(A) Medial pterygoid
(B) Masseter
(C) Temporalis
(D) Lateral pterygoid
(E) Buccinator

67. Which of the following conditions could occur if the lesser petrosal nerve is injured?

(A) Lack of lacrimal secretion
(B) Lack of submandibular gland secretion
(C) Lack of parotid gland secretion
(D) Constriction of the pupil
(E) Ptosis of the upper eyelid

68. A 21-year-old patient has an uvula that deviates to the left side on phonation. Which of the following nerves is injured?

(A) Left hypoglossal
(B) Right hypoglossal
(C) Left vagus
(D) Right vagus
(E) Left trigeminal

69. During palatine tonsillectomy, a surgeon ligates arteries to avoid bleeding. Which of the following arteries is spared?

(A) Lesser palatine
(B) Facial
(C) Lingual
(D) Superior thyroid
(E) Ascending pharyngeal

70. The nasal cavity is chronically dry due to a lack of glandular secretions, indicating lesions of which of the following structures?

(A) Superior cervical ganglion
(B) Lesser petrosal nerve
(C) Facial nerve in the facial canal
(D) Greater petrosal nerve
(E) Deep petrosal nerve

Questions 71–72

A 12-year-old girl suffers from a type of neural tube defect called tethered cord syndrome, a congenital anomaly that results from defective closure of the neural tube. This syndrome is characterized by an abnormally low conus medullaris, which is tethered by a short, thickened filum terminale, leading to progressive neurologic defects in the legs and feet.

71. Which of the following defects is commonly associated with the tethered cord syndrome?

(A) Spina bifida occulta
(B) Kyphosis
(C) Meningomyelocele
(D) Herniated disk
(E) Scoliosis

72. The girl has strong muscle function of the flexors of the thigh, but she has weakness of the extensors (hamstrings). A lesion has occurred at which of the following spinal cord levels?

(A) T12
(B) L1
(C) L3
(D) L5
(E) S5

Directions: Each set of matching questions in this section consists of a list of four to twenty-six lettered options (some of which may be in figures) followed by several numbered items. For each numbered item, select the ONE lettered option that is most closely associated with it. To avoid spending too much time on matching sets with large numbers of options, it is generally advisable to begin each set by reading the list of options. Then, for each item in the set, try to generate the correct answer and locate it in the option list, rather than evaluating each option individually. Each lettered option may be selected once, more than once, or not at all.

Questions 73–75

Match each statement below with the muscle it describes.

(A) Pectoralis major
(B) Latissimus dorsi
(C) Anterior serratus
(D) Infraspinatus
(E) Long head of triceps brachii

73. Forms the anterior axillary fold; functions to flex and adduct the arm

74. Arises from the scapula; is innervated by branches from the radial nerve

75. Helps stabilize the glenohumeral joint; is innervated by a branch from the suprascapular nerve

Questions 76–80

Match each statement below with the muscle it describes.

    (A) Interossei
    (B) Lumbrical muscles
    (C) Flexor digitorum profundus
    (D) Flexor digitorum superficialis
    (E) Extensor digitorum

76. Flexes interphalangeal joints; is innervated by the median and ulnar nerves

77. Originates from the radial side of tendons of another muscle

78. Flexes interphalangeal joints; is innervated solely by the median nerve

79. Extends interphalangeal joints when metacarpophalangeal joints are flexed

80. Inserts into extensor expansion; adducts and abducts the fingers

Questions 81–85

Match each statement below with the nerve it describes.

    (A) Femoral nerve
    (B) Obturator nerve
    (C) Pudendal nerve
    (D) Superior gluteal nerve
    (E) Sciatic nerve

81. Innervates the adductor magnus that also receives innervation from the sciatic nerve

82. Enters the gluteal region through the greater sciatic foramen and exits this region at the inferior border of the gluteus maximus

83. Enters the gluteal region through the greater sciatic foramen and exits this region through the lesser sciatic foramen in close proximity to the ischial spine

84. Innervates the tensor fascia lata

85. Innervates the gracilis

Questions 86–90

Match each statement below with the artery it describes.

    (A) Right coronary artery
    (B) Superior intercostal artery
    (C) Left coronary artery
    (D) Internal thoracic artery
    (E) Pulmonary artery

86. A branch of the costocervical trunk

87. Gives rise to the superior epigastric artery

88. Carries the major blood supply for the anterior portion of the interventricular septum

89. Gives rise to anterior intercostal arteries

90. Usually carries the major blood supply for the posterior portion of the interventricular septum

Questions 91–95

Match each statement below with the ligament it describes.

(A) Broad ligament
(B) Round ligament of the uterus
(C) Ovarian ligament
(D) Suspensory ligament of the ovary
(E) Cardinal ligament

91. Enters the deep inguinal ring

92. A double layer of mesentery that attaches to the lateral surface of the uterus

93. Homologous to the most superior portion of the gubernaculum in males

94. Extends from the ovary to the dorsolateral body wall

95. A uterine support that extends from the cervix and the lateral fornices of the vagina to the pelvic wall

Questions 96–100

Match each statement below with the nerve it describes.

(A) Hypoglossal nerve
(B) Recurrent laryngeal nerve
(C) Chorda tympani
(D) Lingual nerve
(E) Glossopharyngeal nerve

96. Provides motor innervation to the intrinsic muscles of the larynx

97. Carries general sensation from the anterior two-thirds of the tongue

98. Carries special visceral (taste) sensation from the anterior two-thirds of the tongue

99. Provides motor innervation to the intrinsic muscles of the tongue

100. Carries sensation from pressure receptors in the carotid sinus

Questions 101–105

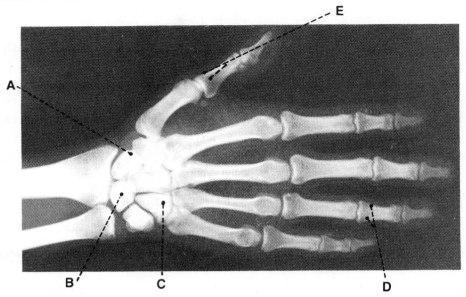

Match each description below with the appropriate lettered site or structure in this radiograph of the bones of the hand.

101. Lunate bone

102. Hamate bone

103. Site of attachment of the muscles that form the thenar eminence

104. Site of tendinous attachment of the flexor digitorum superficialis

105. Floor of the anatomical snuff-box

Questions 106–110

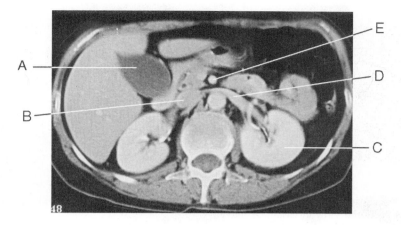

Match each description below with the appropriate lettered structure in this computed tomography (CT) scan—a sectional view of the abdomen.

106. Receives the left testicular vein

107. Concentrates and stores bile

108. Gives off the middle colic artery

109. Produces and excretes urine

110. Receives the right suprarenal vein

Questions 111–115

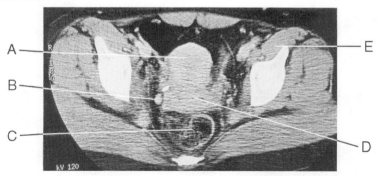

Match each description below with the appropriate lettered structure in this computed tomography (CT) scan—a sectional view of the female pelvis.

111. Is a common site of uterine cancer

112. Descends retroperitoneally on the psoas muscle and runs under the uterine artery

113. Has venous blood that returns to the portal and caval (systemic) venous systems

114. Has a detrusor muscle that is innervated by autonomic nerves

115. Inserts on the lesser trochanter

Questions 116–118

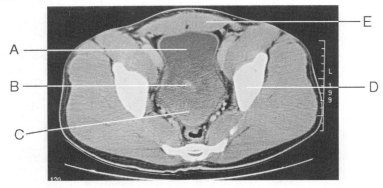

Match each description below with the appropriate lettered structure in this computed tomography (CT) scan—a sectional view of the male pelvis.

116. Forms a medial boundary of the inguinal triangle

117. Secretes a fluid that produces the characteristic odor of semen

118. Receives the ejaculatory duct

Questions 119–120

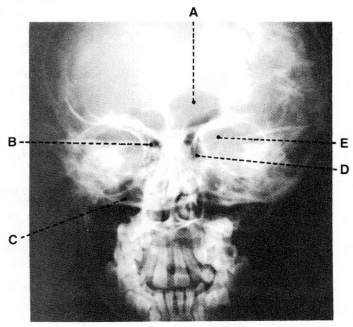

Match each description below with the appropriate lettered structure in this radiograph—a frontal view of the head.

119. Frontal sinus

120. Superior orbital fissure

Answers and Explanations

1-B. The axillary nerve runs posteriorly to the humerus, accompanying the posterior humeral circumflex artery through the quadrangular space and innervating the teres minor and deltoid muscles.

2-D. The abductors of the arm are the deltoid and supraspinatus muscles. The deltoid is innervated by the axillary nerve, which arises from the posterior cord of the brachial plexus. The supraspinatus is innervated by the suprascapular nerve, which arises from the upper trunk of the brachial plexus.

3-B. The brachioradialis is innervated by the radial nerve and functions to flex the elbow. The biceps brachii and brachialis muscles flex the elbow and are innervated by the musculocutaneous nerve. The flexor digitorum longus and extensor digitorum longus do not act in the elbow.

4-E. The radial nerve innervates the extensor muscles of the hand. The skin on the medial side of the forearm is innervated by the medial antebrachial cutaneous nerve. The opponens pollicis, pronator teres, and pronator quadratus muscles are innervated by the median nerve. The abductors of the arm (deltoid and supraspinatus muscles) are innervated by the axillary nerve and upper trunk of the brachial plexus, respectively.

5-E. Fracture of the medial epicondyle of the humerus might injure the ulnar nerve, which supplies the skin of the medial side of the hand; thus a lesion of the ulnar nerve would cause no cutaneous sensation and lack of sweating in that area. The muscles involved in abduction of the hand are the flexor carpi radialis and the extensor carpi radialis longus and brevis, which are innervated by the median and radial nerves, respectively. Carpal tunnel syndrome and thenar atrophy result from a lesion of the median nerve, whereas wrist drop results from a lesion of the radial nerve.

6-A. The ulnar nerve innervates the dorsal interossei, which are the only abductors of the fingers.

7-C. The radius and the articular disk articulate with the scaphoid, lunate, and triquetrum at the radiocarpal (wrist) joint. However, the triquetrum does not articulate with the radius, but instead articulates with the articular disk on the head of the ulna.

8-D. The thoracodorsal nerve innervates the latissimus dorsi, which adducts, extends, and medially rotates the arm. The arm is abducted by the supraspinatus and laterally rotated by the infraspinatus, teres minor, and deltoid (posterior part) muscles. The scapula is elevated by the trapezium and levator scapulae muscles and adducted by the rhomboid and trapezius muscles.

9-C. The lateral antebrachial cutaneous nerve contains general somatic afferent (GSA) fibers, which have cell bodies located in the dorsal root ganglia, and sympathetic postganglionic (general visceral efferent [GVE]) fibers, which have cell bodies located in the sympathetic chain ganglia.

10-C. The proximal and distal interphalangeal joints of the ring finger are extended by the extensor digitorum, which is innervated by the radial nerve. When the metacarpophalangeal joint of the ring finger is extended by the extensor digitorum, the interphalangeal joints can be extended by the dorsal and palmar interossei and lumbrical muscles, which are innervated by the ulnar nerve.

11-D. The metacarpophalangeal joint of the ring finger is innervated by the extensor digitorum, which is innervated by the radial nerve. This joint is flexed by the lumbrical and interossei muscles, abducted by the dorsal interosseous, and adducted by the palmar interosseous. The medial two lumbricals and both the dorsal and palmar interossei are innervated by the ulnar nerve.

12-A. In Erb-Duchenne paralysis (or upper trunk injury), the nerve fibers in the roots of C5 and C6 of the brachial plexus are damaged. The infraspinatus, a lateral rotator muscle, is innervated by the suprascapular nerve (C5 and C6). The ulnar nerve (C8 and T1) innervates the flexor carpi ulnaris, palmar interossei, adductor pollicis, and palmaris brevis muscles.

13-C. In carpal tunnel syndrome, structures entering the palm deep to the flexor retinaculum are compressed; these include the median nerve and the tendons of the flexor pollicis longus, flexor digitorum profundus, and flexor digitorum superficialis muscles. The flexor carpi radialis runs lateral to the carpal tunnel and inserts on the bases of the second and third metacarpals. Structures entering the palm superficial to the flexor retinaculum include the ulnar nerve, ulnar artery, and palmaris longus tendon (which inserts on the palmar aponeurosis).

14-B. The anterior cruciate ligament of the knee joint prevents posterior displacement of the femur on the tibia and limits hyperextension of the knee joint. This ligament becomes taut when the knee is extended and lax when the knee is flexed. It inserts into the lateral femoral condyle posteriorly within the intercondylar notch.

15-B. The deep peroneal nerve innervates the dorsiflexors of the foot, which include the tibialis anterior, extensor hallucis longus, extensor digitorum longus, and peroneus tertius muscles.

16-E. An embolus from the deep veins of the lower limb would travel through the femoral vein, the external and common iliac veins, the inferior vena cava, the right atrium, the right ventricle, the pulmonary trunk, and into the pulmonary arteries, where it could obstruct and occlude these vessels.

17-A. Flat foot is characterized by disappearance of the medial portion of the longitudinal arch, which appears completely flattened. The plantar calcaneonavicular (spring) ligament supports the head of the talus and the medial side of the longitudinal arch. The planar calcaneocuboid (short plantar) ligament supports the lateral portion of the longitudinal arch. Other ligaments support the ankle joint.

18-D. The posterior cruciate ligament prevents forward displacement of the femur on the tibia when the knee is flexed. The medial meniscus acts as a cushion, or shock absorber, and forms a more stable base for the articulation of the femoral condyle. The tibial and fibular collateral ligaments prevent medial and lateral displacement, respectively, of the two long bones. The anterior cruciate ligament prevents backward dislocation of the femur on the tibia when the knee is extended.

19-E. The lateral longitudinal arch is formed by the calcaneus, cuboid bone, and lateral two metatarsal bones, whereas the medial longitudinal arch of the foot is formed by the talus, calcaneus, navicular bone, cuneiform bones, and medial three metatarsal bones.

20-E. The deep iliac circumflex artery does not supply the hip joint, which receives blood from branches of the medial and lateral femoral circumflex, superior and inferior gluteal, and obturator arteries.

21-D. The lateral meniscus, like the medial meniscus, lies outside the synovial cavity but within the joint cavity. However, the lateral meniscus is nearly circular, while the medial meniscus is C-shaped or forms a semicircle. The lateral meniscus is smaller than the medial meniscus and less frequently torn in injuries than the medial meniscus. In addition, the lateral meniscus is separated from the fibular collateral ligament by the tendon of the popliteal muscle, while the medial meniscus attaches to the tibial collateral ligament.

22-C. The ventral root of a thoracic spinal nerve contains sympathetic preganglionic fibers, which have cell bodies located in the lateral horn of the gray matter of the spinal cord, and general somatic efferent (GSE) fibers, which have cell bodies located in the anterior horn of the gray matter of the spinal cord.

23-B. The azygos vein receives the hemiazygos and accessory hemiazygos veins and drains into the superior vena cava. The internal thoracic vein drains into the subclavian vein. The right superior intercostal vein drains into the azygos vein, while the left superior intercostal vein drains into the left brachiocephalic vein.

24-C. The great cardiac vein is accompanied by the anterior interventricular artery, which is a branch of the left coronary artery. The circumflex branch of the left coronary artery runs along with the coronary sinus. The right marginal artery is accompanied by the small cardiac vein, and the posterior interventricular artery is accompanied by the middle cardiac vein.

25-B. The right and left coronary arteries arise from the ascending aorta, and reduced blood flow in the ascending aorta means that these arteries receive much less blood. Blockage of the pulmonary trunk or coronary sinus minimally affects blood flow in the coronary arteries. Blockage of the origin of the aortic arch or the descending aorta increases blood flow in these arteries.

26-B. The right lymphatic duct drains the right sides of the thorax, upper limb, head and neck, while the thoracic duct drains the rest of the body.

27-D. The third rib articulates with the body of the sternum rather than the manubrium. The manubrium of the sternum articulates with the body of the sternum, the first and second ribs, and the clavicle.

28-D. Gray rami communicantes contain postganglionic sympathetic nerve fibers, whose cell bodies are located in the sympathetic chain ganglia, and no other nerve fibers.

29-B. The dorsal root contains both general somatic afferent (GSA) and general visceral afferent (GVA) fibers. The sympathetic trunk, greater splanchnic nerve, and white rami communicantes contain GVA fibers. The gray rami communicantes contain sympathetic postganglionic (GVE) fibers.

30-C. Because the anterior cardiac vein drains directly into the right atrium, its diameter is unchanged. However, all other cardiac veins drain into the coronary sinus, and they are dilated.

31-D. The mediastinum does not contain the lungs; it contains the thymus, esophagus, trachea, and heart.

32-D. The carina is the point where the trachea divides into the right and left main bronchi. The left lung has a lingula and has a smaller volume than the right one. The trachea contains C-shaped cartilaginous rings, and the main bronchi contain cartilaginous rings. The right lung usually receives one bronchial artery, and the left lung receives two bronchial arteries.

33-D. The pulmonary veins carry oxygenated blood, while the pulmonary artery carries deoxygenated blood. The right atrium, which contains the crista terminalis and pectinate muscle, and the right ventricle, which contains the septomarginal trabecula, both carry deoxygenated blood.

34-C. The falx inguinalis (conjoint tendon) is formed by the aponeuroses of the internal abdominal oblique and transverse abdominal muscles. The floor of the inguinal canal is formed by the inguinal and lacunar ligaments, and the posterior wall of the canal is formed by the aponeurosis of the transverse abdominal muscle and the transversalis fascia. There is no posterior layer of the rectus sheath below the arcuate line, and the rectus abdominis muscle is in contact with the transversalis fascia. The internal spermatic fascia is derived from the transversalis fascia.

35-C. The anterior wall of the inguinal canal is formed by the aponeuroses of the external and internal abdominal oblique muscles. The posterior wall is formed by aponeurosis of the transverse abdominal muscle and transversalis fascia. The superior wall (roof) is formed by arching fibers of the internal oblique and transverse muscles. The inferior wall (floor) is formed by the inguinal and lacunar ligaments. The falx inguinalis is formed by the aponeuroses of the internal abdominal oblique and transverse abdominal muscles.

36-A. An indirect inguinal hernia occurs lateral to the inferior epigastric vessels. A direct inguinal hernia arises medial to these vessels.

37-B. The vagus nerve supplies parasympathetic fibers to the thoracic and abdominal viscera, including the transverse colon. The descending and sigmoid colons and other pelvic viscera are innervated by the pelvic splanchnic nerves.

38-C. The bile duct traverses the head of the pancreas, and thus a tumor located there could compress this structure. The gastroduodenal junction comes into contact with the tip of the uncinate process and the interior portion of the body of the pancreas. The other structures are not closely associated with the head of the pancreas.

39-C. The arterial supply to the pancreas is from both the celiac trunk and superior mesenteric artery. Other organs, including the liver, spleen, gallbladder, and stomach, receive blood from the celiac trunk.

40-C. The superior rectal vein is part of the portal venous system. All the other veins belong to the systemic (caval) venous system.

41-E. The sigmoid colon drains its venous blood into the portal venous system, has its own mesentery, receives parasympathetic fibers from the pelvic splanchnic nerve, receives blood from the inferior mesenteric artery, and converts the liquid contents of the ileum into semisolid feces by absorbing water and electrolytes.

42-C. The deep perineal space, a space between the superior and inferior fasciae of the urogenital diaphragm, contains a segment of the dorsal nerve of the penis in males. The superficial transverse perineal muscles and the greater vestibular glands are found in the superficial perineal space.

43-D. Extravasated urine can pass into the superficial perineal space. The urine could spread inferiorly into the scrotum, anteriorly around the penis, and superiorly into the abdominal wall, but it could not spread into the thigh because the superficial fascia of the perineum is firmly attached laterally to the ischiopubic rami and connected with the deep fascia of the thigh (the fascia lata).

44-B. The inferior hypogastric (pelvic) plexus contains preganglionic parasympathetic fibers from the pelvic splanchnic nerves. The lumbar and sacral splanchnic nerves contain preganglionic sympathetic fibers. The vagus nerve does not supply parasympathetic nerve fibers to the pelvic organs.

45-B. The urinary bladder receives parasympathetic fibers from the pelvic splanchnic nerve, not the vagus nerve. The greater, lesser, lumbar, and sacral splanchnic nerves contain sympathetic preganglionic fibers.

46-C. Carcinoma of the uterus can spread directly to the labium majus through the lymphatics that follow the round ligament of the uterus. This ligament extends from the uterus, enters the inguinal canal at the deep inguinal ring, emerges from the superficial inguinal ring, and merges with the subcutaneous tissue of the labium majus. Other structures do not reach the labium majus.

47-C. The iliohypogastric nerve does not supply the scrotum. The scrotum is innervated by the anterior scrotal branch of the ilioinguinal nerve, the genital branch of the genitofemoral nerve, the posterior scrotal branch of the perineal branch of the pudendal nerve, and the perineal branch of the posterior femoral cutaneous nerve.

48-C. Although the pubic crest forms a part of the pelvic inlet (pelvic brim), it does not contribute to the formation of the pubic outlet. The pelvic outlet (lower pelvic aperture) is bounded posteriorly by the sacrum and coccyx; laterally by the ischial tuberosities and sacrotuberous ligaments; and anteriorly by the pubic symphysis, the arcuate ligament, and the rami of the pubis and ischium.

49-A. Compared to the male pelvis, the female pelvis is characterized by presence of the oval inlet, larger outlet, larger pelvic angle, shorter and wider sacrum, and wider and shallower cavity.

50-E. The cauda equina is formed by dorsal and ventral roots of the lumbar and sacral spinal nerves. So it is crushed at the level of the L5 vertebra, whereas the other structures are not. The vertebral artery, which arises from the subclavian artery, ascends through the transverse foramina of the upper six cervical vertebrae. The spinal cord ends at the level of the L2 vertebra. The filum terminale externus (filum of the dura) extends from the apex of the dura at the level of the S2 vertebra to the dorsum of the coccyx. The denticulate ligament, a lateral extension of the pia between the dorsal and ventral roots of the spinal nerves, consists of 21 pairs of processes, the last one lying between the twelfth thoracic and first lumbar spinal nerves.

51-C. The suboccipital nerve supplies the rectus capitis posterior major and minor, the obliquus capitis superior and inferior, and the semispinalis capitis. The dorsal primary rami of the spinal nerves innervate the deep muscles of the back, including the splenius capitis and iliocostalis muscles. The spinal accessory nerve innervates the trapezius muscle, and the dorsal scapular nerve innervates the levator scapulae muscle; these are the superficial muscles of the back.

52-C. To obtain cerebrospinal fluid (CSF) contained in the subarachnoid space, penetration of the dura mater and arachnoid mater is necessary. The denticulate ligament, pia mater, anulus fibrosus, and nucleus pulposus should not be penetrated during a lumbar puncture.

53-D. The levator scapulae is attached to the transverse processes of the upper cervical vertebrae. All other muscles are attached to the spinous processes.

54-B. The transverse cervical nerve innervates the skin over the anterior cervical triangle; the great auricular nerve innervates the skin behind the auricle and over the parotid gland. The ansa cervicalis innervates the infrahyoid muscles, including the sternohyoid, sternothyroid, and omohyoid muscles.

55-D. The common carotid artery normally bifurcates into the external and internal carotid arteries at the level of the superior border of the thyroid cartilage.

56-D. The lateral pterygoid muscle inserts on the articular disk and capsule of the temporomandibular joint. The temporalis muscle inserts on the coronoid process, and the medial pterygoid and masseter muscles insert on the medial and lateral surfaces of the ramus and angle of the mandible, respectively.

57-C. Damage to the oculomotor nerve results in ptosis (drooping) of the eyelid, because the levator palpebrae superioris is innervated by the oculomotor nerve. The trochlear nerve innervates the superior oblique, and the abducens nerve innervates the lateral rectus. The oculomotor nerve innervates the remaining ocular muscles. The facial nerve innervates the orbicularis oculi, which functions to close the eyelids.

58-A. The superior petrosal sinus lies in the margin of the tentorium cerebelli. The falx cerebri contains the inferior and superior sagittal sinuses, and the falx cerebelli encloses the occipital sinus. The diaphragma sellae forms the dural roof of the sella turcica. The straight sinus runs along the line of attachment of the falx cerebri and tentorium cerebelli.

59-A. Arachnoid granulations are tuft-like collections of highly folded arachnoid that project into the superior sagittal sinus and other dural sinuses. They absorb the cerebrospinal fluid (CSF) into dural sinuses and often produce erosion or pitting of the inner surface of the calvaria.

60-E. The great cerebral vein of Galen and the inferior sagittal sinus unite to form the straight sinus.

61-B. The tendon of the tensor veli palatini curves around the pterygoid hamulus to insert on the soft palate. The tensor tympani inserts on the handle of the malleus, the levator veli palatini on the soft palate, the superior pharyngeal constrictor on the median raphe and the pharyngeal tubercle, and the stylohyoid on the body of the hyoid.

62-C. The pterygomandibular raphe serves as a common origin for the superior pharyngeal constrictor and buccinator muscles.

63-D. The tensor tympani and the tensor veli palatini are both innervated by the trigeminal nerve, the palatoglossus by the vagus nerve, the cricothyroid by the external laryngeal branch of the superior laryngeal nerve, and the geniohyoid muscle by the first cervical nerve through the hypoglossal nerve.

64-E. The mylohyoid muscle indents the submandibular gland and divides it into superficial and deep parts.

65-B. The auditory (eustachian) tube connects the nasopharynx with the middle ear cavity. The vestibule and semicircular canals are parts of the inner ear.

66-D. The action of the lateral pterygoid muscles opens the jaws. The medial pterygoid, masseter, and temporalis muscles are involved in closing the jaws.

67-C. Parasympathetic preganglionic fibers in the lesser petrosal nerve enter the otic ganglion, where they synapse, and postganglionic parasympathetic fibers join the auriculotemporal nerve to supply the parotid gland for secretion of saliva.

68-D. The musculus uvulae is innervated by the vagus nerve. A lesion of the vagus nerve results in deviation of the uvula toward the opposite side of the injury. An injury of the right vagus nerve causes paralysis of the right uvular muscle, which means that the uvula deviates toward the left.

69-D. The superior thyroid artery does not supply the palatine tonsil. The palatine tonsil receives blood from the lesser palatine branch of the maxillary artery, the ascending palatine branch of the facial artery, the dorsal lingual branches of the lingual artery, and the ascending pharyngeal artery.

70-E. The parasympathetic secretomotor fibers for mucous glands in the nasal cavity run in the facial nerve, the greater petrosal nerve, the nerve of the pterygoid canal, and the pterygopalatine ganglion. The facial nerve in the facial canal does not contain parasympathetic fibers for mucous glands in the nasal cavity but instead motor [special visceral efferent (SVE)] fibers to innervate the muscles of facial expression. The lesser petrosal nerve contains parasympathetic preganglionic fibers for the parotid gland. The superior cervical ganglion and the deep petrosal nerve contain sympathetic postganglionic neuron cell bodies and/or fibers, which supply blood vessels in the lacrimal gland and the nasal and palate mucosa. Sympathetic fibers are not secretomotor fibers, but they supply blood vessels in the nasal mucosa.

71-C. Tethered cord syndrome is frequently associated with meningomyelocele or intraspinal lipomatous growth. Meningomyelocele is a protrusion of the spinal cord and the meninges through the unfused arch of the vertebra. Spinal bifida occulta is a condition caused by failure of the vertebral arch to fuse, with no protrusion of the spinal cord and the meninges. Kyphosis is an abnormal accentuation of lumbar curvature. Herniated disk represents a protrusion of the nucleus pulposus through the anulus fibrosus of the intervertebral disk into the intervertebral foramen or into the vertebral canal, compressing the spinal nerve roots. Scoliosis is a lateral deviation of the spine due to unequal growth of the vertebral column.

72-D. The quadratus femoris muscles, the flexors of the thigh, are innervated by the femoral nerve, which originates from the spinal cord at L2–L4. In contrast, the hamstring muscles, the extensors of the thigh, are innervated by the sciatic nerve, which originates from L4–S3. Therefore, the lesion occurs at the level of L5 (between L4 and S3).

73-A. The pectoralis major adducts and medially rotates the arm. The clavicular part rotates the arm medially and flexes it, and the sternocostal part depresses the arm and shoulder. The lateral border of the pectoralis major forms the anterior axillary fold.

74-E. The long head of the triceps brachii, which is innervated by branches from the radial nerve, originates from the infraglenoid tubercle of the scapula.

75-D. The tendon of the infraspinatus, which is innervated by a branch from the suprascapular nerve, forms the rotator (musculotendinous) cuff and thus helps stabilize the glenohumeral joint.

76-C. The flexor digitorum profundus, which is innervated by the median and ulnar nerves, can flex the distal interphalangeal joints.

77-B. The lumbricals arise, which are innervated by the median and ulnar nerves, arise from the radial side of the tendon of the flexor digitorum profundus.

78-D. The flexor digitorum superficialis, which is innervated solely by the median nerve, flexes the proximal interphalangeal joints.

79-E. The extensor digitorum communis extends the proximal and distal interphalangeal joints when the metacarpophalangeal joints are flexed by the interossei and the lumbricals.

80-A. The dorsal and palmar interossei, which are innervated by the ulnar nerve, insert into the extensor expansion. The dorsal interossei abduct the fingers, and the palmar interossei adduct the fingers.

81-B. The obturator and sciatic nerves innervate the adductor magnus.

82-E. The sciatic nerve enters the gluteal region through the greater sciatic foramen, has no branches in the gluteal region, and exits this region at the inferior border of the gluteus maximus.

83-C. The pudendal nerve enters the gluteal region through the greater sciatic foramen and exits this region through the lesser sciatic foramen in close proximity to the ischial spine.

84-D. The superior gluteal nerve innervates the gluteus medius, gluteus minimus, and tensor fascia lata muscles.

85-B. The obturator nerve innervates the medial muscles of the thigh.

86-B. The superior intercostal and deep cervical arteries branch from the costocervical trunk.

87-D. The internal thoracic artery gives rise to the anterior intercostal arteries and then terminates at the sixth intercostal space by dividing into the superior epigastric and musculophrenic arteries.

88-C. The anterior interventricular artery, which branches from the left coronary artery, supplies the anterior portion of the interventricular septum.

89-D. The anterior intercostal arteries are branches of the internal thoracic artery.

90-A. The right coronary artery gives rise to the posterior interventricular artery, which provides the major blood supply of the posterior portion of the interventricular septum.

91-B. The round ligament of the uterus enters the deep inguinal ring, runs through the inguinal canal, emerges from the superficial inguinal ring, and becomes lost in the labium majus.

92-A. The broad ligament is a double layer of mesentery that attaches to the lateral surface of the uterus.

93-C. The ovarian (proper) ligament is homologous to the most superior portion of the gubernaculum in males.

94-D. The suspensory ligament of the ovary, which is composed of the connective tissue around the ovarian vessels, extends from the ovary to the dorsolateral body wall.

95-E. The cardinal (lateral cervical) ligament, an important uterine support, is composed of fibro-muscular condensations of pelvic fascia from the cervix and the lateral fornices of the vagina that extend to the pelvic wall.

96-B. The recurrent laryngeal nerve provides motor innervation to the intrinsic muscles of the larynx.

97-D. The lingual nerve carries general sensation from the anterior two-thirds of the tongue.

98-C. The chorda tympani carries special visceral sensation from the anterior two-thirds of the tongue.

99-A. The hypoglossal nerve provides motor innervation to the intrinsic muscles of the tongue.

100-E. The glossopharyngeal nerve carries sensation from pressure receptors in the carotid sinus.

101-B. The structure is the lunate bone.

102-C. The structure is the hamate bone.

103-E. This structure is the base of the proximal phalanx of the thumb and is the site of attachment for the for the flexor pollicis brevis, which, along with the opponens pollicis, form the thenar eminence. It is also the site of attachment for the adductor pollicis brevis.

104-D. This structure is the middle phalanx of the ring finger, which is the site of attachment for the flexor digitorum superficialis.

105-A. The scaphoid bone forms the floor of the anatomical snuff-box.

106-D. The left renal vein receives the left testicular vein.

107-A. The gallbladder receives bile and concentrates and stores it.

108-E. The superior mesenteric artery gives off the middle colic artery.

109-C. The kidney produces and excretes urine.

110-B. The right suprarenal vein drains into the inferior vena cava. However, the left renal vein receives the left suprarenal vein.

111-D. The uterine cervix is the common site of uterine cancer.

112-B. The ureter descends retroperitoneally on the psoas muscle in the abdomen and runs under the uterine artery in the pelvis.

113-C. The rectum returns its venous blood to the portal vein via the superior rectal vein, and to the caval (systemic) venous system via the middle and inferior rectal veins.

114-A. The detrusor muscle in the wall of the bladder is innervated by the sympathetic nerve.

115-E. The iliacus muscle together with the psoas major muscle inserts on the lesser trochanter.

116-E. The margin of the rectus abdominis forms the medial boundary of the inguinal triangle.

117-C. The prostate gland secretes a fluid that produces the characteristic odor of semen.

118-B. The prostatic urethra receives the ejaculatory duct.

119-A. The structure is the frontal sinus.

120-E. The structure is the superior orbital fissure.

Index

437

90 - 10%.
78 - 17%.
94 - 25%.
    - 20%.
    - 25%.